Van Allen's Pictorial Manual of Neurologic Tests

Third Edition

Robert L. Rodnitzky, M.D.
Professor, Department of Neurology
University of Iowa College of Medicine
Iowa City, Iowa

Illustrated by
George Buckley

Van Allen's Pictorial Manual of Neurologic Tests

A Guide to the Performance and Interpretation of the Neurologic Examination

Third Edition

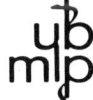

Year Book Medical Publishers, Inc.
Chicago   London   Boca Raton

Sponsoring Editor: Richard H. Lampert
Associate Managing Editor, Manuscript Services: Deborah Thorp
Production Project Manager: Gayle Paprocki
Proofroom Supervisor: Shirley E. Taylor

Copyright © 1969, 1981, and 1988 by Year Book Medical Publishers, Inc. All rights reserved. No part of this publication may be reproduced, stored in a retrieval system, or transmitted, in any form or by any means—electronic, mechanical, photocopying, recording, or otherwise— without prior written permission from the publisher. Printed in the United States of America.

1 2 3 4 5 6 7 8 9 0 M R 92 91 90 89 88

Library of Congress Cataloging-in-Publication Data

Van Allen, Maurice W., 1918-
 Van Allen's pictorial manual of neurologic tests.

 Rev. ed. of: Pictorial manual of neurologic tests / Maurice W. Van Allen, Robert L. Rodnitzky. 2nd ed. c1981.
 Bibliography: p.
 Includes index.
 1. Neurologic examination—Handbooks, manuals, etc.
I. Rodnitzky, Robert L. II. Title. III. Title:
Pictorial manual of neurologic tests. [DNLM:
1. Nervous System Diseases—diagnosis. 2. Neurologic Examination—atlases. WL 17 V217p]
RC348.V35   1988   616.8′04754   87-23213
ISBN 0-8151-8961-3

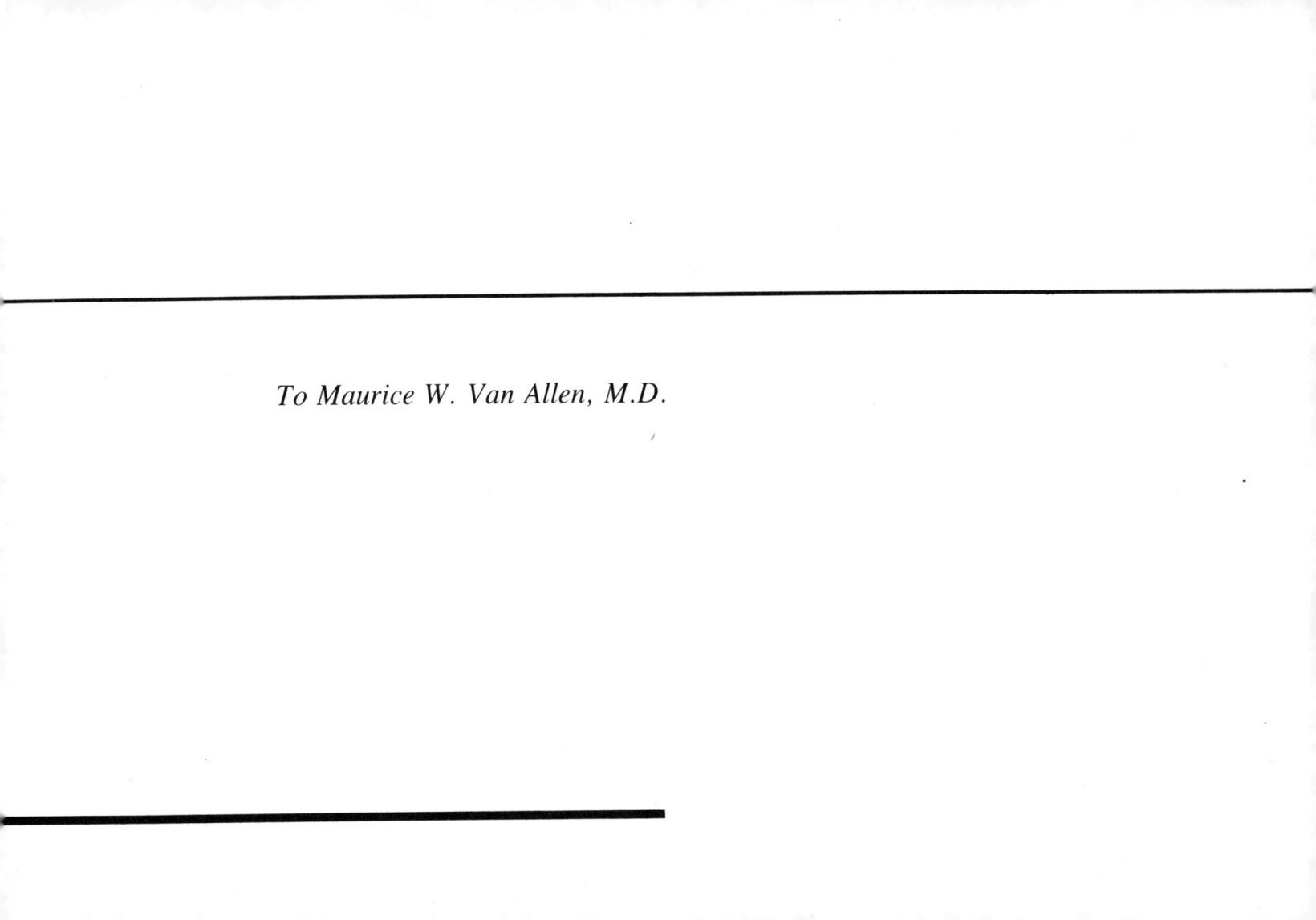

To Maurice W. Van Allen, M.D.

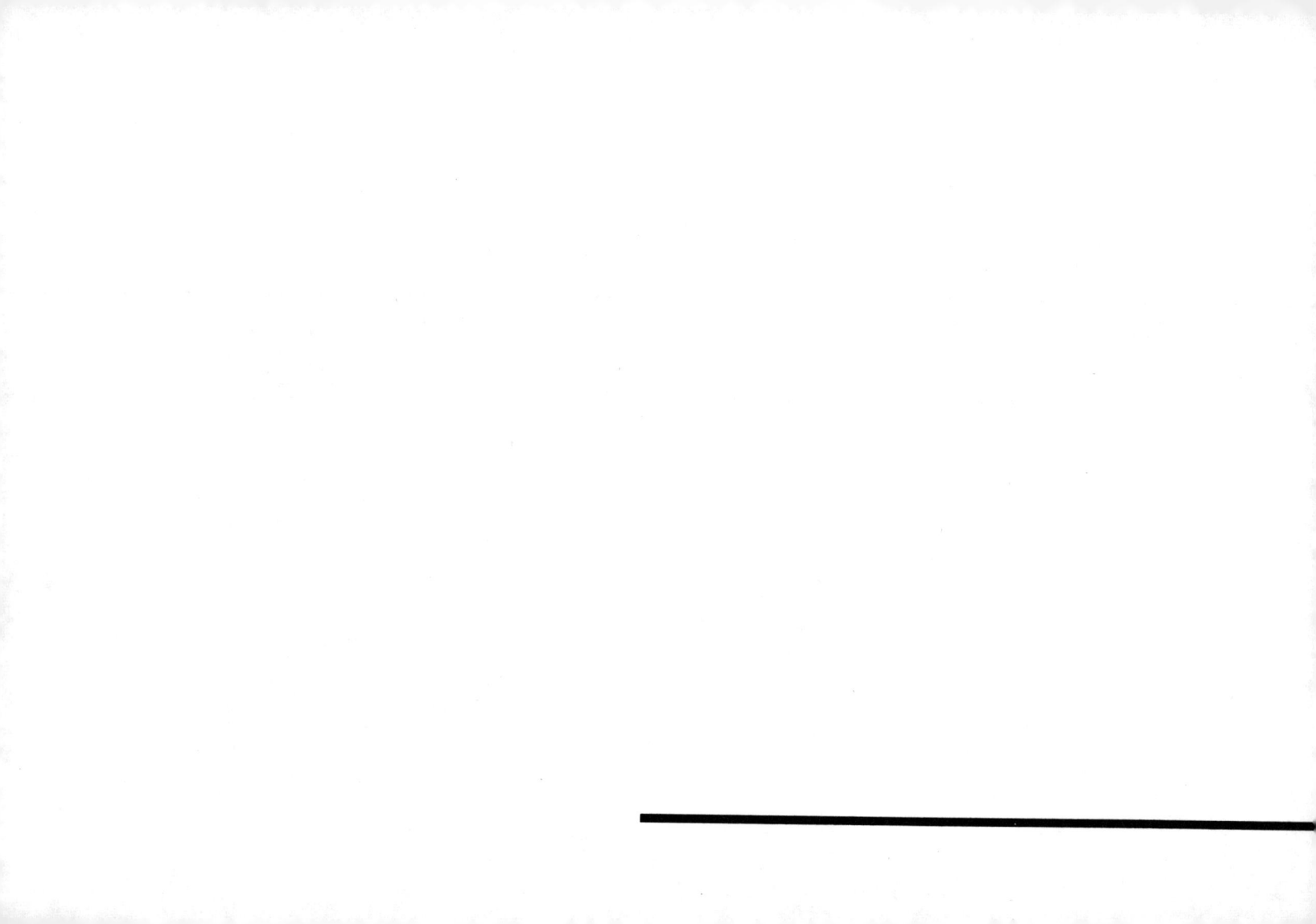

Preface

Dr. Maurice W. Van Allen conceived the format and content of the first edition of *Pictorial Manual of Neurologic Tests* and was its sole author. I was fortunate to have joined him in authoring the second edition. In his long and distinguished career, up to the time of his death, he personally taught neurology to thousands of students and house staff officers. This teaching emphasized careful observation, alertness to subtle clinical clues, and the importance of placing those clues in the context of the global impression gained from the patient. Dr. Van Allen was not only a coauthor, but also my mentor and friend. Our long association impressed upon me the wisdom of this approach to neurology, and I have strived to adhere to it in preparing new material for this edition.

In preparing the third edition of *Pictorial Manual of Neurologic Tests*, I have refined and amplified, wherever possible, material contained in the previous edition and introduced new material reflecting the continued evolution of techniques for neurologic examination. Since the last edition of this book, there have been significant advances in laboratory neurodiagnostic tests, especially electrophysiologic tests and neuroimaging procedures. While these innovations have, in some respect, simplified the task of those who make neurologic diagnoses, they have not diminished the importance of a logically planned and carefully performed clinical examination. Still paramount to the intelligent diagnosis of neurologic disease is the correlation between objective demonstration of neurologic dysfunction and abnormalities found on laboratory or radiologic tests. In this edition, as described more fully below, a section describing the techniques, indications, and findings of the major neurodiagnostic laboratory and neuroimaging procedures has been included. The modern neurologic diagnostician can use these tests to great advantage, but it must always be remembered that the results cannot be properly interpreted in the absence of solid clinical information gained from a careful personal examination of the patient.

This book is intended primarily to supplement the instruction of medical students and residents and to be an aid to physicians in fields other than neurology. The practitioner may find it useful to reinforce occasionally used knowledge and to improve efficiency and technique in neurologic diagnosis.

The manual differs from others in several respects. It is extensively illustrated with line drawings. Whenever a drawing could shorten description, facilitate understanding, or reinforce memory, it was used. Although some may doubt the need to illustrate a test of strength of the grip, the format is based on the belief that proximity of pictures, description, and emphasis on meaning serve to hasten the acquisition of clinical skills. The manual is almost exclusively a guide to examination and the use of ancillary laboratory tests. However, the temptation to include practical applications of the information obtained from examination has not been entirely resisted.

The organization of the first section, "The Basic Neurologic Examination," reflects a personal approach to the examination and departs slightly from the more traditional sequence. However, all of the traditional components of the examination are included.

The majority of patients requiring neurologic examination are able to walk into the physician's office, and many will not have discernible signs of organic disorder of the nervous system. Hence, the manual is organized so that the examiner may begin with a screening examination of such patients that is sufficiently searching to uncover significant evidence of dysfunction and yet is practical in terms of ordinary limitations of time and energy. This first section is designed to encourage and facilitate a more thorough examination than is commonly done and one that, if negative, would more reliably rule out the presence of neurologic disease. One should be aware, however, that major disease of the nervous system may be present without discernible functional alteration, no matter how searching the examination. The examination should, of course, be regarded as preliminary to a regional or local examination when symptoms call for more detailed inspection of a symptomatic area or a disturbed function.

Some will find it advantageous to combine the neurologic examination with the general physical examination, while others may find analysis easier by performing the neurologic examination separately. Many symptomatic disorders of the nervous system are usually related to disorders not primarily neurologic, e.g., atherosclerosis, valvular heart disease, metastatic malignancy, diabetes, and uremia. The possible relationship of nonneurologic findings to neurologic symptoms should always be kept in mind.

The second section describes common abnormal signs and syndromes of disease to help the examiner identify and interpret the significance of abnormalities disclosed by regional examination. The next sections are concerned with special problems in examining infants, diagnosing seizure disorders, and examining comatose patients.

An entirely new section on neurodiagnostic tests follows. This encompasses electromyography and nerve conduction tests, visual, auditory, and somatosensory evoked potential studies, electroencephalography, and the entire spectrum of modern neuroimaging procedures ranging from plain x-rays, cerebral angiography, and myelography to computer tomography and magnetic resonance imaging. This new section is not intended to be an encyclopedic discourse, but rather an introduction to these diagnostic aids that will enable the reader to understand how they are performed, what information can be gained from them, and ultimately, which should be requested in specific situations as an adjunct to the clinical examination. In keeping with the pictorial format of the book, this new section is amply illustrated with both normal and abnormal tracings and images.

Special supplementary diagnostic procedures that can be carried out on the ward or in the office are then described. These are followed by a section covering the mental status examination including specific techniques for evaluating memory, orientation, higher intellectual functions, spoken language and reception, writing, and reading.

Some repetition of text has been a natural consequence of the organization of the book. Some has been purposeful for emphasis. The methods and signs selected for description reflect a preference based on their usefulness in actual daily practice.

The neurologic examination and its related special sensory and performance tests are the most precise parts of a physical examination. The charm and unique value of the neurologic examination will not fade with progress in laboratory medicine. The examiner is able to go far beyond percussion, palpation, and auscultation. By observing function firsthand, he secures evidence of a quality not available to other disciplines except by laboratory studies. The more and greater variety of function that he can observe, the more evidence he can gather.

Robert L. Rodnitzky, M.D.

Acknowledgments

The contribution of Mr. George Buckley, who prepared the illustrations included in all three editions, is again gratefully acknowledged. Several colleagues were instrumental in the genesis of this text. Dr. Arthur Benton provided invaluable assistance in the original preparation of the section on mental status examination and in the subsequently expanded version that appears in the second and current edition of this book. Similarly, Dr. William Bell was very helpful in the genesis of the section on neurologic evaluation of the infant. Dr. James Corbett made valuable suggestions on neuro-ophthalmologic topics. Drs. Neill Graff-Radford, James Seabold, and Steven Cornell provided neuroradiologic illustrations for this edition. Drs. Thoru Yamada and Jun Kimura reviewed the sections on clinical electrophysiology and made many important suggestions.

I also wish to thank Mrs. Bernadette Spurgeon for her competent secretarial assistance in preparing the text.

ROBERT L. RODNITZKY, M.D.

Table of Contents

Preface vii

History 1
Preliminary Evaluation of Mentation and Speech 2

The Basic Neurologic Examination 5
Cranial Nerve Function 17
Strength and Function of the Extremities 35
The Reflexes 46
The Sensory Examination 58

Abnormal Signs and Syndromes—Basis and Interpretation 75
The Cranial Nerves: Their Relationships and Disorders 76
"Cerebellar Signs" 108
Hemiplegia and Hemiparesis 108
Dyskinesias 112
Parkinson's Disease 114
Motor Neuron Disease: Amyotrophic Lateral Sclerosis 116
Fasciculations 116
Spinal Paraplegia 117
Signs of Meningeal Irritation 119
Peripheral Neuropathy 119
Root Compression Syndromes 120
Paralysis of Peripheral Nerves 128
Disorders of Muscle 137
Polymyositis and Dermatomyositis 144
Myasthenia Gravis 144
Neurocutaneous Syndromes 147
Neurologic Disorders of Urinary Control 148
Rectal and Pelvic Examinations 148

Disturbances of Consciousness 151
Examination of the Patient in Coma 152
Seizures 156

Neurologic Evaluation of the Infant 161
Neurologic Examination of the Infant 162
Examination and Measurement of the Head 171

Laboratory Neurodiagnostic Aids 175
Electrophysiologic Tests 176
Neuroradiologic Tests of Skull and Brain 191
Neuroradiologic Tests of Spine and Spinal Cord 206

Supplemental Diagnostic Procedures 213
Brief Tests of Mental Status 214
Higher Intellectual Functions 216
Caloric Test for Vestibular Function 223
Lumbar Puncture 224

Index 232

History

Although the separation of history and examination is essential for record keeping, in fact the examination starts as soon as one sees the patient, and the history often is supplemented during the course of examination with unexpected findings.

Begin the history with age, occupation, handedness, residence, marital status, and military service of the patient. Then, with only the principal symptoms of the present illness in mind, establish the family and medical background to determine the setting of these symptoms. Inquire about surgical procedures, trauma and hospitalizations, parenthood, menstrual history, and yearly time on sick leave. Because of the potential of AIDS (acquired immune deficiency syndrome) to cause neurologic disease, it is more important than ever to ask about the patient's sexual preference and proclivity and use of intravenous drugs. Considerable tact and good judgment must be used in obtaining this information so as to avoid insulting or embarrassing the patient.

In the system review, ask especially about diabetes, heart and lung disease, hypertension, gastrointestinal complaints, and urinary function. Questions about neurologic disorders of parents and siblings may give revealing answers. Faced with a complex problem, one may plan to question the patient further at a later time.

When the patient is an infant or child, probe into the circumstances of gestation and delivery, attainment of standard landmarks of achievement, rate of gain in weight and height, and curve of continued progress. Ask about childhood diseases, serious illnesses, and trauma.

Having established the background, proceed to reconstruct the story of the present illness. Here instruction can have only limited value to the examiner. One learns from experience how to question people about disease. It will not always be clear when symptoms pertinent to the illness at hand actually started. Often a bit of probing will reveal that symptoms are of longer duration than at first stated. Be skeptical when serious symptoms are dated to an improbably related accident and especially a compensable one. When the neurologic symptoms are obviously secondary to a general disorder, develop the story of that disorder, chronologically fitting in the occurrence of neurologic symptoms. Note what previous treatment has been received—especially the kind and amount of drugs. Drug-induced disorders are frequently seen.

Some common symptoms of disease of the nervous system should be reviewed with each case:

1. Loss of interest, drive, and energy
2. Disorders of memory and thought
3. Headache
4. Seizures with convulsive activity, loss or alteration in consciousness, with details of aura and character of the episode
5. Visual changes (dimness, diplopia, and monocular or binocular acuity changes)
6. Loss of hearing and tinnitus
7. Loss of balance and vertigo
8. Change in speech and difficulty in swallowing
9. Clumsiness or weakness of the extremities, tremors, and involuntary movements
10. Spinal pain

11. The distribution, nature, and duration of pain, with its aggravating and ameliorating factors
12. Sensory distortions (paresthesias) or sensory loss in face, extremities, or trunk
13. Impotence or difficulty in urination

An accurate history is often worth many hours and much money spent on supplemental procedures. Pay particular attention to the proper chronology of events and to the time relationships of the various symptoms. The aim is to reconstruct an accurate picture of the appearance, regression, progression, and modification of symptoms, properly ordered in time.

Repeat questions concerning the various organ systems as each is examined or when abnormalities are uncovered. The examiner's inquisitiveness and the patient's memory will be stimulated during examination. For example, a scar found on the scalp may lead to reiteration of a previous question about head injury. The patient may then recall the details of forgotten trauma. The interrogation is likely to be more of an ordeal for the patient than the physician realizes, and important facts may be forgotten in the anxiety of an initial interview. Continued questioning during the course of examination will often produce significant information.

Always try to assess the reliability of sources of information and to check important points with as many observers as possible, particularly in regard to episodes of disturbed behavior, mental changes, periods of altered consciousness, or convulsions.

In puzzling cases, sit down with the patient or his relatives after a day or so and review the history at leisure. New information or corrections in the temporal order of events may then further elucidate the problem and lead to a correct diagnosis.

Preliminary Evaluation of Mentation and Speech

The mental examination begins with the first meeting and handshake. The grooming, dress, carriage, and, with women, make-up and accessories give some immediate insight into the patient's self-image. Later the physician will be able to determine how appropriate this self-image is and can then estimate the stresses that plague the patient. Poor grooming, careless dress, and indifferent posture, if inappropriate to the patient's background, raise the question of mental deterioration or depression.

The patient requires a fair degree of savoir faire to maintain poise and operate efficiently if he is unaccustomed to the role of patient. Hence he is apt to display less than his best ability at organization, recall, and understanding. This is not necessarily disadvantageous since the stressful situation, while reducing the efficiency of the normal person, will often uncover deficiencies of mentation in the ill that were not evident previously to either patient or family. The inability to do simple arithmetic or to carry out consecutive commands may be exposed as an unpleasant surprise to all concerned.

First impressions are not always sufficient to evaluate the normality of performance, considering the wide range of normal behavior and mental capacities of the patients encountered. Usually, however, when the initial interview is completed the physician will have formed a fairly accurate estimate of the patient's mental capabilities. The ability to recognize the content of questions put to him, to formulate a reasonable and fairly precise answer, and to stay on the subject without too much circumstantiality are all factors that go into judgment of normalcy of mental functioning. Alacrity in verbal response is characteristic of normal alertness, mental drive, motivation, and mood.

As the dialogue continues, the patient's level of education, vocabulary, and word usage will be evident. Only the more subtle forms of dysphasia are likely to escape the close attention to conversation that should be employed in history taking.

Do not attempt a detailed mental examination before rapport is established, usually after the physical examination or perhaps not until a second visit. A less rigorous mental examination obviously will be in order for the alert, fluent, and disgruntled patient with sciatica, whereas a more detailed study will be appropriate for the patient who is slow and vague in responding, uncertain in choosing common words, or lacking in spontaneity. The patient may be deceptively alert, however, and still have appreciable specific deficits. See Supplemental Diagnostic Procedures (p. 213) for the examination for aphasia and tests for determining mental status.

The Basic Neurologic Examination

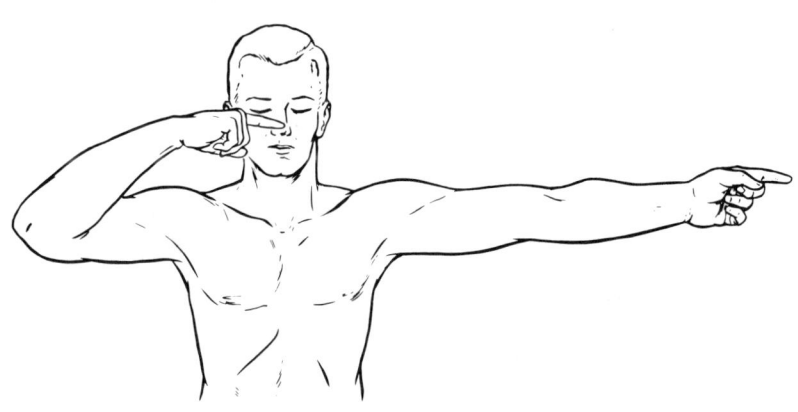

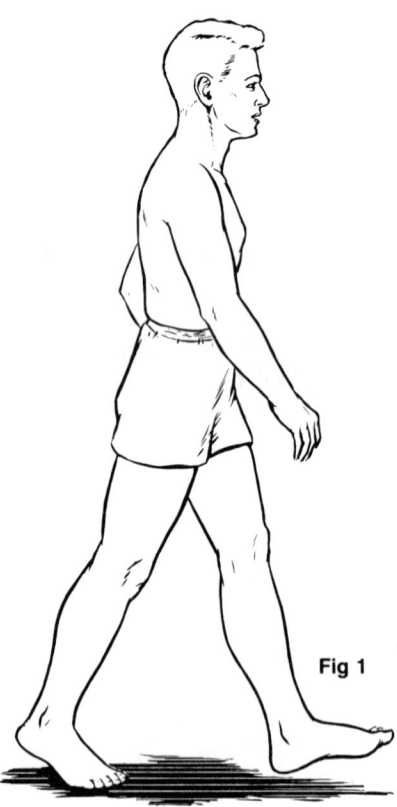

Fig 1

The energy, speed, and agility with which the patient rises and walks about provide important initial clues to his general health, his mood, and the status of his musculoskeletal and nervous systems. Maintenance of upright posture and walking bring into action a substantial portion of the nervous system, both motor and sensory. To see the patient get up and move about is as important in general orientation as the background history. Prior to the formal assessment of gait, it is worthwhile to observe the patient as he walks to the examining room. Often more can be learned while the patient is unaware that his gait is under scrutiny.

Walking is not a delicate function, however, and compensatory mechanisms can mask deficiencies. Moreover, disorders of gait caused by nonneurologic conditions, especially joint disease, may be misleading. Nevertheless, close observation of walking may yield important evidence of dysfunction of the nervous system. Ask the patient to walk back and forth several times and observe successively his posture, balance, arm swinging, and leg movement. As in almost any aspect of the examination, allowance must be made for age and obvious nonneurologic disability. If the gait seems unusually slow and cautious, encourage the patient to walk more rapidly since this may uncover subtle abnormalities not seen when he is moving at a slower pace. Common sense must be used in asking an ill or decrepit patient to walk. Sometimes it is fitting to assist a partially disabled patient to walk when this can be done safely.

The normal person progresses with only casual observation of the floor and a brief survey of the range of the area. Balance is normally achieved with no apparent attention or correction, with appropriate arm swinging, and with slightly flexed posture of elbows and fingers, palms facing thighs. As weight is shifted from one leg to the other, the heel of the weight-carrying foot lifts from the floor. The other foot swinging through is kept at right angles to clear the floor, and the pelvis remains parallel to the floor without tilting. The "springiness" of this normal gait is recognized as a sign of health and energy. Observe the hands for tremors and disturbed posture (dystonia), which may become more evident when the nervous system is occupied with the task of walking.

A cautious, short-stepped gait may be due to weakness, pain, disturbed sense of balance, disease of basal ganglia, or diffuse cerebral disease. A waddling gait results from weakness of the glutei, usually due to muscular dystrophy. A scraping toe may be due to footdrop of central or peripheral origin, in which case elevation of the leg to swing through is accompanied by a slapping of the foot. The spastic leg is characterized by limited swing, tendency to adduction, and loss of free joint movement.

In cases of spastic paraparesis, the legs of the patient may actually scissor and tend to trip him. The unilateral spastic leg in patients with hemiparesis may be pulled forward, with outward circling (circumduction) and stiffness and with dragging of the toe. Parkinsonism is characterized by stooped posture, loss of free swinging of the arms, a turning in one piece (en bloc) with stiff trunk and neck, and, often, shuffling. The depressed patient's slumped shoulders and slow gait may simulate Parkinson's disease. In patients with disease of the cerebellum, upright posture may be maintained only with difficulty, and often the excessive corrections for threatened loss of posture result in reeling and staggering. The hysterical patient may adopt bizarre postures and progression, often with dramatic values.

Accumulated deficits from lesions in several parts of the nervous system contribute to loss of function. The free-swinging, springy gait of

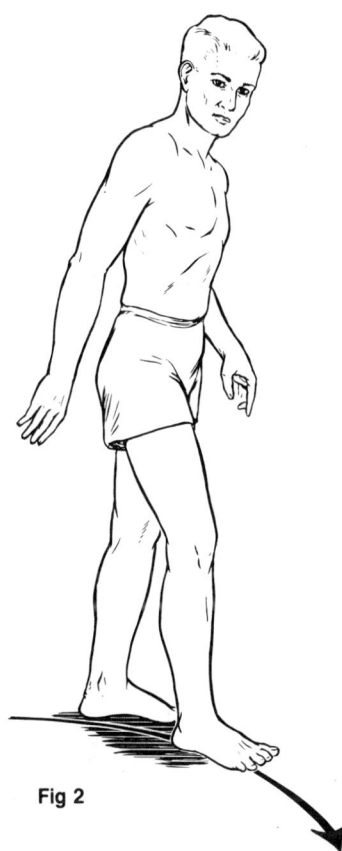

Fig 2

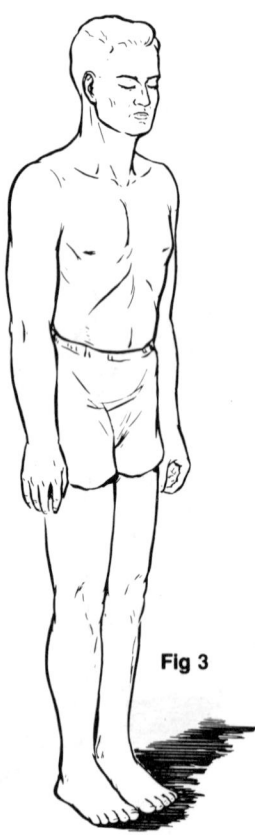

Fig 3

youth may give way in the aged to stiffer and slower, even shuffling, steps. Arthritic joints and loss of musculature add further to the decrepitude.

Ask the patient to turn rapidly as he walks. The face and head should lead, and balance should be well maintained. Ataxia may be betrayed by missteps or lurching. Failure to swing the arm and to turn head and trunk successively suggests parkinsonism or spinal arthritis. Running is more demanding, but it is usually neither possible nor wise to test this. Inquiry about this ability in the young is always appropriate.

The Romberg test assesses the ability of the patient to maintain upright posture while standing on a narrow base. This ability rests on sufficient strength for the job, on accurate information about position and about rate and direction of deviations in position as they occur, and on ability to make quick and appropriate compensations for threatened loss of balance. The patient stands erect, with feet approximated, looking straight ahead. Erect posture can be maintained with little swaying by most normal people. Young patients should be able to maintain balance with their feet in tandem position. *Always stand near the patient.*

Vision, even if defective, compensates substantially for deficits in posterior column and peripheral nerve function. When the eyes are closed the visual guide to posture is lost, and swaying and even falling may occur if the other sensory systems are diseased. When inability to balance well is caused by cerebellar disease, for example, vision is less able to correct for the difficulty in maintaining posture, and the patient will sway with eyes opened or closed. When there is a unilateral lesion of the cerebellum, the patient tends to fall toward the side where the lesion is located.

Swaying occurs in tense and hysterical patients; occasionally a hysterical patient will consistently fall into the arms of the examiner, whether the examiner stands to the right or the left. However, be careful, for such patients may also fall if the examiner is not close by. The test may have to be repeated to determine consistency of performance. Sometimes performance will improve if the test is repeated while the patient is distracted with another task. The Romberg test is not especially sensitive, and the range between normal and abnormal is broad. A subtle appeal to the patient's ego will elicit his maximal performance. Time is saved and more information gained by testing arm posture (p. 36) at the same time this test is done.

Standing on either leg alone is a much more demanding test of ability to maintain balance but is done poorly by many normal people. To do this for more than a few seconds with the eyes closed is difficult, and the test is chiefly of value in younger patients.

Tandem walking is a much more sensitive test of balance than the Romberg test. It is done as shown in Figure 4. Ask the patient to walk heel to toe down a line on the floor. The patient should be able to proceed without side steps or loss of balance. This test in effect narrows the base for maintaining balance and demands greater ability to compensate for changes in posture as walking proceeds. The patient normally will watch the line and the floor. Visual control will in part compensate for dystaxia based on afferent nerve, root, or posterior column lesions. The patient with disease of the cerebellum will have considerable difficulty with this test. Normal older people sometimes have difficulty in tandem gait, as may very obese patients. If the patient can perform this test well, other tests for body posture and dystaxia and the heel-to-knee test will usually be negative.

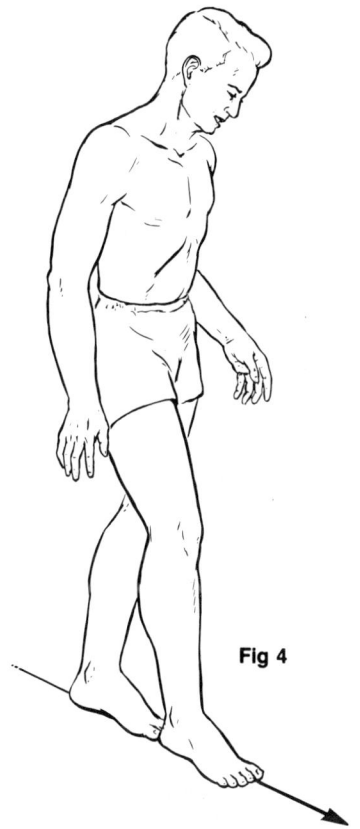

Fig 4

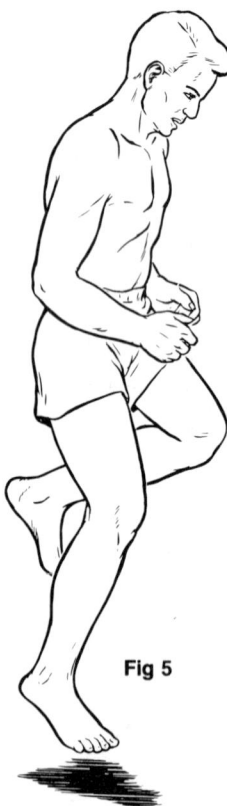

Fig 5

Hopping in place on either leg is one of the best screening tests for function that can be used for the ambulatory patient. Obviously it should not be requested of those whose general state of health or apparent disability make attempted hopping unwise. Elderly, arthritic, or obese patients would not perform well and might find the exercise impossible. Use caution and common sense in deciding which patients should perform this test, and routinely steady those who perform by holding one elbow lightly.

Hopping with agility requires intact function of much of the nervous system. If the patient can hop well on either foot, springing up and down in one spot on his toes while maintaining balance, he has little dysfunction of the long motor and sensory tracts, the cerebellum, the basal ganglia, the peripheral nerves, or the muscles of the hip and lower extremity. Hitting the heel hard, losing balance, being unable to get off the floor, or landing more than a few inches from takeoff serve notice of some disorder. A low, heavy, flat-footed hop is typical of upper motor neuron disorders. Slight awkwardness in hopping on one side often will be the only functional evidence of early paresis due to a lesion of cord or brain. Hopping may occasionally be done well in the presence of pathologic hyperreflexia and the Babinski sign if the patient is young and athletically accomplished. In patients with ataxia of posterior column or cerebellar origin, the performance will be awkward, with a poor springing action and inability to drop the foot at the point of takeoff. The cautious patient may refuse to perform, while the more cooperative and less judicious (e.g., occasionally a patient with multiple sclerosis) may try, with rather wild and frightening incoordination.

Although hopping is an excellent screening test for function, analysis of difficulties in performing this act can give only a general idea of the nature of the functional disorder.

While the patient is on his feet, it is convenient to proceed to other examinations of function of the legs, especially those testing the strength of muscle groups. These can instead be deferred to the time of examination of the lower extremities (p. 42). However, some of the muscle groups are so strong originally that in the early stages of disease weakness will not be detected on direct examination. Hence, whenever possible, test the strength of the leg muscles while the patient is standing upright and bearing weight.

Even though the musculature that extends the knee has already been tested in hopping, it is good to stress it more vigorously by requesting a *shallow* squat and rise, with the patient bearing the entire weight on one leg. The squat is then repeated on the other leg. This is the best and safest way to discover minor degrees of weakness. It is at the same time a test of the musculature that stabilizes the pelvis and that extends the thigh on the hip while engaging the back and hip-girdle musculature and hamstrings in the activity. Light support at the patient's elbow is appropriate. The normal person can easily squat and rise on one leg with only a little help in balance. Any differences between the performances of the right and left sides will be readily apparent. Difficulty in rising indicates weakness, and if the quadriceps is very weak, the patient will collapse to the floor. Arthritis, deformity of knee or ankle, primary muscle weakness, or a lesion at any level in the nervous system will interfere with performance of this maneuver. A less demanding test that is more suitable for the elderly patient is to have him step up on a footstool. In cases of

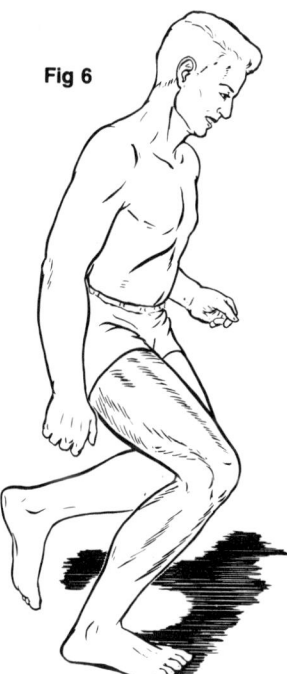

Fig 6

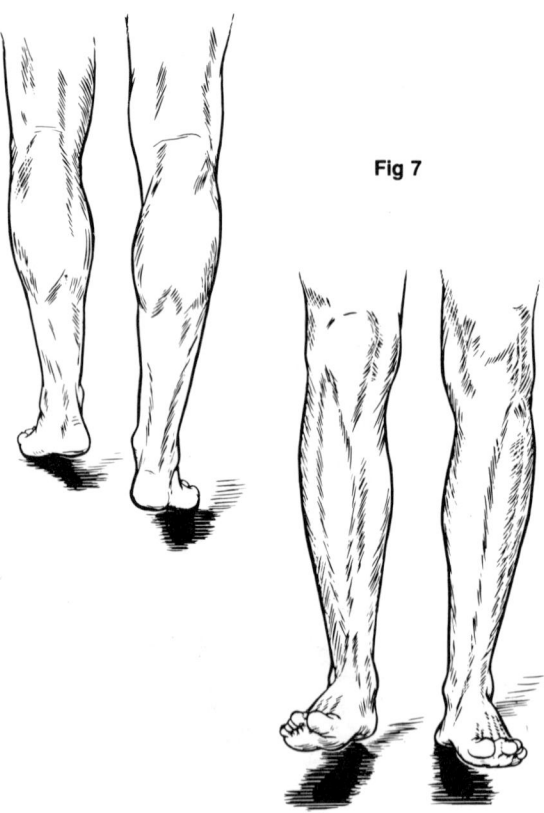

Fig 7

patients with proximal muscle weakness it is useful to observe the patient's attempt at squatting on both legs simultaneously.

When weakness is apparent, look for atrophy that may signify a lower motor neuron lesion or muscular disorder. However, disuse of a muscle from any cause—pain, immobilization, or paralysis of central origin—will result in some loss of muscle mass. The quadriceps, for example, is notoriously prone to disuse atrophy.

The patient who hops well does not have serious weakness of the gastrocnemius. This is a strong muscle and difficult to evaluate by direct testing. Watch the patient walk on his toes as he supports his entire weight on first one foot and then the other. Weakness will be evident if the heel drops in walking. Observe the contours of the musculature for atrophy and for hypertrophy. The patient who has suffered a stroke and has a moderate degree of spasticity and increased tone in antigravity muscles may still be able to rise on his toes. When weakness is evident on attempting this maneuver, look first for a primary disorder of root, nerve, or muscle.

Having the patient walk on the heels is an especially valuable screening test, since dorsiflexion of ankle and toes is weakened in many muscular and neural disorders. (Help the patient to maintain balance if necessary.) The normal person can hold the anterior foot and toes off the floor, strongly dorsiflexing the great toe as he walks on his heels. If he can do this, he does not have footdrop. He could, however, still have some minor weakness of the muscles of the anterior compartment, and these should be tested directly (p. 44). Footdrop may be of either central or peripheral origin. The severe footdrop of peripheral origin is clearly revealed by the abnormal nature of the gait and by an observable loss of dorsiflexion of the ankle and toes. If footdrop of peripheral origin (lower motor neuron) has been present several weeks, shrinkage and softness of the anterior compartment also will be apparent. When the leg is shaken, as in the test for alternating motion rate, the foot will be unstable and flop about. The foot is less floppy in central disorders (upper motor neuron lesions) and may be relatively fixed in plantar flexion. The toes of the spastic leg, when dorsiflexion of ankles and toes is weak, are dragged in walking. Before the examiner concludes that there is weakness of dorsiflexion, the foot should be passively dorsiflexed to be certain that previous weakness, now healed, did not permanently shorten the gastrocnemius.

These introductory tests serve as a valuable survey for screening in the ambulatory patient. The same principles should be applied throughout the examination. Elicit as much movement as is possible and sensible, patterned movement as well as isolated movement. Test strength against gravity whenever possible and applicable.

The term "upper motor neuron paralysis" refers to supranuclear disorders in which weakness, slowness, incoordination, and incompleteness of movement are due to lesions above the lower motor neuron. Atrophy of muscle can result from disuse but is seldom conspicuous. Stretch reflex pathways remain intact, and reflex responses are often exaggerated. The Babinski sign is usually present (p. 55). The motor system is so complex that the pattern of malfunction may vary greatly depending on the location and multiplicity of lesions. However, typical patterns can be found in conditions such as hemiplegia (p. 108) and spinal paraplegia (p. 117).

In lower motor neuron paralysis, weakness of movement is, by definition, due to a lesion of the motor cell or its axon, and diminished tonus is characteristic. The muscle shrinks and becomes soft and the reflex arc is interrupted, resulting in diminished or absent stretch reflexes. The Babinski sign is not present. Fasciculations of muscle may be present (p. 117). This pattern of malfunction is seen in poliomyelitis, motor neuron disease (p. 116), peripheral neuropathy (p. 119), and peripheral nerve injuries (p. 128).

In some conditions, notably amyotrophic lateral sclerosis and some spinal cord neoplasms, upper and lower motor neuron paralysis may coexist, and the clinical signs of each are found together, sometimes even in the same extremity.

Examination of the scalp provides clues to inflammatory or suppurative conditions, abnormalities of the underlying cranium, and previous cranial trauma or surgery. If the patient wears a hairpiece or wig it should be removed. It is surprising how much may be hidden by a heavy growth of hair. Palpating both sides simultaneously for comparison, move your fingers systematically over the entire scalp beginning at the occiput and progressing forward.

A horseshoe-shaped, surgical scar with small depressions of burr holes or larger defects of bone indicates a previous craniotomy. This finding is of special importance in the comatose or epileptic patient. Scars of old or recent trauma may be important.

Occasionally, a tumor of bone or an underlying meningioma will cause a hard, palpable elevation under the scalp (Fig 8,A). Sometimes enlarged scalp arteries will enter such an area. Listen for a bruit of increased blood flow. The metastases of hypernephroma and multiple myeloma may be associated with bruits. The external occipital protuberance is located in the midline posteriorly as shown in Figure 8,A. It may be ridgelike and quite large and is subject to considerable normal variation. It is occasionally mistaken for a neoplasm.

The scalp often contains small, movable tumors, usually inclusion cysts. Metastatic carcinoma may seed the scalp, and recently appearing tumors should be suspect. Lytic lesions of the skull due to metastatic tumors may not cause palpable elevation of the scalp but will transmit the patient's vocally produced sound in a manner distinguishable from that of the normal skull. When such lesions are suspected, use a stethoscope over the skull while having the patient say "ninety-nine" (Green-Joynt sign).

Always examine areas of pain, and gently percuss the scalp for focal tenderness. In acute sinusitis, tenderness will be present over frontal and maxillary sinuses. In some cranial neuralgias, tenderness will be found over the larger nerves of the scalp in occipital, temporal, and supraorbital locations. Local tenderness is common over scars in instances of post-traumatic headache.

Intense local or diffuse headache in the elderly patient may be associated with tender, hardened scalp arteries (giant-cell arteritis). Palpable arteries are shown in Figure 8,C.

The superficial temporal artery pulse may be asymmetrically bounding on one side, suggesting that, as part of the external carotid system, it is carrying collateral flow to compensate for internal carotid artery stenosis or occlusion on that side.

Many headaches are of extracranial origin, and some are associated with tightness and tenderness of posterior cervical muscles and the trapezii ("muscle-contraction" headaches). Often there is also point tenderness in the cervico-occipital region mesial to the mastoid.

Auscultation of the head and neck may reveal the sound of vascular turbulence. Areas of auscultation are shown in Figure 8,D. Compression of a normal artery by the stethoscope bell may sometimes produce a bruit. Bruits continuous over the full pulse cycle may be heard where peripheral resistance is low, as in arteriovenous malformations of the brain. Some bruits in infancy and childhood may not be pathologically based. In the neck, a venous hum can be distinguished from an arterial bruit by applying light pressure over the internal jugular vein above the point of auscultation. This will completely silence a hum but have no significant effect on an arterial bruit.

When examining comatose patients, look through the hair for signs of blood, scalp lacerations, and contusions. After proper preparation of the wound edges, one may use a sterile-gloved finger to search larger lacerations for fracture. When infection is found in a wound several days after trauma, the presence of a foreign body should be suspected. If hematomas are present, palpation of the scalp can yield misleading information, since the configuration of the swollen and infiltrated tissues may suggest a depressed fracture. Bleeding from an ear or drainage of cerebrospinal fluid from the ear, blood behind an eardrum, or ecchymosis over the mastoid process (Battle's sign; Figs 8,A and B), when not the result of direct trauma, are signs strongly indicative of a basal skull fracture.

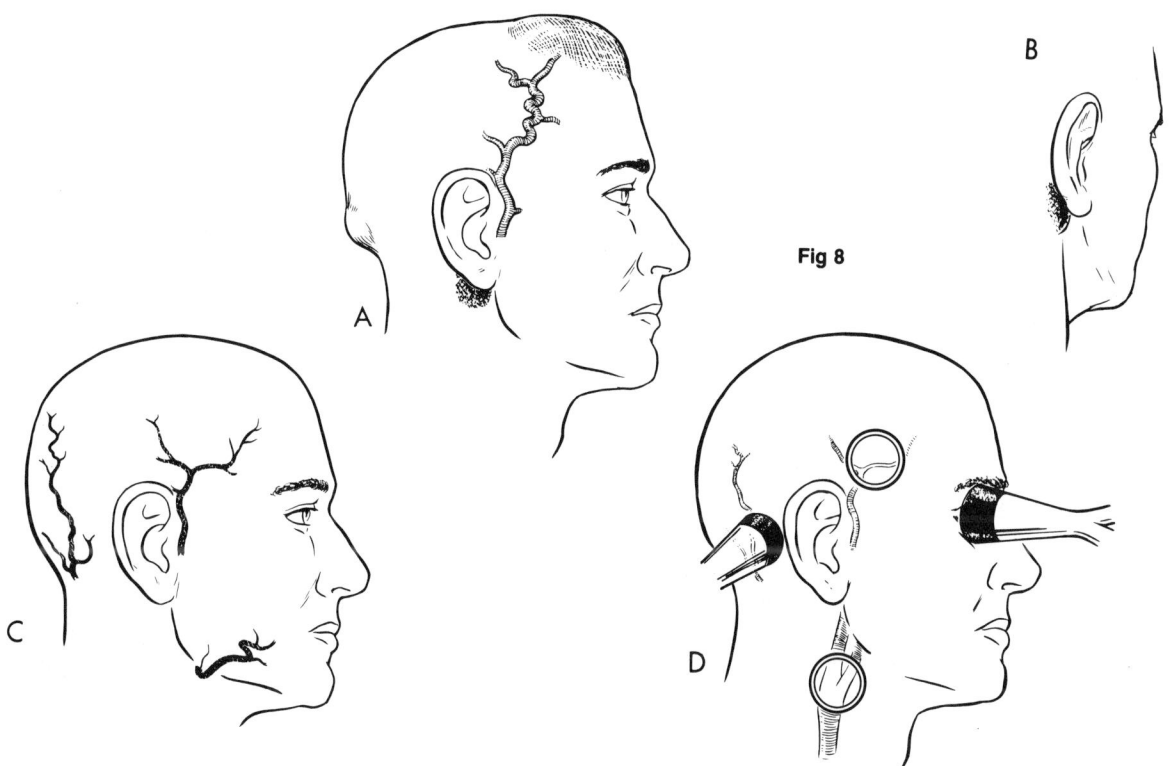

Fig 8

The Head / 15

Palpate the cervical spine posteriorly for local tenderness or deformity, especially when pain is a complaint. Move the neck *gently* through a full range of motion, flexing, extending, and rotating the head to either side and tilting it laterally (use caution in cases of trauma and of acutely acquired neck pain where there might be cervical instability due to fracture or neoplastic destruction of spinal elements). If pain on movement is severe, wait for roentgenograms of the cervical spine before proceeding with further manipulation. Cervical arthritis commonly limits lateral and twisting movements but seldom limits anteflexion. Meningitis limits forward flexion more than other movement (p. 119). Ask whether flexion of the neck causes tingling in arms, trunk, or legs (Lhermitte's sign), indicating cervical myelopathy. This sign is suggestive of multiple sclerosis but sometimes is present with other intraspinal disease.

When pain in the shoulder or arm is aggravated by neck movement or by pressure over the spine posteriorly (Fig 9,B), suspect nerve root impingement (p. 120).

If movements of the neck are not painful, grasp the patient's head, placing your hands on his forehead and occiput, and after assuring that the patient is relaxed, flex and extend his neck with smooth but moderately rapid movements. Resistance to forward flexion, especially a ratchetlike sensation ("cogwheel" rigidity), is seen in parkinsonism. However, this finding is not pathognomonic and is present in emotional tension states.

Flexion of the neck is not a strong function and is often weakened in patients with muscular dystrophies, motor neuron disease, and myasthenia gravis. Ask the patient to press his forehead into your palm, as shown in Figure 9,A, bending, not thrusting, the head forward and resisting your efforts to straighten the neck. One must, of course, have

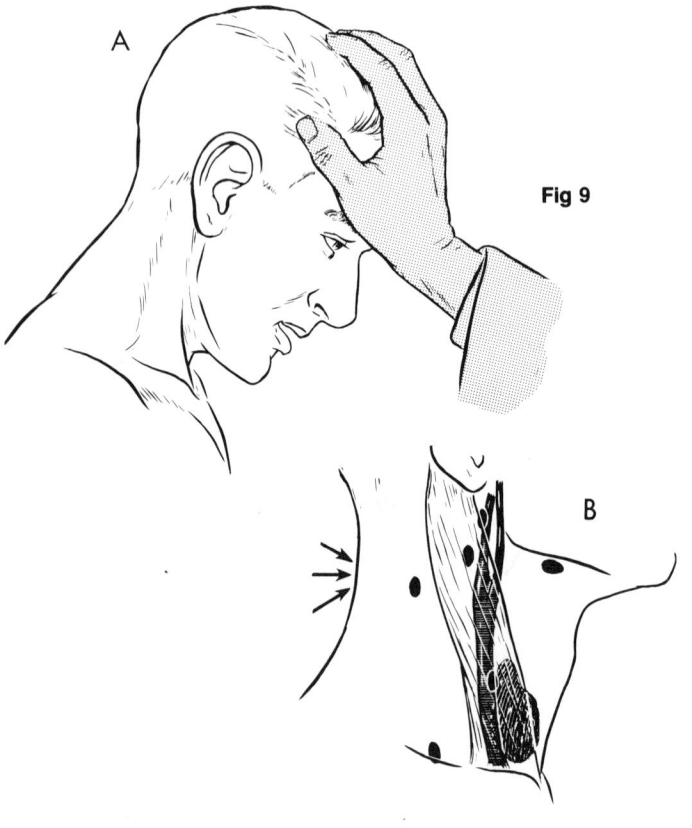

Fig 9

16 / The Neck

some knowledge of the normal range of strength. This test is a valuable part of the examination when muscular weakness is found elsewhere, especially weakness of ocular movement or of the lids. Weakness of the neck indicates a more diffuse disorder. Weakness without atrophy is seen in myasthenia gravis. As elsewhere, pain will inhibit full application of strength.

Palpate for the carotid pulses gently and listen for bruits (p. 14). Estimation of the degree of patency is not reliable, but absence of the pulse may indicate common carotid occlusion. Bruits over the bulb are an important sign of extracranial vascular disease. They are due to constriction of the lumen, usually of atherosclerotic origin, but occasionally are due to a kink or redundant coil in the vessel. Always listen below the carotid bulb over the common carotid artery, at the supraclavicular notch, over the upper chest and the heart, since bruits may be transmitted upward.

Avoid compression of the carotid arteries, which may cause syncope or convulsion. Carotid compression tests are not part of an initial examination and should be performed only by those able to deal with the consequences of untoward results.

Look for lymphadenopathy of infectious or neoplastic origin. Enlargement of the thyroid may indicate malignancy or thyroid disease.

Cranial Nerve Function

The 12 pairs of cranial nerves with their several end organs gather and conduct to the central nervous system much of the information that it receives from the outside world and much of what it receives from the viscera as well. The motor functions are devoted to positioning and adjusting the organs of the special senses, vocalizing, chewing and swallowing food, and controlling and adjusting the reflex of respiratory and visceral functions.

The physiologic and anatomic implications of disturbed function in the cranial nerves are so important to clinical diagnosis that a substantial portion of the examination is devoted to them. This is particularly true of the visual system and its subservient oculomotor apparatus.

Olfaction, a function of the first cranial nerve, may be tested using a variety of odors. Usually aromatic, nonirritating materials are used.

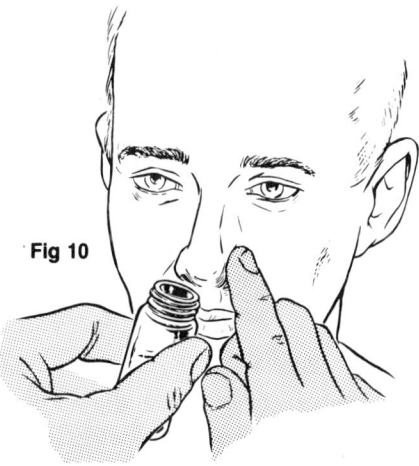

Fig 10

Oil of pine, oil of wintergreen, oil of rose, and oil of cinnamon are readily available and may be kept in small vials. Soap, tobacco, and coffee may also be used, care being taken to avoid giving a clue as to the substance employed. Test each olfactory nerve separately by closing one of the patient's nostrils while he sniffs the odor through the other. Both acuity of smell and ability to identify odors accurately are quite variable in normal people. The average adult person who is free of nasal obstruction and acute or chronic disease of the nasal mucosa will sense the odors mentioned. He should also be able to categorize the general nature of the odor, as, for example, perfume, candy, soap, seasoning, or the like.

The most telling finding is unilateral loss of smell with no evident nasal disease. This should be especially sought when other findings suggest a frontal neoplasm. Unilateral or bilateral loss of smell is a classic symptom of meningioma of the olfactory groove, may follow trauma, may accompany meningitis, and occasionally occurs for no apparent reason in elderly people, who also sometimes report distortion of smell (parosmia).

The findings on this examination bear no relationship to uncinate seizures or the spontaneous sensing of nonexistent bad odor, which may be a feature of certain convulsive disorders.

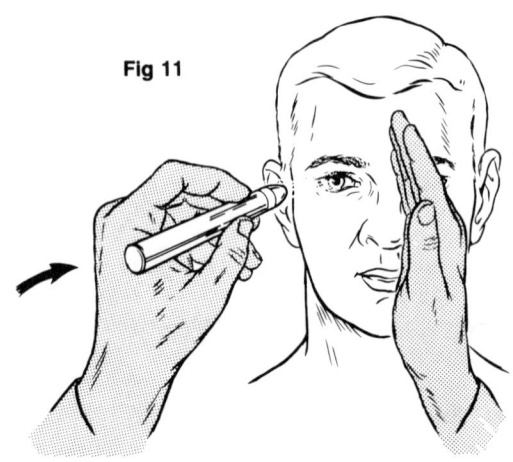

Fig 11

Normally the pupils are round and equal in diameter. Difference in size (anisocoria), if small, may not represent disease and can be evaluated accurately only with reference to other findings, such as ptosis. Pupillary diameter is chiefly dependent on intensity of illumination but is greater in children than in adults and is usually small in the elderly. In ordinary room light the diameter may vary from 2 to 6 mm. Diameter should also be assessed in dim light.

The reaction to light should be tested in diminished illumination. Shield one eye of the patient and swing the light beam from his side onto the pupil. Pupillary constriction based on the near reflex will then be avoided. Contraction will normally be prompt and maintained if the light is bright, and dilation will be prompt when the light is removed. Avoid thrusts at the eye, which will startle the patient. Watch the opposite pupil while illuminating its fellow. It should constrict as quickly and as extensively as the directly tested eye. This is the *consensual* light reaction.

Ask the patient to look at the end of your finger (or, better, his finger) as it is brought toward the nose in the midline. As the eyes converge, the pupils should constrict. This miosis is part of the near reflex, which includes convergence and accommodative changes in the lens for focus.

The pupillary size results from the balance between sympathetic and parasympathetic innervation. Drugs, such as atropine, that act on the autonomic nervous system therefore profoundly affect pupil size and reaction. Startle (e.g., to a loud noise), fear, or pain dilate the pupil unless its sympathetic fibers are interrupted (pp. 77; 98).

It may be difficult to see the pupil because of reflection from the cornea or, in some patients, because of a deeply pigmented iris. The ordinary otoscope attachment on a battery handle can be used to advantage. Take off the speculum, focus on the pupil through the viewing lens, and turn on the light. The pupillary reaction can then be followed easily.

Visual acuity should be measured in all patients. This is customarily done by having the patient read the lines of a well-illuminated Snellen chart (Fig 12) at 20 ft (6 m). Determine the acuity for each eye alone with the other covered. If the line designed to be read at 20 ft is read at that distance, the vision is recorded as 20/20. If at 20 ft the patient can read no line lower than that which the normal person can read at 40 ft, the visual acuity is recorded as 20/40. OD designates the right eye, OS the left. When acuity is so reduced that the patient can read none of the letters at any distance, he should be requested to count the number of fingers that the examiner holds up. If he cannot do this, he may be able to tell whether the room is light or dark or may sense a light flashed in his eye, in which case he is said to have light perception only.

Because measurement of visual acuity is so often neglected, the chart below is furnished. This chart is to be read at 5 ft and has been reduced to one fourth the size intended to be read at 20 ft. Five feet is approximately the distance from the eyes of a patient in bed with head elevated

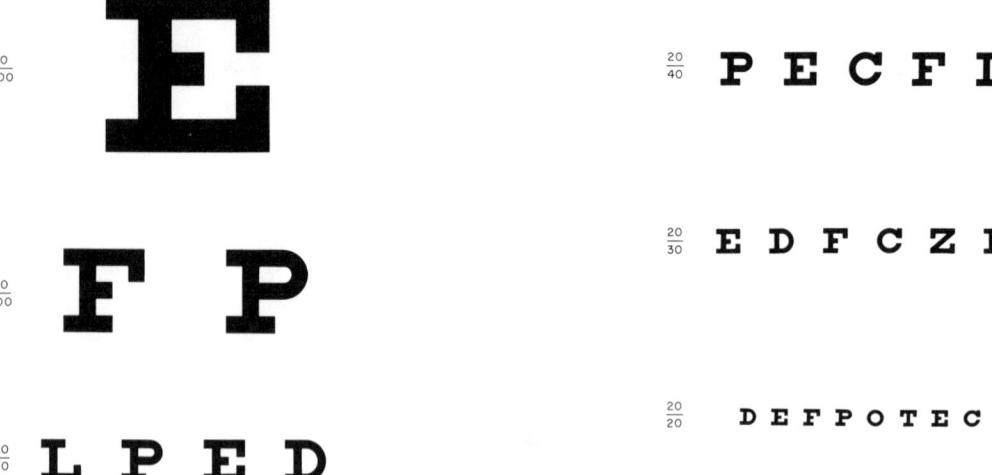

Fig 12

20 / The Second Cranial Nerve

to the book held by the examiner standing at the foot of the bed. This distance is also appropriate for a small examining room. When possible, determine the distance with a tape measure. The chart page should be well lighted and held as flat as possible. The eyes are tested alternately, the patient covering one eye with a card. If he ordinarily uses glasses to improve vision at this distance, he should wear them for the test. After the first eye is tested, the second should be tested by asking the patient to read the line in reverse. The fraction on the left of each line indicates the visual acuity necessary to read this line under the conditions just stated. The fractional notation of the smallest line that can be read is the visual acuity of the examined eye. If only the large E can be read, then acuity is 20/200. If the smallest line, DEFPOTEC, can be read at 5 ft, the acuity is normal, or 20/20. Some degree of accommodation is involved in reading at 5 ft, but the error so introduced will be small and usually negligible except in the elderly patient with severe presbyopia. When in doubt, resort to the standard chart under standard conditions.

When an uncorrected refractive error is a possible explanation for poor acuity, the pinhole test is used. Viewing the chart through a pinhole eliminates much of the optical problem in refractive abnormalities. With a common pin, make eight or ten holes near the corner of a card (preferably one with a dark surface). This makes it easy for the patient to find a hole and to hold it in front of the pupil while he repeats the test. Acuity will be improved if visual loss is due to a refractive error but not if it is due to disease of the retina or visual pathways.

Normal central acuity may remain even when there are substantial defects in the peripheral fields.

Observe the eyes for normal relationship of lids to cornea (Fig 13,A), for possible dropping of an upper lid (ptosis), and for the close following of the lids in vertical movements (Figs 13,B and D). Contraction of the frontalis is a normal synkinesis of strong vertical gaze upward (Fig 13,B).

Observe for parallelism of the visual axes in forward gaze and for conjugate movements in lateral and vertical gaze necessary to the maintenance of this parallelism (Figs 13,B-F). Ask the patient to follow a moving object with his eyes. His fixation should be directed to a finger or an object held several feet from the eyes to avoid convergence. The eyes should be able to follow smoothly and conjugately without jerking. Ask the patient if he has double vision (diplopia) and, if he does, determine by moving the finger about where diplopia is most evident. When visual acuity in one or both eyes is much reduced or when such an extreme gaze position is elicited that the adducting eye is covered by the nose, diplopia will not be reported even though there is weakness of one or more ocular muscles.

Hold the patient's thumb and ask him to focus on it as you move it in the midline toward his nose from a distance of 2 ft. The eyes should converge (Fig13,G) and the pupils constrict (p. 77). The ability to converge is quite variable, and very limited convergence may be normal. Fair visual acuity in each eye is usually necessary for convergence.

The illustrations show the eyes carried into vertical and horizontal gazes only. This is usually sufficient for a screening examination because diplopia will be elicited by these maneuvers and, when present, can be analyzed in more detail later. Severe paralysis of an eye muscle or of one of the three cranial nerves subserving eye movement will reveal itself in a deficiency of movement or lack of parallelism of the eyes (pp. 86; 88).

Vertical and horizontal gazes are subserved by different mechanisms, and selective involvement of one pattern of movement has interpretable significance. Vertical gaze upward is commonly reduced in the aged.

Many disorders of eye position and movement are congenital. In ordinary strabismus, the movements of each eye tested alone are of full range and the dysconjugate position of the eyes is constant in all directions of gaze. This is called concomitant strabismus and is not attributable to neurologic disease. Always inquire about the duration of any deviation seen.

Usually, any recently acquired paresis of extraocular muscles will cause diplopia. Later, vision in one eye may be suppressed, and this symptom will be lost. A head tilt may be present to compensate for a weakened ocular muscle or gaze paralysis.

After observing for defects in ocular movement and for diplopia in the several gaze positions noted, repeat the maneuvers to observe for jerky movements of the eyes (nystagmus), an abnormality usually aggravated by gazing away from the midline. A few low-amplitude jerks at extremes of gaze position are usually not evidence of abnormality (p. 94).

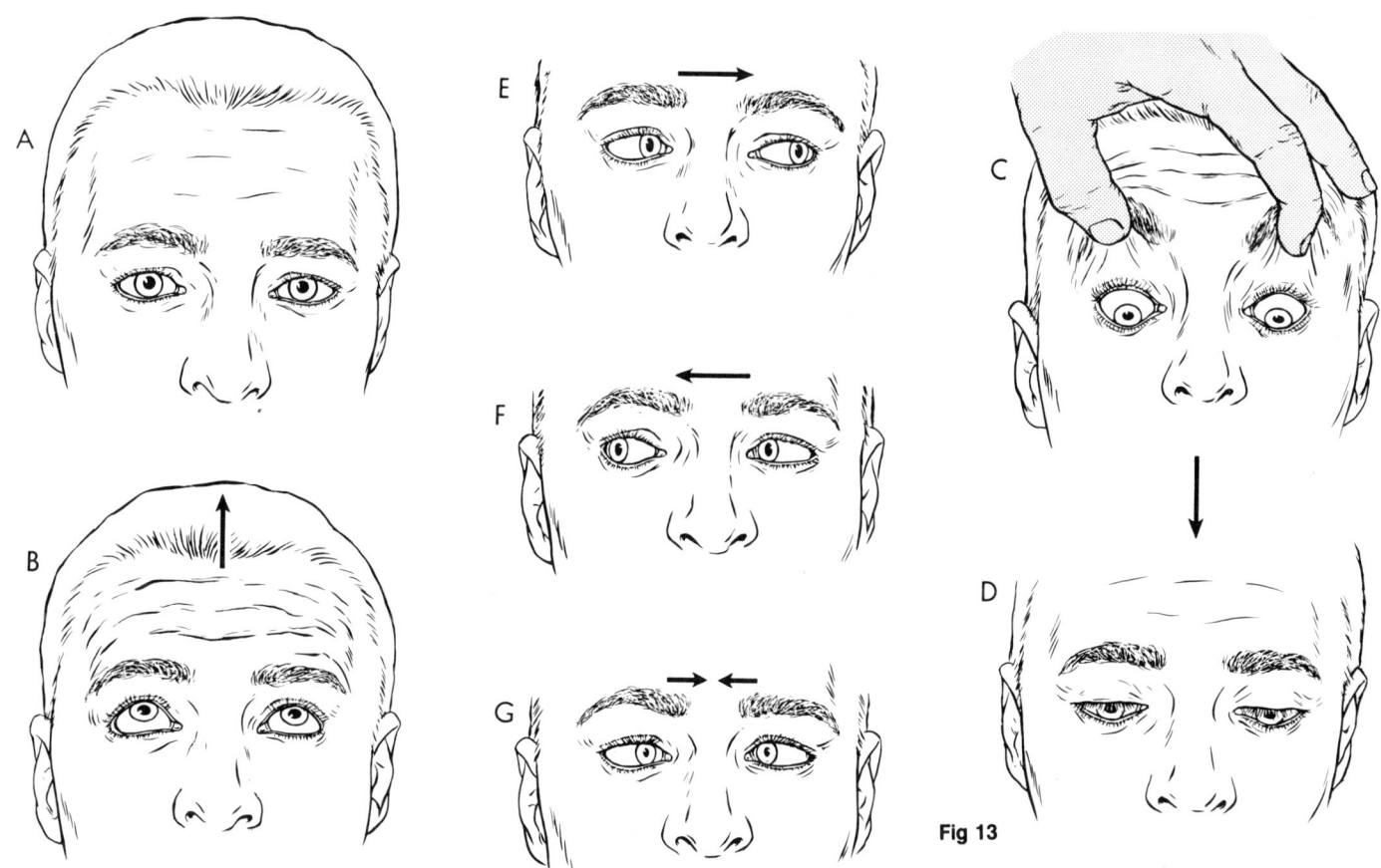

Fig 13

The Third, Fourth, and Sixth Cranial Nerves (Oculomotor, Trochlear, and Abducens) / 23

The method of visual field estimation shown here is that of confrontation. The field of each eye alone extends about 60 degrees nasally, 100 degrees temporally, and 130 degrees vertically. One eye is tested at a time, with the other covered. The physician and patient focus on the opposite eye of one another at distance of about 3 ft. Then the examiner, with arms outstretched, simply asks the patient if both hands can be seen and if they appear identical. A difference in clarity, brightness, size, or color, or simply a response that one hand looks "different," should be regarded as a clue to a possible visual field defect. Often such nondescript alterations in perception in one field are the only clue to a visual field loss later evidenced on formal perimetry. Next, the patient is asked to point to the finger that is being moved slightly and irregularly from side to side and up and down. If the movement is not seen, the examiner's finger is slowly brought toward the center of vision, moving slightly all the while, until it is seen. Usually such movements are made in radii, as though the pupil were the center of a wheel. Areas of lost vision should be checked several times and charted on paper for analysis (pp. 82–84).

Another useful way of testing is to ask the patient to count the number of fingers being held up by the examiner in each of the four visual field quadrants. This test can be made more sensitive by the method of simultaneous stimulation. Fingers are presented at the same time in areas on either side of the midpoint or above and below the horizontal axis. When vision is defective in one area, the fingers in that field may not be detected though the other fingers are seen in the normal part of the field.

Sensitivity to red is reduced in areas of visual field depression. Use the basic confrontation technique and slowly move a red test object (e.g., a red plastic picnic spoon) across the field from normal to suspected abnormal side. Inquire if and where the red color is lost or takes on a different shade. Do this in several radii, searching for regions of loss of redness perception. This test adds further sensitivity to confrontation testing. Sensitivity to red is normally reduced in the peripheral field beyond the central 20 degrees of vision.

When there is a defect on the same side of the field in **each eye,** the test should be repeated with the patient using both eyes. **In cases of** homonymous defects, the same deficit will be found **whether the patient** uses both eyes or each eye alone. Bitemporal defects **will not be found** when both eyes are used because of overlapping in the binocular field.

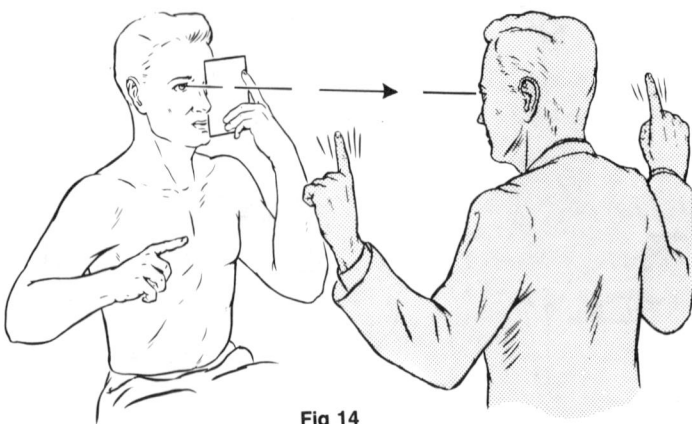

Fig 14

Ophthalmoscopy provides a fascinating, direct view of the complex neural tissue of the retina and its rich blood supply. Most of the abnormalities of the retina, whether secondary to systemic diseases or apparently primary within the retina, are of potential importance to neurologic diagnosis.

The optic nerve head with its adjacent vessels is the primary focus of the neurologist's attention (Fig 15). This area can usually be seen through the normal pupil. Have the patient seated or reclining in a darkened room and staring straight into the distance. Often it will be necessary to point out some object for fixation if his eyes wander. Normal variations are considerable, but one soon learns to expect to see a reasonably sharp outline of the disc with a normal complement of fine intrinsic vessels and a pinkish color. The pallor of primary optic atrophy is associated with disappearance of this vasculature. A poorly outlined disc with swollen fibers radiating out in all directions and apparently elevated above the fundus is characteristic of papilledema. Usually the veins appear congested and enlarged. Often small striate hemorrhages are seen if intracranial hypertension is severe or has increased rapidly (p. 79).

The major retinal vessels should be closely inspected for irregularity, segmental spasm, or reduction in size. Some estimation of the severity of general vascular disease can be made on the basis of these changes, together with evidence of any hemorrhages or exudates seen in patients with malignant hypertension.

Pigmentary degeneration of the retina may be associated with degenerative or inflammatory disease of the nervous system. The student is referred to standard texts for further study of this important area in diagnosis.

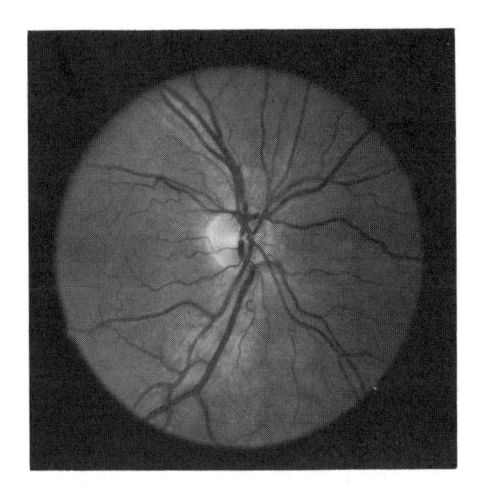

Fig 15

The motor branch of this nerve supplies the muscles used in mastication but does not innervate the muscles used in facial expression. It innervates temporal, masseter, and pterygoid muscles. Observe first the contours of the temporal and masseter muscles. Nerve injury, motor neuron disease, and muscle dystrophies result in weakness and atrophy, with hollowing out of these areas. Some hollowing, but not weakness, is normal in the aged and those who have lost weight. Ask the patient to simulate a bite, bringing the jaws together, while you palpate the masseters with your fingers and attempt to open the patient's jaw with your thumbs (Fig 16,A). The normal strong contraction and bulging of the masseters will be apparent. No tolerable force can spring the normal jaws apart. Differences in the two sides are usually easy to detect but should be evaluated bearing in mind that asymmetry of bite can cause uneven contraction. Slipping a tongue blade between the molars will enable the patient to execute a full bite on that side. Pterygoid strength can be tested by having the patient forcefully deviate the jaw to each side against the examiner's hand. It is important to remember that the pterygoids subserve jaw deviation to the contralateral side.

The sensory portion of the nerve innervates much of the scalp and most of the face (Fig 16,D), overlapping with branches of the cervical nerves and plexus. It conveys sensation from the gums, buccal mucosa, and anterior tongue. The ophthalmic division (*I*) conducts sensation from the eye and from the cutaneous area shown. It also supplies the tentorium of the cerebellum. The maxillary division (*II*) conducts sensation from the facial area shown in Figure 16, from the upper jaw, gums, teeth and nasal mucosa. The mandibular division (*III*) carries sensation from the face, tongue, lower jaw, gums, and teeth.

Carefully prick the face with a pin on one side and then the other, asking for the patient's sensation and comparison. Always show the patient the pin first. It is very easy to suggest differences, and reports of minor differences are common (pp. 58–60). The ophthalmic branch does not end at the normal hairline but will continue far posteriorly, so the pin should be advanced posteriorly on the side of the suspected deficit. If the patient notes a change at the end of the nerve distribution, this strongly suggests that sensory loss is authentic.

An excellent and more objective method of comparing pain sensation in the ophthalmic division of the two sides is to elicit the blink reflex to corneal stimulation. Tell the patient you are going to touch the eye. Ask him to look to one side (Fig 16,B) while you touch the cornea gently with a wisp of cotton (Fig 16,C), approaching the cornea laterally so the cotton is not seen. It is wise to apply a test stimulus to the relatively insensitive sclera first to be certain that any blink observed is not in response to the threat of the moving cotton wisp perceived in the periphery of vision. Upon stimulating the cornea, compare the promptness and completeness of lid closure and ask for the patient's subjective comparison. Presence of a weak orbicular muscle will diminish the motor response, but otherwise the patient's reactions of lid closure and withdrawal of the head should be executed promptly if sensory function is intact.

Ask for the feeling produced by light application of cotton to the face in all divisions, comparing the two sides. Usually one is misled less by ignoring minor differences.

Diseases of the fifth cranial nerve may cause only pain and not any of the motor or sensory findings here described. Trigeminal neuralgia is such a condition.

Fig 16

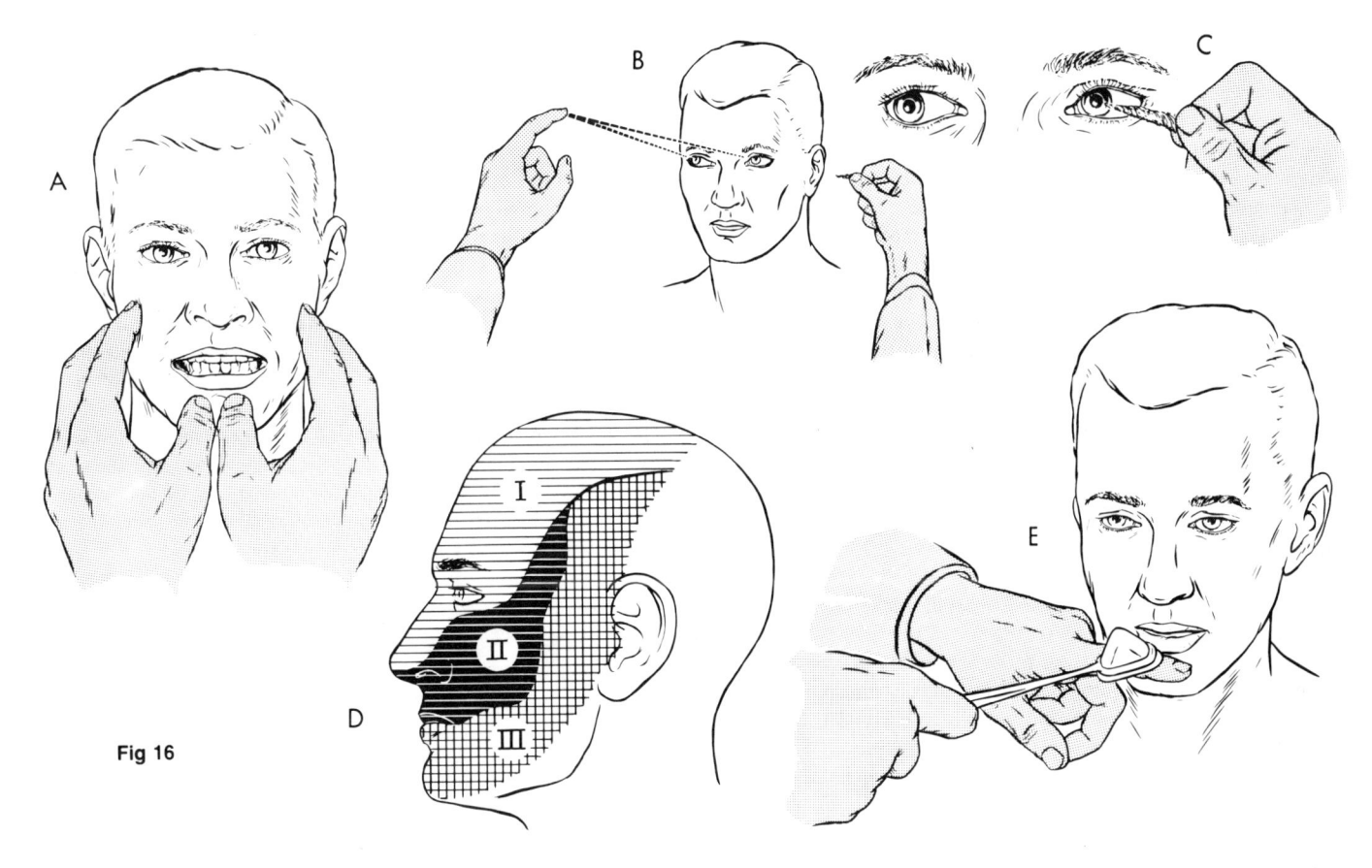

The Fifth Cranial Nerve (Trigeminal) / 27

The jaw jerk or stretch reflex of the muscles of mastication is mediated by the fifth nerve. Elicit this reflex as shown in Figure 16,E, asking the patient to relax and slightly open the jaw. Exaggeration of this reflex is evidence of bilateral corticobulbar disease.

Study the patient's face carefully while taking the history. With experience, impressions of prime importance may be gained from noting facial color, texture, and mobility while appraising mood, state of health, and intelligence.

The musculature of the face and the platysma are innervated by the seventh cranial nerve. Observe the play of expression and look for symmetry of movement, abnormal movements, tics, grimaces, and tremors. Note the degree of expressional change or its absence; watch for the slack-jawed loss of expression seen in patients with dystrophies and pseudobulbar palsy, and for the immobility with infrequent blinking symptomatic of parkinsonism. Minor degrees of unilateral weakness are often best seen when the patient is at rest or during expressional changes of conversation, with blinking.

The extent of normal facial mobility varies widely. Some people are unable to make relatively isolated movements such as a wink. Ask the patient to direct his gaze strongly upward and at the same time to wrinkle his forehead (Fig 17,A). The strength of the frontalis can then be estimated by smoothing the wrinkles with your fingers. Have the patient close his eyes tightly. Look for asymmetry in the ability to bury the eyelash under the folds of the contracting upper and lower lids (Fig 17,B). Next, try to open the patient's eyelids gently (Fig 17,C). Ask him, "Show me your teeth," so that you can check retraction of the corners of the mouth (Fig 17,D). Many patients are either sensitive about the appearance of the teeth or preoccupied with their dentures; if this movement is tested after several others, the patient will know the examiner's interest is in his face, not his teeth, and inappropriate responses may be avoided. Request that he blow out his cheeks, containing the air with pursed lips (Fig 17,E). Then squeeze the cheeks in to force expulsion of the air. Weakness will be apparent if present, compared with the response in a patient with normal strength. Ask the patient to pout the lips as shown in Figure 17,F. Test the platysma by asking the patient to pull down the corners of his mouth (Fig 17,G). It may be necessary to demonstrate this maneuver. This musculature is poorly developed in some people; nevertheless, minor degrees of unilateral facial weakness may sometimes be displayed first in this muscle. One may have the reluctant patient exhibit expression while testing the grips and thus take advantage of the synkinesis produced by grimacing on effort.

Remember that the entire face may be weak, hence the importance of A, C, and E in Figure 17. If part of the face is weak, estimate whether this weakness is only in the lower face or is shared by both upper and lower parts (p. 99). The facial nerve via its division, the chorda tympani, conveys taste from the anterior tongue (p. 103).

28 / The Seventh Cranial Nerve (Facial)

Fig 17

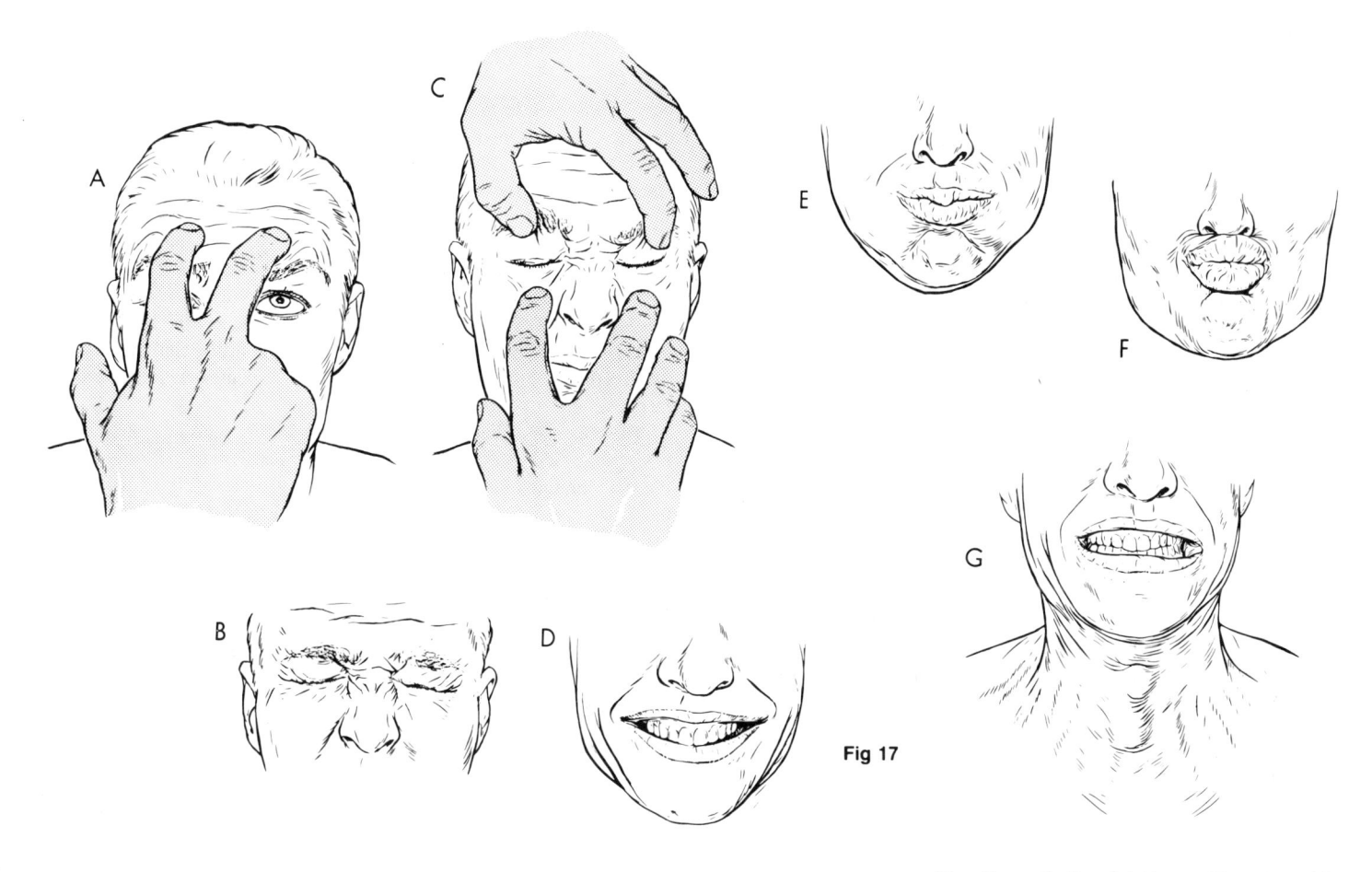

The Seventh Cranial Nerve (Facial) / **29**

The eighth cranial nerve has two divisions, the auditory and the vestibular. Only the auditory division is tested in the usual clinical examination. Evaluation of the vestibular portion will be described in the section on Supplemental Diagnostic Procedures.

Always reiterate questions about hearing when this part of the examination starts. If ordinary conversation can be heard in a noisy room (excepting cases of otosclerosis, in which hearing loss is paradoxically improved in a noisy environment) and if the telephone can be used with either ear, the degree of loss is not great. The complaint of tinnitus should always alert one to the likelihood of hearing loss.

Examination of the external ear canal and tympanum is, of course, routine. Infection of the middle ear must be looked for in any case of meningitis. Evidence of old, healed middle-ear disease suggests that hearing loss is due to that past disease rather than to a present neural deficit. Chronic suppuration of the middle ear and mastoiditis are classically, although no longer commonly, complicated by an abscess of the cerebellum or of the temporal lobe.

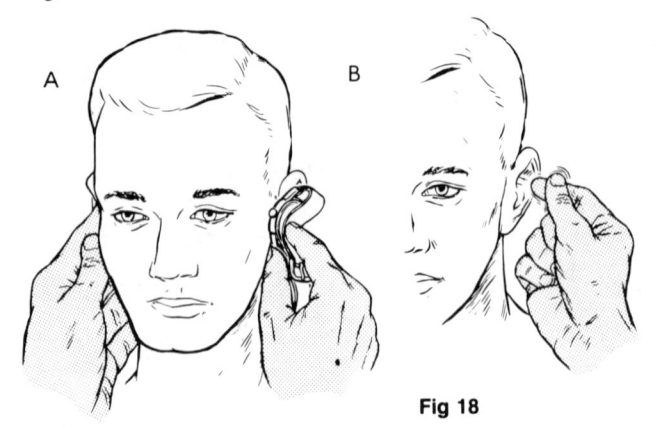

Test the hearing by determining if the patient can hear a wristwatch tick with either ear (Fig 18,A). The tick of any watch (other than electronic watches, which hum rather than tick) can be heard by the patient with normal hearing. Rub the fingertips together lightly at varying distances from the external meatus (Fig 18,B) to compare the acuity of the patient's hearing on the right and left sides. One may quantitate this test rather crudely by comparing the patient's responses with one's own responses or with those of normal patients.

The Rinne and Weber tests are of value in distinguishing nerve deafness from middle-ear deafness. The Rinne test is done on both sides. Place a vibrating tuning fork (256 cps) on the mastoid (Fig 19,B). When the sound ceases, hold the tines near the acoustic meatus (Fig 19,A). In the normal ear the waning vibrations will still be audible. This result is termed a positive Rinne test. In cases of middle-ear deafness, air conduction is not louder than bone conduction, so the waning vibrations will not be audible at the acoustic meatus, and the Rinne test will be termed negative. A hearing loss of approximately 10 to 20 dB or more will be detected by this test.

The Weber test is performed by placing the vibrating tuning fork (256 cps) firmly on the scalp at the vertex (Fig 19,C) and asking the patient if he hears the tone and if it is more evident in one ear than in the other. In the normal patient the sound will be sensed in the midline area. When unilateral hearing loss is due to middle-ear disease, the patient reports

Fig 18

hearing a louder tone on the diseased side—presumably because of diminished competition from extraneous, air-conducted noise on that side. Check this by doing the same test on yourself while closing one ear with a finger. A conductive hearing loss of only 7 to 12 dB is sufficient to cause a lateralization of sound to the abnormal ear. When there is nerve deafness on one side, the sound will be louder in the normal ear.

When performing tuning-fork tests, it is important to be certain that the patient can distinguish between the sound of the fork and the tactile sensation of vibration. Though a 256-cps fork is more effectively used than a 512-cps fork in uncovering mild hearing loss, it also results in a more prominent sense of vibration. If it is not clear that the patient is responding to the sound of the fork rather than to its vibration, it is useful to attempt to educate the patient about the difference between sound and vibration by applying a 512-cps fork, which produces a tone with very little sense of vibration.

Loss of hearing in children or young adults is usually due to infection, noise exposure, trauma, or otosclerosis. Loss of hearing is almost never due to brain-stem, thalamic, or cortical lesions. In adults, middle-aged or older, vascular disease, presbycusis or Meniere's disease may be responsible. Toxic agents such as streptomycin and other aminoglycoside antibiotics may cause hearing loss and/or vestibular damage at any age. A tumor of the eighth nerve may cause unilateral loss of hearing, tinnitus, and loss of vestibular nerve function at any age, but typically after adolescence.

Whenever detailed information about the auditory division of the eighth nerve is desirable, audiometry must be used. Similarly, electronystagmography is helpful in investigating the function of the vestibular

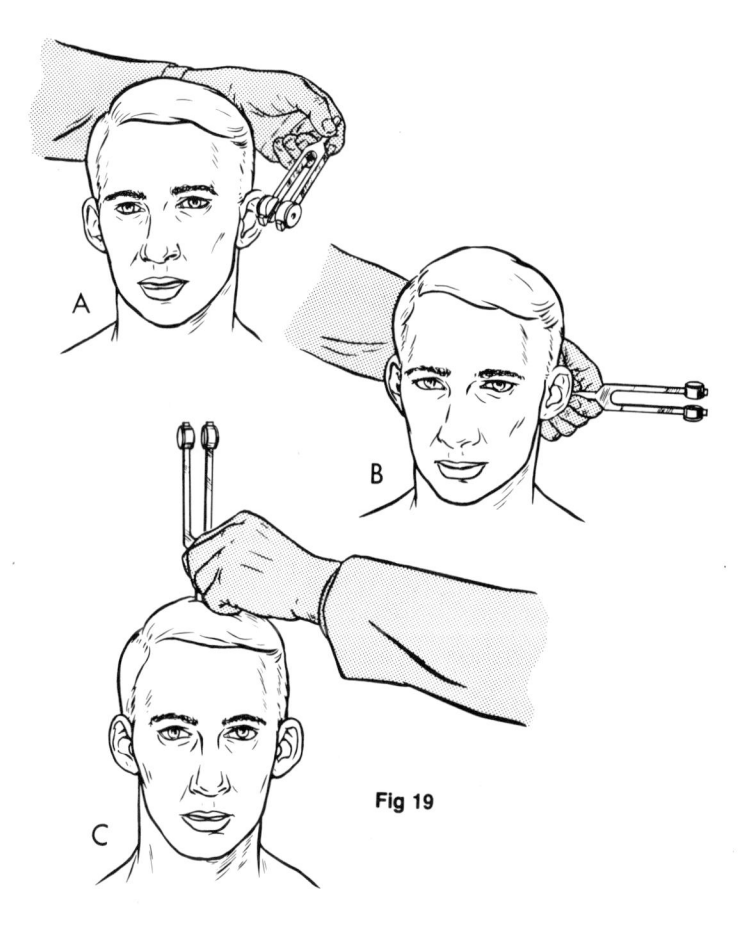

Fig 19

The Eighth Cranial Nerve (Auditory Division) / 31

division. These techniques provide precise information about the relative involvement of vestibular and auditory functions, including, in audiometry, localization to the cochlea, cochlear nerve, or middle-ear ossicles. Both tests are particularly useful in the diagnosis of tumors of the eighth nerve.

The origins and the courses of the ninth and tenth cranial nerves from the medulla through the base of the skull are closely proximate, and their testable functions are not entirely separable. Thus, it is logical to discuss them together.

The ninth (glossopharyngeal) nerve conveys taste from the posterior tongue and contributes to the sensory innervation of the tonsillar pillars, soft palate, and pharyngeal wall. It innervates musculature that elevates and constricts the pharynx. Because it is afferent for baroceptors in the carotid bulb, conditions in which the nerve is stimulated, such as glossopharyngeal neuralgia, may be associated with bradycardia, whereas neuropathies, such as the Guillain-Barré syndrome, can produce tachycardia.

The functions of the tenth, or vagus, nerve overlap those of the ninth; in addition, this nerve innervates the larynx in part by recurrent branches that loop around the aorta on the left and the subclavian artery on the right in long and somewhat vulnerable courses. Its extensive visceral functions are not tested in the ordinary neurologic examination. Recently and suddenly acquired noninfectious hoarseness suggests paralytic involvement of a vocal cord, in which case the strength of coughing will be reduced. An otolaryngologist should be consulted to confirm any suspicion of vocal-cord paralysis.

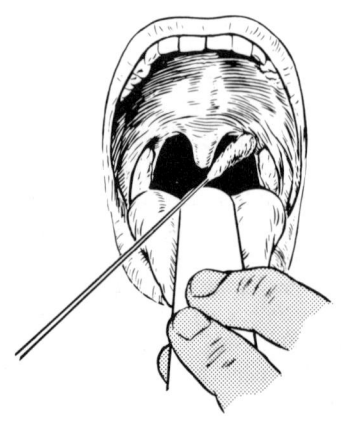

Fig 20

Otherwise, clinical examination is largely limited to observing elevation of the palate and contraction of the pharyngeal wall in phonation and gagging. Elevation of the palate should be strong and symmetric. If there is weakness on one side, the palate will be pulled to the normal side (p. 105). Slight asymmetry of the soft palate at rest is often seen in patients who have had tonsillectomy and is not necessarily indicative of neurologic dysfunction. The gag reflex is tested by touching either the tonsillar pillars or posterior pharyngeal wall with an applicator. It may be absent in elderly people.

The 11th cranial nerve innervates the sternocleidomastoid muscle and the upper portion of the trapezius muscle. Inspect the contour of these muscles and palpate the upper edge of the trapezius muscles for normal mass. As usual, comparison of the two sides is essential. Test the trapezius as shown in Figure 21,A by asking the patient to lift his shoulders up toward his ears while you resist his movement from above.

The sternocleidomastoid muscle is tested by asking the patient to force his face to one side against the resistance of your hand on his chin (Fig 21,B). The left sternocleidomastoid muscle turns the head to the right, and vice versa. Observe the contour and mass of this muscle when it is contracted.

These tests are important not only for assessing function of the 11th nerve but also for determining involvement by motor neuron disease or dystrophy. Since the nuclei of origin of the various parts of this nerve are not adjacent, differential paresis may occur from central nuclear lesions. The tests of function shown here will expose weakness of either central or peripheral origin.

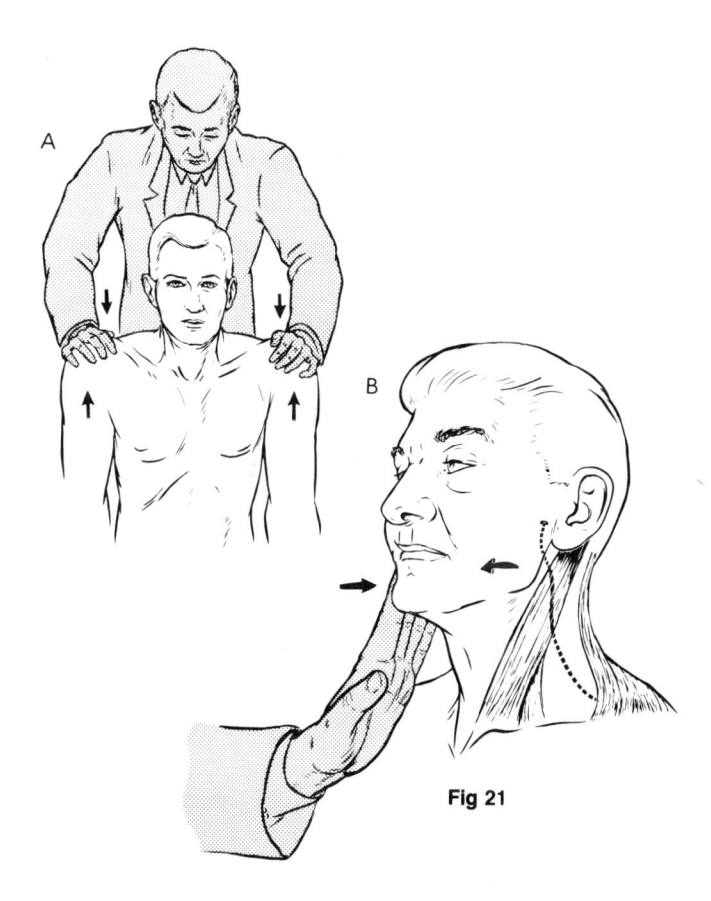

Fig 21

The Eleventh Cranial Nerve (Spinal Accessory)

The 12th cranial nerve emerges from the lower medulla and leaves the skull via the hypoglossal foramen in the occipital condyle. It courses along the floor of the skull externally and is in close relationship to the 9th, 10th, and 11th nerves before traveling forward between the internal and external carotid arteries. The function is motor, primarily to the ipsilateral part of the tongue.

Ability to protrude the tongue varies considerably, but normally the tongue can be moved quickly and strongly and protruded far from the mouth (Fig 22,A). The contour and mass of the normal tongue will quickly become familiar. Although the tongue should be protruded in the midline, minor deviations are usually best ignored. Consistent protrusion to one side suggests ipsilateral weakness.

The patient should also be asked to press the tongue forcefully against the inside of first the right cheek and then the left, allowing the examiner to compare the strength on the two sides by palpating from the outside (Fig 22,C). Look closely for atrophy and for fasciculations (p. 107). The tongue is a restless muscle, and tremors are normal when the tongue is protruded. Observe it at rest on the floor of the mouth.

Ask the patient to flip the tongue rapidly in and out of the mouth (Fig 22,B). Often it is necessary to demonstrate this. Some normal people do it poorly, but fair facility should be evident after brief practice. Slowed alternating motion rate (AMR) usually indicates bilateral upper motor neuron (supranuclear) dysfunction. Some experience in observing the normal range of performance is necessary for the examiner to evaluate the results of this test.

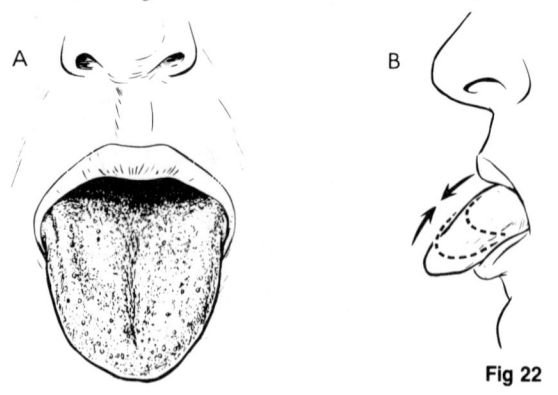

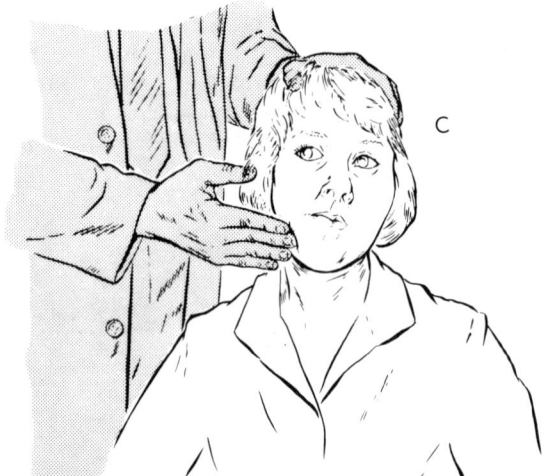

Fig 22

34 / *The Twelfth Cranial Nerve (Hypoglossal)*

Strength and Function of the Extremities

Muscular weakness is a cardinal sign of dysfunction in many parts of the nervous system. The degree of weakness present can be judged about as accurately as most other abnormalities, but experience must be gained in learning what is normal strength for men, women, and children of various ages, states of health, and responsiveness. Pain and fear of pain will inhibit maximum effort, and anxiety, indifference, hysteria, and, rarely, malingering may cause reduced effort. Strength of the extremities is tested by directly opposing the action of various muscle groups, as well as by utilizing various functional tests (see pp. 37–45). Cajole or tease the patient, as appropriate, to maximum exertion, but use restraint and consideration in testing the injured, debilitated, or elderly.

Evaluation of the central nervous system is concerned with patterns of movement rather than contraction of isolated muscles. For application of maximum strength of a muscle or muscle group, contraction of many other groups must occur contemporaneously to provide a stable base for the movement being studied. In analyzing peripheral nerve and root lesions, one may attempt to appraise the involvement of a single muscle, but this is not appropriate in most disorders.

Whenever possible, observe and record the ability of the patient to move a part against gravity. Can he raise his head from a firm surface when supine? Can he elevate the straightened leg from the bed, and can he lift the heel from the bed with the leg flexed and supported at the knee? Can he swing the leg up at the knee in the sitting position? Such observations are especially useful when judging whether the seriously weakened patient is improving or worsening.

The method of quantitation of muscle strength most commonly employed is based on an index of 0 to 5:

5 Normal strength
4 Full normal movement possible, but strength of contraction can be overcome by examiner
3 Normal range of movement against gravity but not against added resistance
2 Movement when gravity does not act in opposition
1 Flicker of movement only
0 No movement

A plus or minus is often used to indicate a score in between these grades.

Always observe and palpate the musculature being tested. Often dysfunction is immediately proclaimed by odd posture or loss of normal muscle contour. Atrophy is difficult to evaluate in the aged or malnourished patient; when it is asymmetric or restricted to a specific area or muscle group, then disorder of the nervous or muscular system should be strongly suspected—unless local pain, joint disease, or immobilization provides a possible explanation.

Fig 23

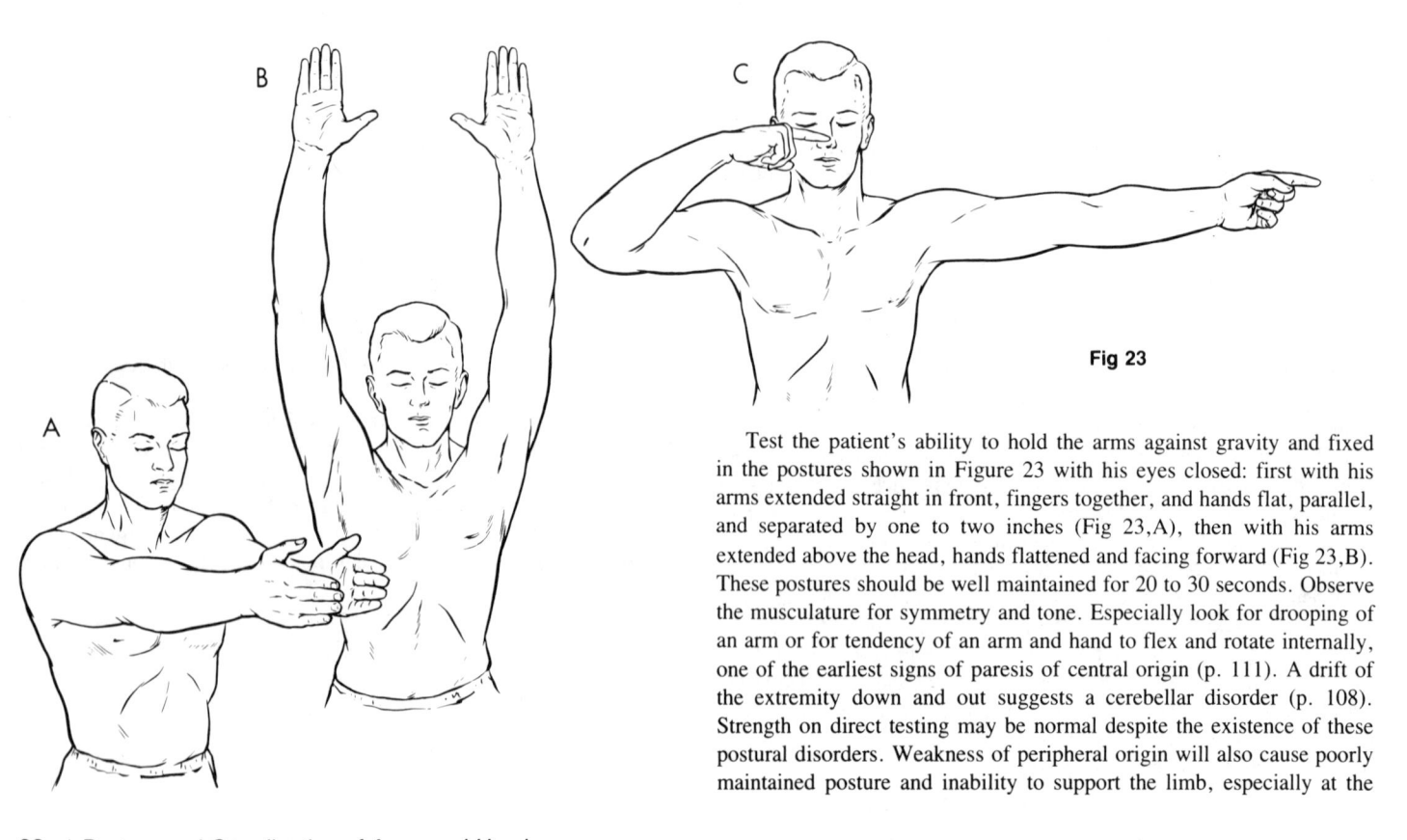

Test the patient's ability to hold the arms against gravity and fixed in the postures shown in Figure 23 with his eyes closed: first with his arms extended straight in front, fingers together, and hands flat, parallel, and separated by one to two inches (Fig 23,A), then with his arms extended above the head, hands flattened and facing forward (Fig 23,B). These postures should be well maintained for 20 to 30 seconds. Observe the musculature for symmetry and tone. Especially look for drooping of an arm or for tendency of an arm and hand to flex and rotate internally, one of the earliest signs of paresis of central origin (p. 111). A drift of the extremity down and out suggests a cerebellar disorder (p. 108). Strength on direct testing may be normal despite the existence of these postural disorders. Weakness of peripheral origin will also cause poorly maintained posture and inability to support the limb, especially at the

36 / *Posture and Coordination of Arms and Hands*

shoulder. Consistent disturbances in maintenance of posture serve notice of a disorder requiring further attention.

Tremors may appear when the fingers are spread with palms facing the floor, and dyskinesias and dystonic posturing may appear during any of these tests.

The finger-to-nose test (Fig 23,C) is done first with the eyes open, then with the eyes closed, and usually with the patient sitting. The arms should be abducted, and then the forefinger should be moved quickly to the tip of the nose, alternating the sides. The movement should be smooth and accurate with little truncal torsion or disturbance in body posture.

Jerky, uncoordinated movements (dyssynergia) are often seen in cases of disease of the cerebellum or its brachia. Oscillating tremor of the hands may appear as the movement is slowed to stop the finger at the nose (terminal tremor). If unilateral, the tremor is ipsilateral to the side of the cerebellar lesion. When the condition is severe, the hand may strike the face or oscillate wildly as it nears the nose. Persistent inaccuracy (dysmetria) may indicate disturbance of position sense due to peripheral neuropathy or to a lesion of the posterior columns of the cord as well as cerebellar dysfunction. Consistent missing or bizarre performance is seen in cases of hysteria.

The patient may also be asked to approximate but not touch the tips of the forefingers of his hands in the position shown in Figure 24. This maneuver helps contrast function on the two sides.

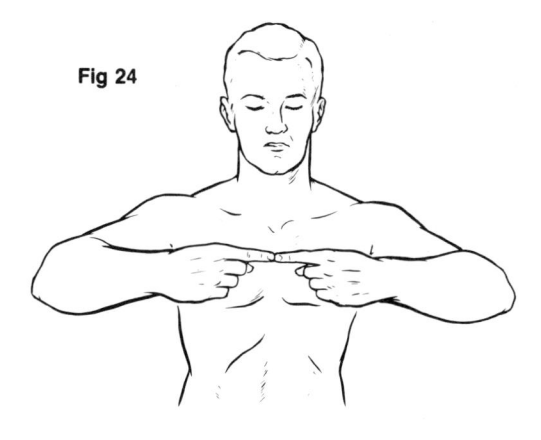

Fig 24

Ability to hold the arms extended above the head (Fig 25,A) is impaired early in hemiparesis or in weakness of the shoulder girdle from any cause. Try to force the patient's arm down against his resistance. The deltoid is the principal muscle tested in the exercise shown in Figure 25,B. Observe the muscle for firmness and contour. Impairment in function of the trapezius, serratus anterior, or other muscles stabilizing the shoulder girdle may compromise the ability of the deltoid to hold this position against the examiner's downward pressure. Painful disorders of the shoulder joint that limit movement will seriously interfere with performance of these tests. Be cautious in diagnosing a neurogenic lesion when the patient has a painful, atrophic shoulder.

Test for scapular winging by depressing the arms while the patient holds them outstretched in front of the body (Fig 25,C) and lateral to the body (Fig 25,B). When the serratus anterior is weak, the *lower angle* of the scapula will wing out and be displaced mesially and up (p. 129). Weakness of the deltoid interferes with testing in this manner, so scapular winging should be looked for by having the patient push against the wall with outstretched arms, first one arm and then the other. If winging is absent, the scapula will remain closely applied to the chest wall. Weakness of the trapezius may also result in scapular winging, which will be displayed by downward and lateral displacement of the scapula on lateral abduction of the arms (p. 106).

Test strength of flexion at the elbow as shown in Figure 25,D. The principal muscles concerned here are the biceps brachii (musculocutaneous nerve), and brachioradialis. The brachioradialis plays a larger role in flexion of the elbow when the palm faces inward. This muscle is innervated by the radial nerve, which mediates both flexion and extension at the elbow.

Extension at the elbows is mediated by the triceps muscle, which is innervated by the radial nerve. An excellent way to test this function is to resist extension while standing behind the patient, as in Figure 25,E. The strength of the two arms is easily compared.

Fig 25

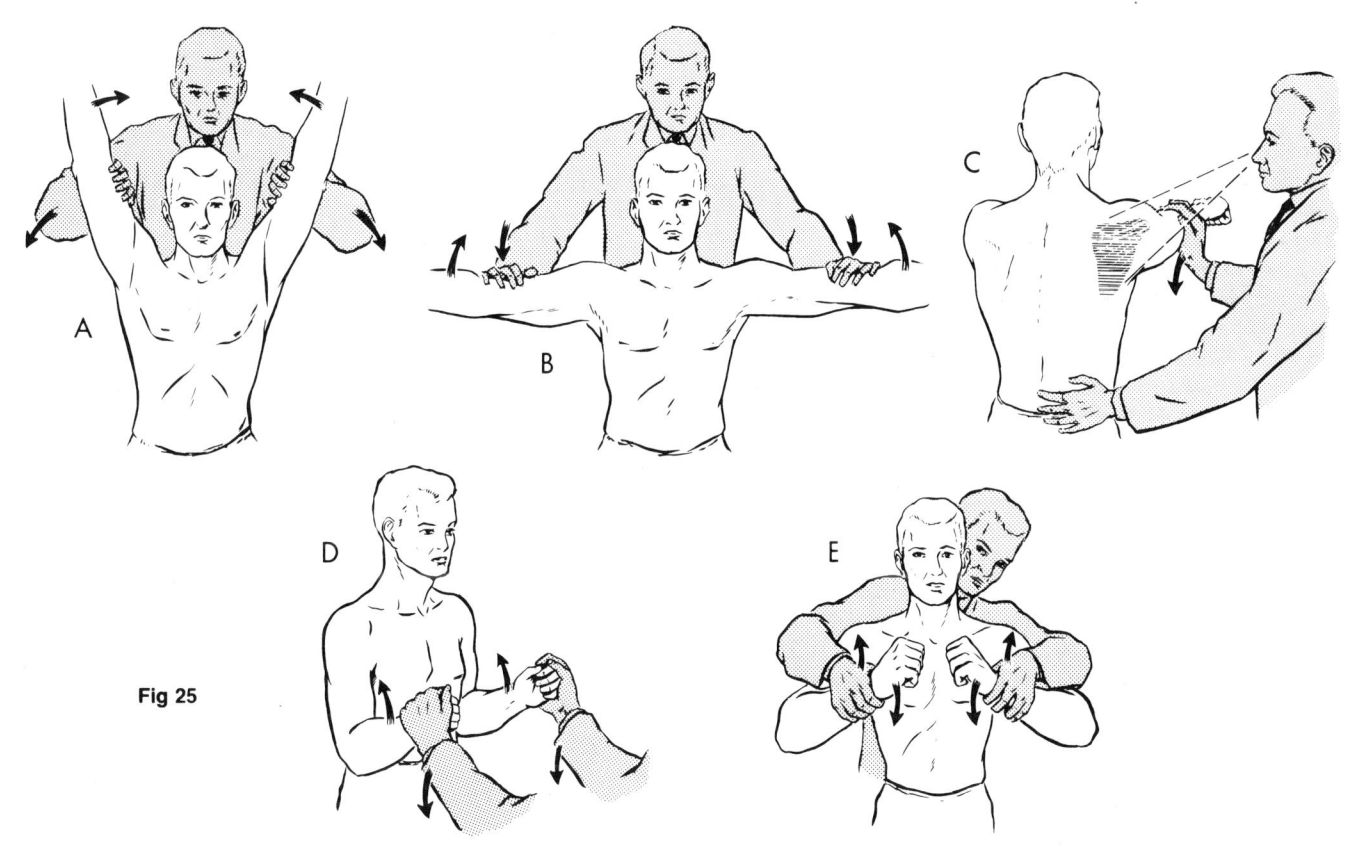

Strength of Shoulders and Arms / 39

Dorsiflexion of the wrist is a vulnerable function and is impaired early in disease of central motor pathways, in radicular compression, in radial nerve paresis, and often in peripheral neuropathy. Ask the patient to make a tight fist and hold it immobile against your attempt to bend the wrist ventrally (Fig 26,A).

A common way to gauge strength is by the force of the grips (Fig 26,B). Two or three fingers may be offered to the patient, two fingers for small hands to give the patient an advantage, and three fingers to powerful hands to reduce discomfort for the examiner. Test the grips of right and left hands simultaneously for easy comparison. Chide the patient into maximum effort and make the test an opportunity for the patient to express a bit of hostility and competitive spirit. Try to withdraw the grasped fingers by twisting and pulling. Some additional estimate of strength and function of arms and shoulders is thus possible. The patient's wrist should not deviate; if it does, weakness of a muscle group in the forearm is probable and effectiveness of the grip is reduced. Strength of the grip can be inhibited by pain anywhere in the extremity. Remember that the grip is largely a function of forearm musculature, which should be observed for contour, symmetry, and tone.

The grips may be strong, even though intrinsic hand muscles are weak. Observe closely for atrophy of these muscles and their distribution. The thenar eminence will give evidence of atrophy in median-nerve disorders, the first dorsal interosseous muscle, in early ulnar-nerve paresis (p. 132). The intrinsic muscles lose mass diffusely in cases of arthritis or other debilitating disease and in cases of disuse or old age. However, strength is retained unless inhibited by pain. In general, loss of strength will accompany visible atrophy if denervation or myopathy is directly responsible for the atrophy. Diffuse atrophy with weakness is seen in patients with some types of neuropathy, myopathy, certain root disorders, and motor neuron disease. However, a lesser atrophy of disuse is common in cases of paresis of upper motor neuron origin, and this finding may be confused with that of atrophy from the other causes just listed. Central lesions producing weakness and secondary atrophy of disuse usually cause hyperreflexia.

Abduction of the fingers is a function that readily loses strength in either central or peripheral disorders, especially ulnar-nerve lesions (p. 133). To assess the strength of this function, attempt to force the patient's fingers together as shown in Figure 26,C. Strength of opposition of the thumb and fifth digit, abduction of the thumb, and flexion of the fingers are tested by pulling one's thumb through the apex of a firmly held cone formed by the patient's digits (Fig 26,D). In most healthy people the fingers will snap back into position.

Fig 26

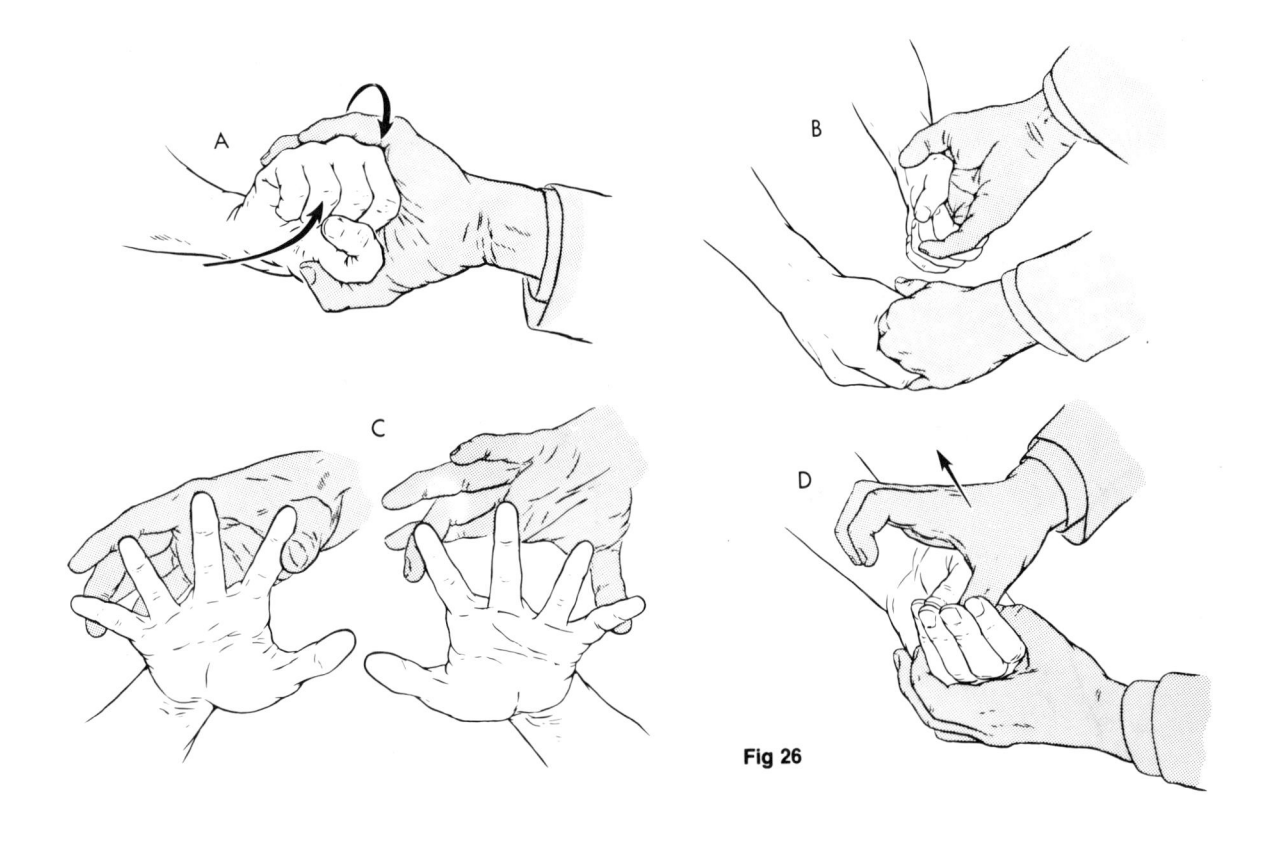

Strength of Wrists and Hands / 41

Ability to perform rapid alternating movement is called diadochokinesia (or AMR). An intact sensorimotor system is essential to the smooth and rapid performance of these tests. The most valuable observations are made when the two sides are compared. The nondominant hand is normally a little slower and less well controlled. Diadochokinesia is less well done by children and old people and is variously well performed by others.

Patting the knee rapidly (Fig 27,B) using wrist motion is a good test, easy to comprehend and to perform. In patients with upper motor neuron lesions or ataxia, this movement will be awkward and slow. A characteristic of central paresis is an inability to stabilize the proximal extremity while attempting to engage in refined and rapid movement distally. Patients with Parkinson's disease may do knee-patting well but be unable to perform rapid pronation and supination of the hand on the knee (Fig 27,A). However, some normal people also perform this poorly. Rapid tapping of the forefinger on the thumb (Fig 27,C) is a good test. Demonstrate the desired movement for the patient. It can be made more demanding by asking him to tap out a specific rhythm.

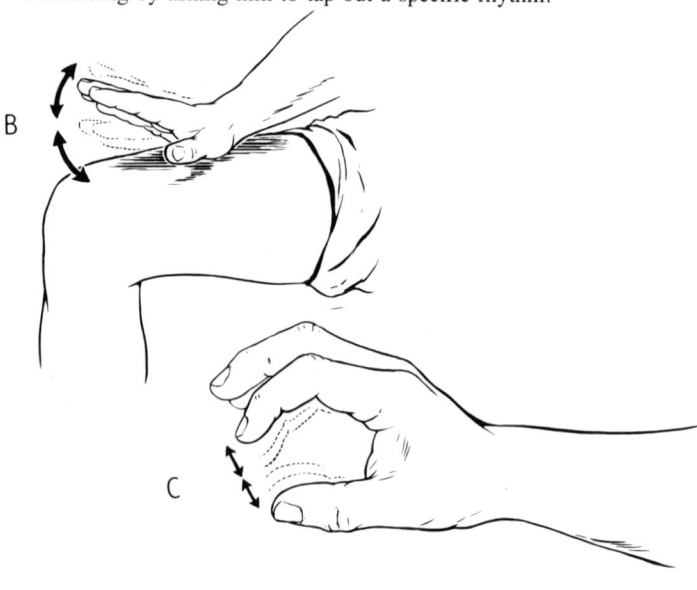

Fig 27

42 / Alternating Motion Rate (Diadochokinesia)

Agility of the hands and fingers is impaired by many disorders. Rapid touching of each finger in succession to the thumb (Fig 28,A) effectively tests this function. Ask the patient to button and unbutton his jacket with the eyes closed (Fig 28,B) or have him pass a safety pin through his pajamas or a sheet, closing and opening it with one hand (Fig 28,C). Such movements are notoriously clumsy when sensation is reduced, as in cases of peripheral neuropathy or demyelination of the posterior columns.

These functions are impaired to various degrees by any motor disorder. Slowed diadochokinesia and loss of finger dexterity are sensitive indicators of motor or sensory disorder. Further examination is necessary to identify the nature of the deficit.

Watch for intention tremors during these maneuvers. Deterioration in handwriting is an early sign of loss of dexterity. Compare old and current signatures, and record for future comparison.

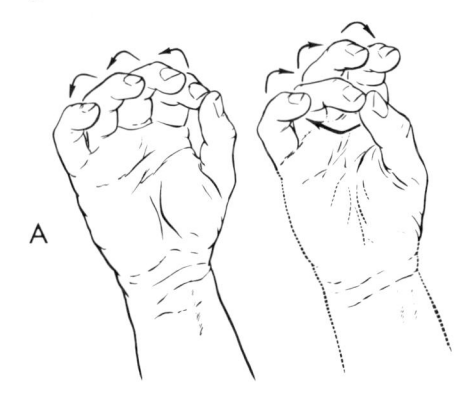

Fig 28

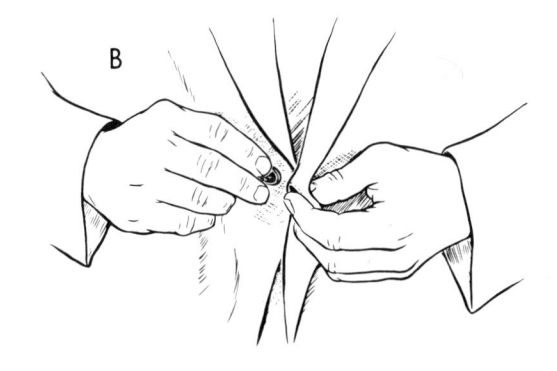

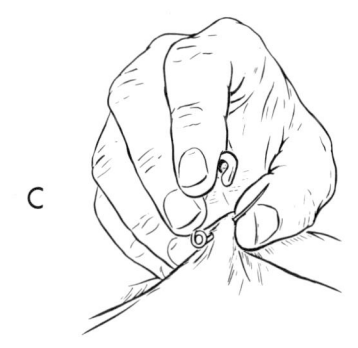

Fine Movements of Fingers / 43

Direct testing is necessary for estimating strength of the lower extremities and hip girdle in the nonambulatory patient and for certain functions in the ambulatory. The movements most vulnerable to impairment are flexion at the hip and dorsiflexion of ankles and toes. Extension of the knee and plantar flexion of the ankle are strong movements mediated by massive musculature and are part of the antigravity functions.

An excellent test is shown in Figure 29,A for determining strength of flexion of the thigh on the abdomen when sitting. This movement is mediated largely by the iliopsoas muscle and is not a strong function. Weakness here is one of the early signs of dysfunction of central motor pathways.

To test flexion of the hip in the supine position, ask the patient to kick, with his knee extended, the examiner's hand held 2 ft above the extremity. Hold your hand so that it will be struck by the shin. The quickness and smartness of such a blow are an accurate index of the strength of the iliopsoas. The patient should also be asked to elevate the leg and hold it against the examiner's downward pressure (Fig 29,B).

Flexion of the knee is largely a function of the hamstring muscles and the sciatic nerve. It is tested as shown in Figure 29,C, with the patient's knee flexed and foot held firmly to the bed while the examiner attempts to straighten the leg. Instruct the patient to hold the foot down. Extension at the knee is tested in the supine position as shown in Figure 29,D. Mild degrees of weakness may not be discerned because of the inherent strength of these muscles (see also p. 35).

Plantar flexion of the ankles and toes may be weakened, yet this weakness may not be easily detected in direct tests of strength. Ask the patient to step down on your hand (Fig 29,E). This function is even better tested by having the patient walk on his toes, as previously described (p. 12).

Dorsiflexion of ankles and toes is tested as shown in Figure 29,F. Most patients understand the instruction to "cock back" the foot.

The AMR of the legs is evaluated by having the patient, if he is able, elevate the leg and shake the foot. The best position to test this function is shown in Figure 30,A. The maneuver can also be done with the patient standing on one leg or sitting. The desired rapidity and amplitude are often best communicated to the patient by asking him to "shake your leg as though you were shaking water off it." Lesions of corticospinal pathways reduce this ability more than do peripheral lesions. However, strength must be fairly well preserved for this test to be done.

Fig 29

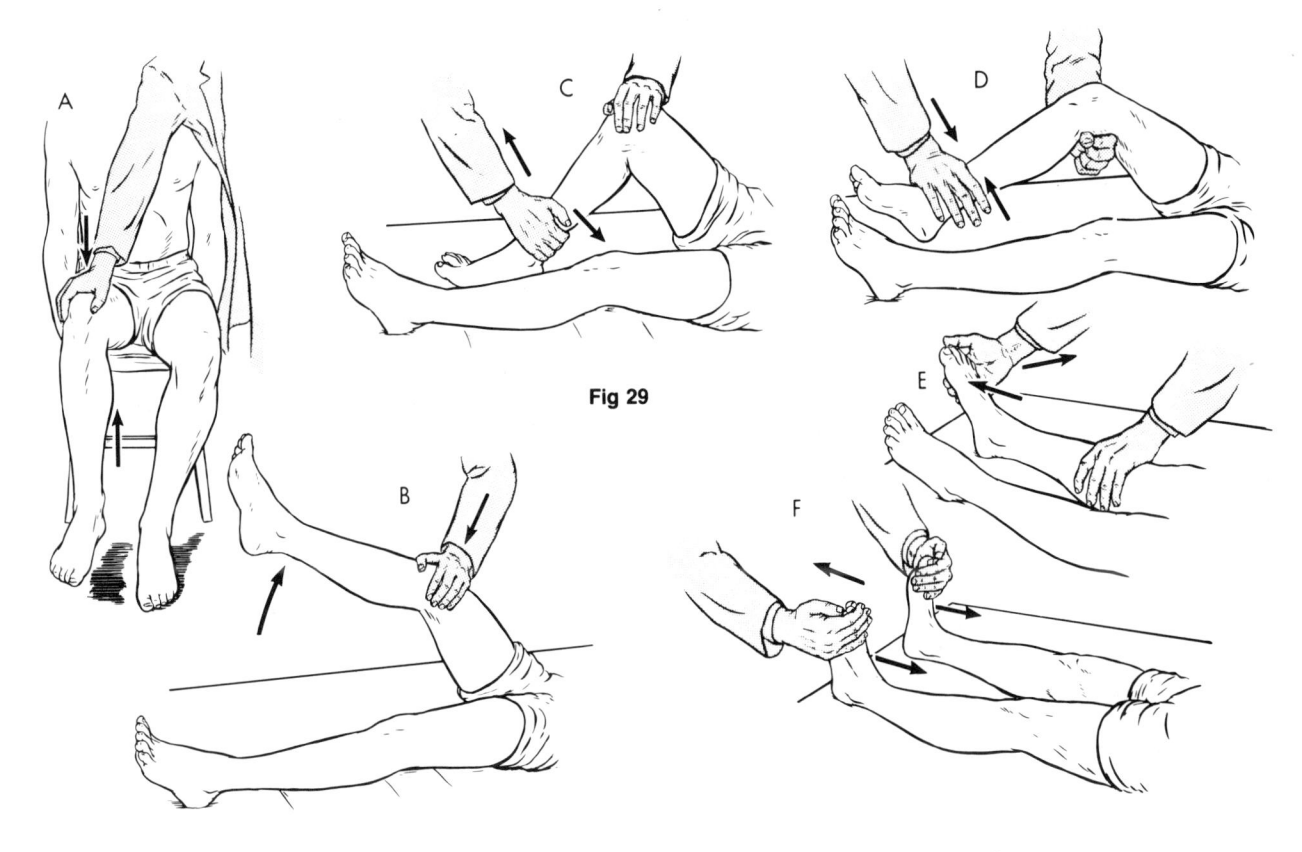

Strength of Lower Extremities / 45

Fig 30

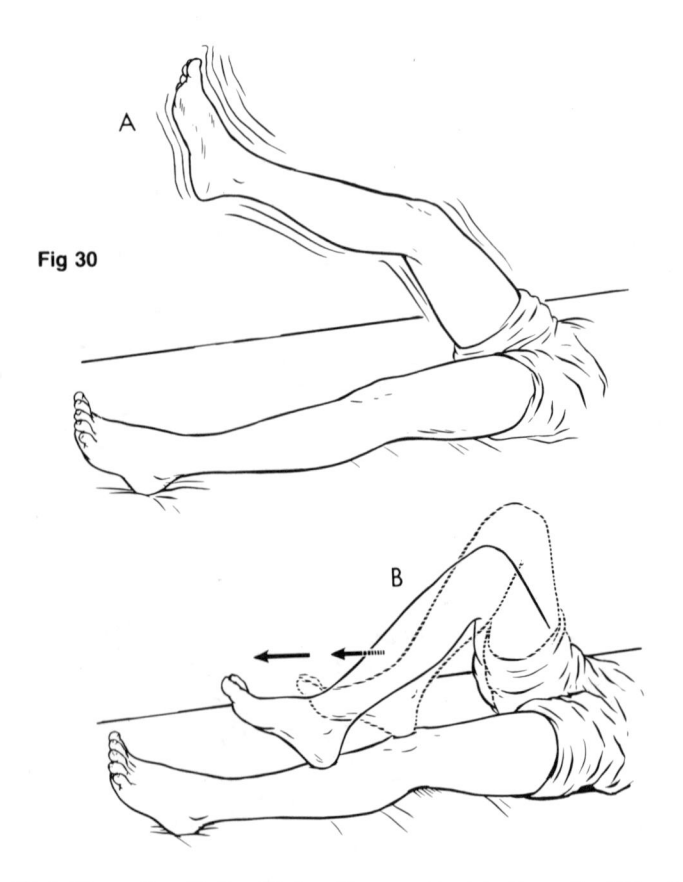

The heel-to-knee test should be done in the position shown in Figure 30,B. Ask the patient to lift one foot and place the heel squarely on the opposite patella without looking and then to slide the heel down the sharp edge of the tibia. The test will be vitiated if the side of the foot is held against the shin. Of course, the legs must be strong enough to accomplish this. If position sense is reduced, the heel will not be placed accurately, nor will its position be held well on the shin. In cerebellar disorders, the original placement may perhaps be fairly well done, with some decomposition of movement, but will be followed by wider and wider oscillations of the heel back and forth across the shin as it slides downward. The position sense should always be checked when the heel-to-knee test is poorly performed, to analyze the nature of the disorder.

If the patient is able to hop well, these two tests will give negative results. If he does not hop well, they will help to identify the nature of the functional loss.

The Reflexes

Sudden stretch of a skeletal muscle results in a reflex contraction of that muscle mediated by a simple and usually monosynaptic reflex arc. The afferent side of the arc begins with muscle stretch receptors, the cell bodies of which are in the dorsal root ganglia. Intramedullary fibers of these cells synapse on the motor neurons in the anterior horns of the spinal cord or on motor nuclei in the lower brain stem. The efferent side of the arc is the motor neuron with its axon and terminal structures that innervate the muscle.

Central influences modify the responsiveness of the motor neuron as well as the complex stretch receptors in the muscle, the latter via the gamma efferent system shown in Figure 31. Hence, the response of the arc depends on its own integrity and on the state of the central nervous system.

When a tendon is tapped, the resulting distortion applies a sudden stretch to the muscle. The response is directly related to the degree of the distortion and its velocity. Slowly applied stretch will cause no detectable response, so the use of a hammer is appropriate since it enables the examiner to place a sudden and well-controlled stimulus.

The elicitation of a motor response means that the arc is intact and conducting impulses. Yet the absence of a response does not have the converse meaning, since normal or abnormal neural influences may suppress the reflex. There is a wide variation in normal amplitude of response with which the student must become acquainted. Moreover, there is variation in response to the same person in both health and disease from time to time.

Because the reflex response is largely beyond voluntary control (when properly elicited), it takes on special value as a manifestation of isolated function subject to objective appraisal. Not only does the presence of involuntary muscle contraction in response to stretch indicate intactness of the arc, but, since the arc itself has a fairly constant path and locus of central connections, the presence or absence of the reflex is helpful in locating the peripheral pathways and vertical levels within the neuraxis. For example, the quadriceps stretch reflex (patellar reflex, knee jerk) is mediated via the femoral nerve peripherally, the lumbar plexus, the lumbar spinal roots (L-2, L-3, L-4), and the cell bodies in the corresponding segments of the spinal cord that lie over the vertebral bodies of the lower dorsal spine (T-11, T-12). Considerable diagnostic significance, moreover, may be assigned to changing reflex responses. For example, progressive diminution or loss of reflexes in poliomyelitis, peripheral neuropathy, and the Guillain-Barré syndrome may be seen within hours or days.

The loss of a reflex in a painful extremity may well mean that nerves or roots innervating the painful area are being impinged. A consistent difference between the two sides of the body in the presence of a disease affecting the reflex arc is evidence of asymmetric involvement and lateralizes the area of greater involvement.

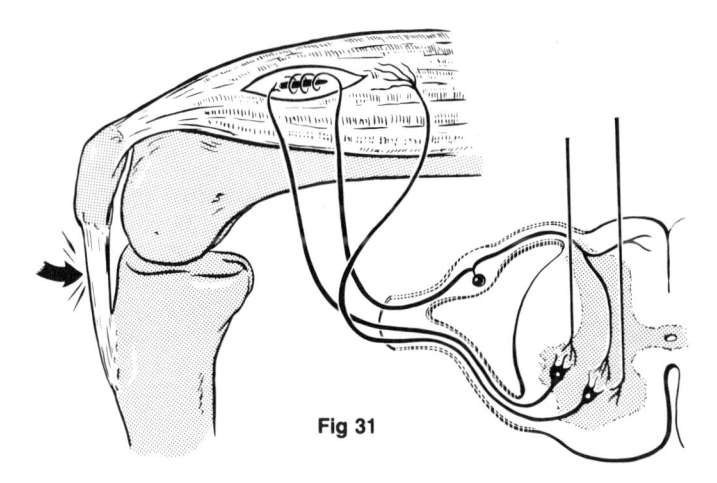

Fig 31

The Reflexes / 47

Classically, the stretch reflex will be exaggerated when normal function of the pyramidal tract above the lower motor neuron is chronically suppressed or destroyed. Thus, enhanced response in the reflex arc may mean disease of the cord, brain stem, or hemispheres and is a basic characteristic of the spastic state. Sometimes other muscles stretched slightly by the maneuver may visibly respond also—a spread of response also typical of the spastic state.

Discretion must be used in evaluating the meaning of uniformly "decreased" or "increased" stretch reflexes, using one's knowledge of normal range as a guide. The normal range is broad. Differences between upper and lower extremities and between the two sides are much more safely regarded as evidence of dysfunction than is the general reflex tonus. At times it may be difficult to decide whether a reflex response is enhanced on one side or decreased on the other. One looks for other evidence of disordered function, e.g., sensory deficits, atrophy, poor motor performance, and the Babinski sign, to integrate with the stretch reflex responses in constructing a concept of pathologic change.

The following system is useful for estimating vigor of reflex muscular contraction to stretch:

4+   Very brisk response—evidence of disease and associated with clonus (p. 54)
3+   A brisk response, possibly indicative of disease
2+   A normal, average response
1+   A response in low-normal range
0   No response and possibly evidence of disease, depending on the circumstances; if reflex response is elicited by reinforcement, then the arc is intact although possibly inhibited
1+(R)   The response of an absent reflex with reinforcement
0(R)   No evident muscle contraction even when reinforced, as in the Jendrassik maneuver; an absent reflex, to be judged as a very likely sign of disease

The wide variation in response in healthy people makes it difficult to determine any absolute value. In recording the reflexes it is useful to use a shorthand system for easy reading and later reference. An example follows:

$$BJ \text{ (biceps jerk)} \quad \frac{2+}{1+} \quad \frac{\text{Right}}{\text{Left}}$$

$$TJ \text{ (triceps jerk)} \quad \frac{2+}{0} \quad \frac{\text{Right}}{\text{Left}}$$

$$KJ \text{ (knee jerk)} \quad \frac{3+}{1+} \quad \frac{\text{Right}}{\text{Left}}$$

When examining the reflexes, position the patient so that he is sitting or reclining with a minimum of effort necessary to maintain balance or position. Then place the extremities in symmetric posture with the muscles to be tested moderately stretched. If the patient is contracting the muscle to be tested, the reflex will be suppressed or absent. Therefore, distract the patient's attention from the region being examined.

Tap lightly but quickly. Use free finger and wrist movement (Figure 32,A). Don't chop with the hammer. The free-swinging movement illustrated in Figure 32 gives a well-regulated, easily duplicated blow of rapidly applied force.

Fig 32

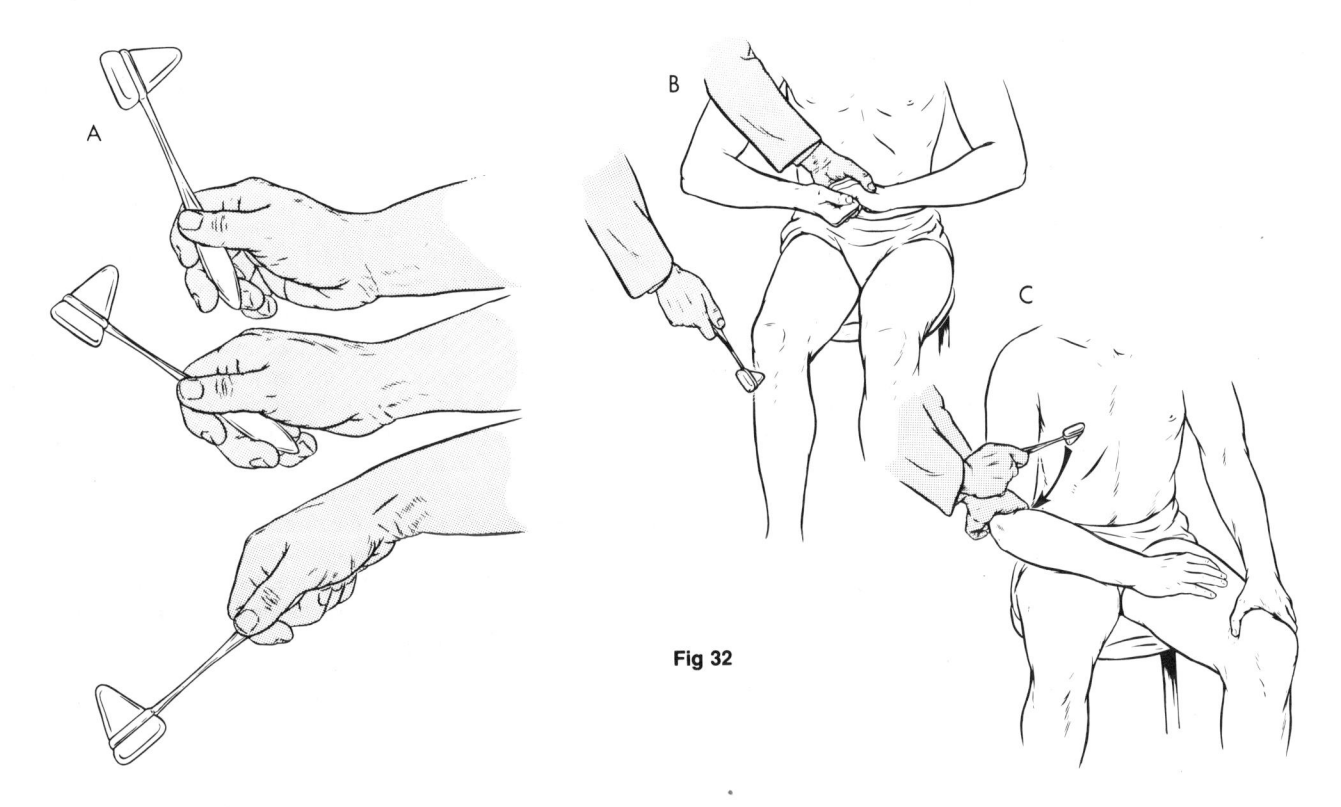

Use of Reflex Hammer / 49

When muscle stretch reflexes are difficult to elicit, determining whether the reflex arc is intact assumes primary importance, especially since many healthy people are hyporeflexic or are flexic to ordinary testing.

Conduction in the arc may be facilitated by isometric muscular contraction elsewhere in the body. Commonly this is done by having the patient lock the fingers of the two hands and pull one against the other while the reflexes of the lower extremities are being elicited (Jendrassik's maneuver; Fig 32,B). For best facilitation of the reflex, the tendon should be struck the moment that suddenly applied tension is detected by the examiner. This can be done if the examiner is holding the patient's arm or the interlocked fingers with one hand and is ready to swing the hammer with the other. The moment that tension is sensed the hammer should be swung. Figure 32C shows a maneuver that may be employed when testing the upper extremity. The patient is instructed to perform some maneuvers with the opposite hand, such as squeezing his thigh or making a fist. (He may, of course, unknowingly influence the reflex response by tensing his muscles.)

The position shown in Figure 33,A is satisfactory for eliciting the biceps stretch reflex. The degree of flexion of the elbow may be varied for best response. Place the thumb on the biceps tendon and strike the thumb. The reflex contraction will be felt by the thumb and should be visible. Note whether contraction of the biceps is indeed responsible for flexion of the elbow, since the brachioradialis, if stretched, also produces this movement. The biceps and the brachioradialis are innervated from the same spinal segments but from different branches of the brachial plexus, the biceps by the musculocutaneous nerve and the brachioradialis by the radial nerve. The C-6 root is primarily involved in this reflex.

A commonly used position for eliciting the triceps reflex is shown in Figure 33,B. This reflex is sometimes difficult to obtain, probably because the disposition of the tendon makes stretching by a laterally displacing force inefficient. The degree of flexion at the elbow should be adjusted for best response, and the triceps should be observed for visible contraction. If the patient can stand, another useful test is to have him place hands on hips with arms akimbo as you stand behind him and strike the triceps tendon 1 to 2 inches above its insertion. The two sides are then easily compared. The C-7 root is primarily involved.

The Hoffmann sign is sought by positioning the patient's hand and wrist as shown in Figure 33,C, the wrist extended a bit beyond the physiologic position of rest. Flick the terminal phalanx of the third digit as shown, snapping it between your thumb and first finger. This maneuver is a convenient way to cause sudden extension of the middle finger, thus eliciting a stretch reflex. The positive sign is said to be present when the patient's thumb and forefinger flex in response. Often the other fingers will flex as well. The Hoffmann sign is often incorrectly considered the upper-extremity equivalent of the Babinski sign. The Babinski sign (see p. 55) is a pathologic reflex, whereas the Hoffmann sign is simply a hyperactive stretch reflex. It has the same meaning as hyperactivity of other stretch reflexes and should be interpreted accordingly.

Another way of eliciting the same reflex response in the thumb and fingers is shown in Figure 33,D and is known as Trömner's sign.

Fig 33

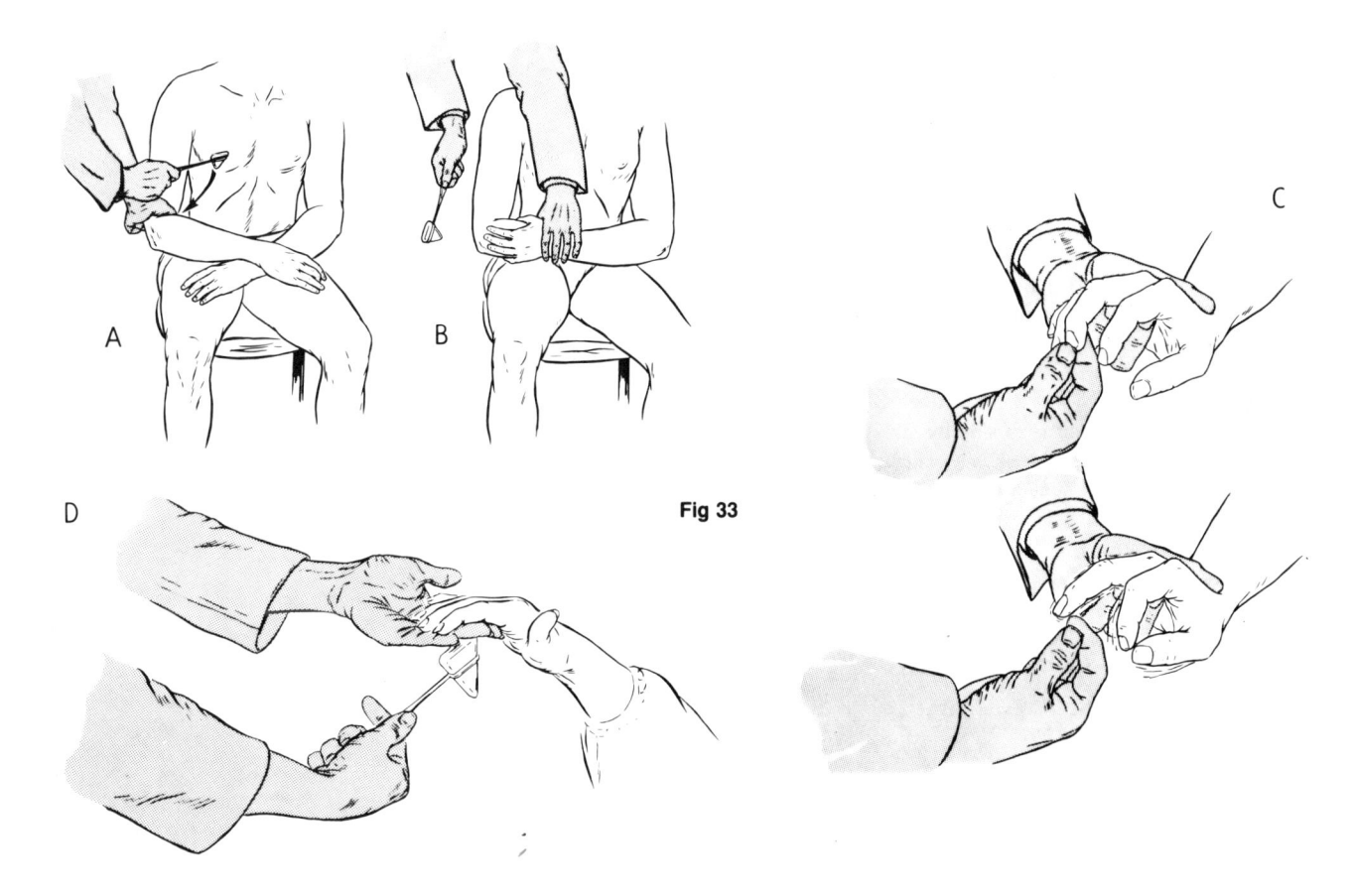

Upper Extremity Reflexes / 51

The patellar reflex or quadriceps stretch reflex is easily elicited with the patient's feet flat on the floor (Figure 34,A). Hold one hand on the distal thigh and strike the tendon just below the patella. The response is both seen and felt. This reflex can be obtained while the patient sits on the edge of the examining table, the response judged from the rapidity and extent of leg movement. The latter method provides an opportunity to observe the poorly damped (pendular) knee jerk of cerebellar disease, but the former method ensures better relaxation. The femoral nerve and the L-2, L-3, L-4 spinal segments and nerve roots are involved. This reflex is obtainable when the patient is supine, as shown in Figure 34,B. The degree of knee flexion varies. If the patient will not relax, ask him to press his heels into the bed.

An excellent way to evoke on each side the Achilles reflex or gastrocnemius and soleus stretch reflex is shown in Figure 34,C. While one hand is positioned as shown to stretch the muscle slightly, tap quickly and gently with the other. A satisfactory horizontal position for obtaining this reflex is seen in Figure 34,D. The sciatic (its tibial branch) nerve and the L-5 and S-1 nerve roots and spinal segments, chiefly the latter, are involved.

Fig 34

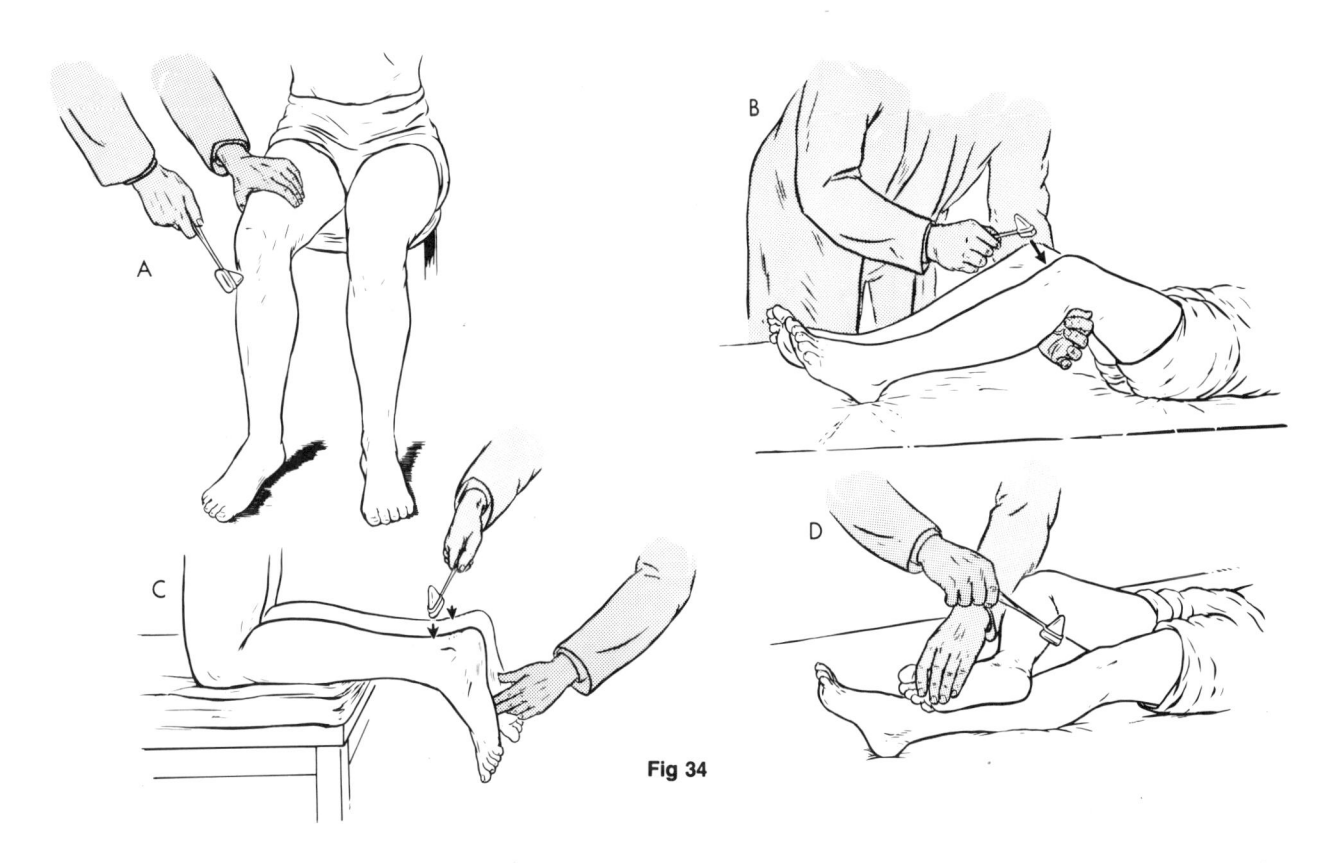

Lower Extremity Reflexes / 53

Fig 35

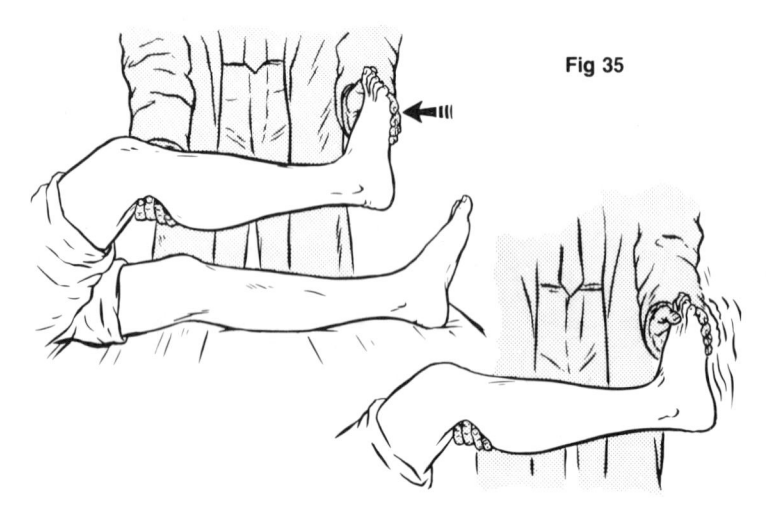

Clonus is elicited by sudden stretch of a muscle that is then maintained by gentle pressure (Fig 35). The ankle is ideally suited mechanically to demonstrate this phenomenon. Hold the limb as shown in the figure and briskly but gently dorsiflex the ankle, maintaining pressure against the sole. The first sudden stretch will bring forth a brisk reflex contraction. Continued applied stretch will cause repetitive reflex responses interrupted by brief "silent periods" in the muscle. As a result, an oscillation can be set up that may continue indefinitely. Sustained clonus usually indicates disease. It is based on hypersynchronization in a poorly inhibited reflex arc and clinically is another sign of hyperreflexia. When spasticity is severe, clonus of the jaw, wrist, and patella may be demonstrable.

The Babinski sign is the most important sign in neurology. When present after age 12 to 16 months, it indicates dysfunction of the corticospinal motor system either by direct involvement or by indirect effect. The lesion, of course, may be old or recent. Absence of the sign is evidence that the corticospinal motor system is not diseased, unless other evidence is strong.

The patient is told that the examiner will stroke or scratch the bottom of his foot and is shown the tool to be used, which should have no sharp edges. The end of an applicator stick is ideal. Begin near the heel and draw the stick up the side of the sole and across the ball of the foot. About 1 second is an appropriate time for this stimulus. The response will not be rapid unless the patient is excessively sensitive and withdraws and wriggles his toes. Reassure him and ask him to avoid movement and to relax the toes; then reduce the strength of the stimulus. The normal response (Fig 36,A) is flexion with adduction of the toes. The abnormal response is dorsiflexion of the great toe and fanning of the others (Fig 36,B), with withdrawal at the knee and hip (Fig 36,C). This is the Babinski sign. Repeated stimuli when the sign is weak will not enhance and may even diminish the abnormal response. Wait a few minutes after several attempts. If the patient is asked to hop and the test then repeated, a latent response may appear. The Babinski sign may also be associated with heavy sedation, and can appear transiently after a generalized or focal seizure.

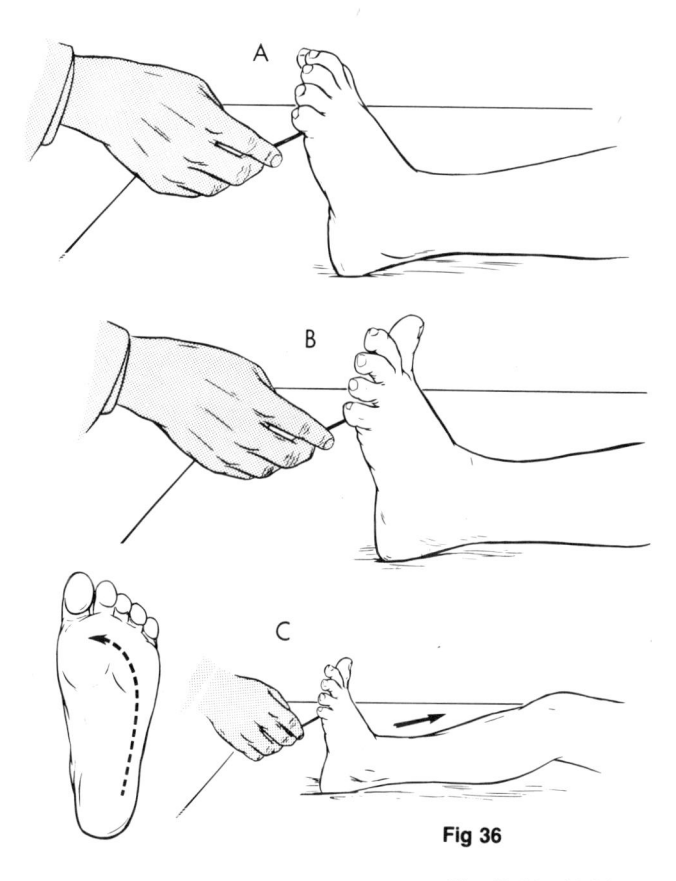

Fig 36

The Babinski Sign / 55

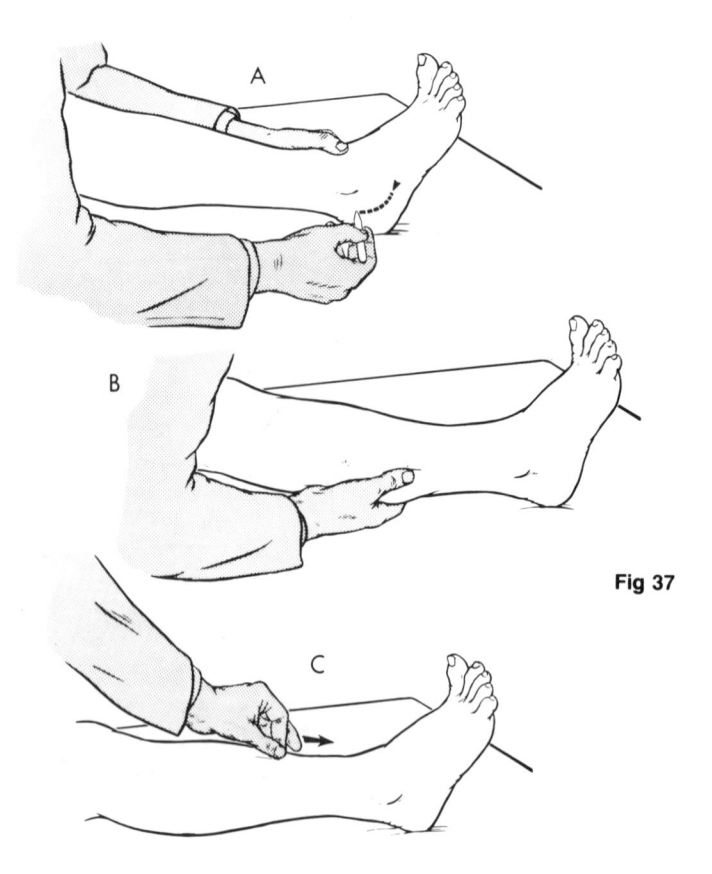

If the sole is unusually sensitive or the response is equivocal, look for other signs by means of the maneuvers illustrated in Figure 37. Stroking the lateral aspect of the foot (Figure 37,A) may elicit the abnormal toe movement of Chaddock's sign; squeezing the calf (Fig 37,B), the toe movement of Gordon's sign; and applying firm pressure on the shin with the fingers positioned and carried downward as shown in Figure 37,C, Oppenheim's sign.

The Babinski sign is referred to as being present or absent, not positive or negative.

Patients with extrapyramidal disorders, particularly Parkinson's disease, may exhibit persistent extension of the great toe. This sign, often called the striatal toe, but more correctly referred to as the dystonic toe, is differentiated from the Babinski sign by its characteristic of prompt flexion of the toe after plantar stimulation.

Fig 37

The abdominal reflexes are referred to as "superficial" reflexes. They are mediated through a spinal arc, but essential facilitation comes from the corticospinal tract above. Properly elicited, they are based not on muscle stretch but rather on cutaneous stimulation. Use an applicator stick and lightly and quickly stroke the skin along the lines shown in Figure 38, with an inward or downward movement. A normal response is for the umbilicus to be deflected toward the side of the stimulus. Peripheral and central sensory pathways must be intact, as must the corticospinal pathways, for this normal response to appear. The reflex response often will not be seen if the abdominal wall is stretched or is

56 / *Other Toe Signs*

covered with a heavy panniculus. This reflex is seldom absent in the healthy person with well-developed abdominal-wall muscles. Sometimes the response is so active that the umbilicus will appear to "follow" the stick if it is drawn around in a circumferential manner.

Absence of the response when the abdominal wall is firm should arouse suspicion of bilaterial cerebral or spinal disease above the T-5 through T-7 area. When only the upper abdominal reflexes (elicited and occurring above the umbilicus) are present, the existence of disease of the spinal cord or, rarely, of the roots in the T-10 region may be inferred. This response is sometimes useful in localizing a cord lesion. When the abdominal reflexes are absent or substantially reduced on one side, one may conclude that there is ipsilateral cord disease or contralateral cerebral disease.

Absence of the abdominal reflexes may be an early sign of corticospinal disease and is regarded as a common sign in multiple sclerosis, yet it is by no means pathognomonic of this disease. Usually hyperreflexia of the lower extremities and the Babinski sign will also be present.

Beevor's sign, though not an abdominal reflex, can be looked for during this part of the examination. Ask the recumbent patient to lift his head off the examining table. Normally, upper and lower abdominal muscles contract equally and the umbilicus does not move. When the lower abdominal muscles alone are weakened, such as in a spinal cord lesion at the T-10 level, the umbilicus will be drawn cephalad by the contraction of the intact upper musculature.

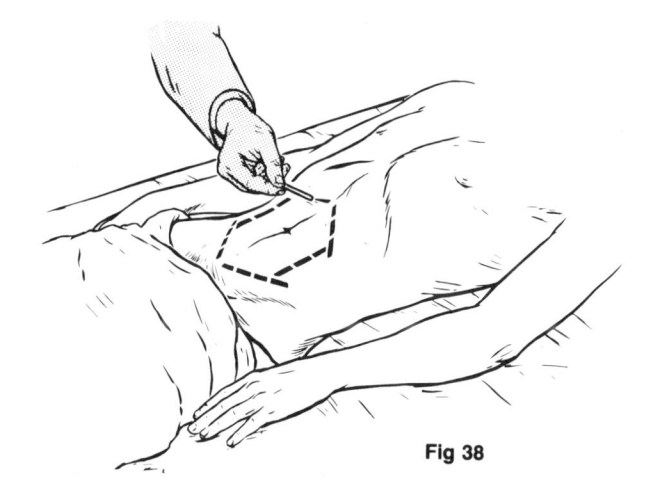

Fig 38

Abdominal Reflexes / 57

The Sensory Examination

The somatic sensory examination is the most difficult and least reliable part of the investigation. It should be left to the end, at which time the examiner will know what specific questions to pose and what findings are realistic. The examiner must be wary of forming hasty conclusions and as open-minded as possible in evaluating responses, since the sensory examination is so prone to bias and suggestion. Often it is best to perform a screening examination at the first visit, with reexamination later of any sensory symptoms or findings.

On reexamination ask again whether the patient is aware of any abnormal sensation or loss of sensation. Paresthesias (tingling, numbness, burning, crawling, coldness, or dead feeling) are common symptoms of disorders of the sensory system at any level. Many people, unfortunately, sue the words "numbness" and "deadness" to refer to weakness or motor dysfunction. Try to determine just what the patient means. Transient paresthesias that appear after unusual posture or pressure on a limb are usually best ignored but may be symptomatic of subclinical neuropathy.

Even when there are no subject complaints, a few tests that are likely to uncover sensory deficits should be included in the screening examination, at least those for pain, touch, vibratory sense, and stereognosis. A prolonged investigation of all modalities of sensation at the first visit is apt to confuse the patient and mislead the physician, so a second visit should be scheduled for a leisurely, detailed sensory examination, if indicated.

Some area of the body must be presumed normal and used to acquaint the patient with the nature of the stimulus. A convenient area of fairly representative sensitivity and one seldom involved in disease is the upper anterior chest or lower neck. Apply the stimulus, e.g., a pinprick, here, and then proceed to other areas, comparing the response of the right with the left sides and of the distal with the proximal extremities. Usually, deficits will be most easily found and most severe in the periphery. Have the patient close his eyes and say "yes" each time you brush the skin with a cotton ball. Ask him to compare the two sides. Test the hands and feet for vibratory sensation and go proximally if necessary until the sensation is detected. Have him identify with his eyes closed a few simple, small objects held in his hands. Finally, outline the margins of a region of sensory loss, if present, with a pinprick, trying to establish the limits of hypalgesia or the level of sensory loss. Further details of testing are given on subsequent pages.

One important technical aspect of sensory testing must be mentioned here. Do not use the same pin on more than one patient since serious infectious diseases, such as hepatitis, can potentially be spread in this fashion.

The student must gain experience in testing all modalities to become acquainted with the vagaries of response that issue from fatigue, misunderstanding, and disinterest, as well as disease. This experience equips one to proceed directly to the areas and modalities most likely to be affected by a suspected disorder. A few generalizations and rules are helpful:

1. Always look for deficits in an area of pain. If hypalgesia can be consistently demonstrated in an anatomically appropriate distribution,

then it may be assumed that the pain is associated with a disorder of the nervous system, often impingement of a root or nerve. A painful area may be hyperalgesic or hyperesthetic, and the patient may overrespond to stimulation. If the patient reports a poorly localized spreading and prolonged unpleasant sensation, i.e., a less than normally discrete response in both space and time, then a deficit in sensory innervation is likely.

2. Look closely for sensory deficit when localized muscular atrophy, weakness, and/or hyporeflexia are found. Examine especially the area of the distribution of the dermatome or nerve that is involved in the motor disorder. Compare the response here with that of areas of presumably uninvolved dermatomes and with that of the other side.

3. Ask the patient to outline areas of sensory loss to orient you and save time.

4. Subjective symptoms of numbness and paresthesia are, unfortunately for the evaluator, much the same qualitatively whether they result from thalamic, spinal, radicular, or peripheral neural deficits. The distribution of symptoms and other findings are helpful in locating the site of disease.

5. Variations in distribution of roots and nerves are common. The patient's nervous system may depart from the usual diagrams by a full dermatome in either direction.

6. Peripheral nerve lesions are often associated with diminished or absent sweating, dry skin, trophic changes in the nails, and loss of subcutaneous tissue. The area of sensory loss may be outlined by such changes in the hand. Occasionally in partial lesions, excessive sweating will take place. The peripheral nerve carries the sympathetic fibers to an area roughly corresponding to its sensory distribution. Hence, a nerve lesion results in both somatic and sympathetic denervation.

7. In root-compression syndromes, in some mononeuropathies, and in the symmetric, diffuse neuropathies, squeeze tenderness of fingers and toes and of paretic musculature may accompany paresthesias and sensory loss.

8. Consistency of findings from several sensory examinations gives some assurance of their validity. However, the suggestible patient may precisely if erroneously report a near-constant line of demarcation. The examiner may wish to precisely outline in ink the area of reported sensory loss for reference on repeated testing. The patient then should be asked to refrain from watching the area being examined. With this visual restriction, his responses, in most cases, will be consistent only if the deficit is organically based.

9. Cutaneous sensitivity is greater on the face, hands, forearms, genitalia, and feet. Calloused areas should be avoided in testing. Allow for denervation distal to scars.

10. The tests ordinarily used for the sensory examination are rather crude and the findings are imprecise; the less complete the lesion, the more imprecise these findings will be.

Although the patient should not watch the examination, when you are attempting to determine a zone or level of sensory loss, he should always first indicate the region where sensation is abnormal and where it becomes normal. He may be able to do this with as much accuracy as can result from examination.

Should it appear that sensation is reduced in some region, start the

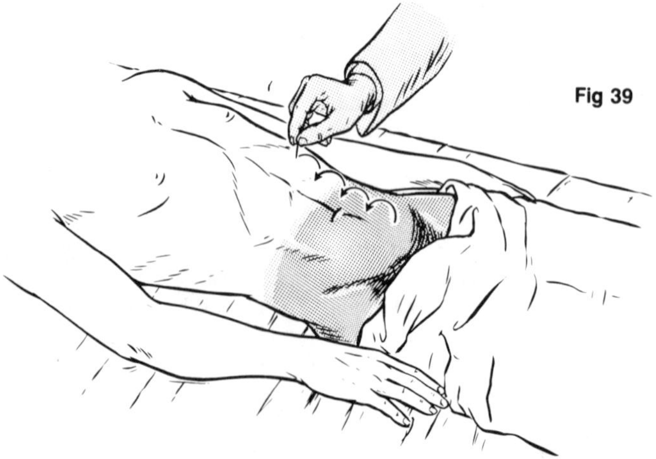

Fig 39

examination in that region and advance to the normal zone by successive, identically applied pinprick stimuli at intervals of about 2 cm as shown in Figure 39. Ask him to tell you when the pinprick sensation changes or when it becomes normal. The level of demarcation between abnormal and normal will be ill defined and variable when sensory loss is not complete. Make notes or drawings of the levels determined, and if responses are inconsistent, repeat the test later. Elicitation of pain, touch, and temperature discrimination are all appropriate for determining a level or zone of denervation.

The history, the subjective complaints, and the motor and reflex findings will often suggest the pattern of sensory loss to be confirmed (p. 62). When root or nerve lesions are suspected, reference to page 69 will be helpful. See also the section on Paralysis of Peripheral Nerves. This approach brings some prejudice to the examination, which is unavoidable, since time and endurance do not allow a complete sensory examination of the entire body of each patient. Try to be as objective as possible. A suggestible patient and a prejudiced physician supplement each other beautifully to the disadvantage of both.

Sensory disturbance that involves one entire side of the body (Fig 40,A), in whatever modality, is referable to cerebral or thalamic disorders, and the lesion will be above the pons. This pattern is also found in cases of hysteria, but then the line of demarcation usually is precisely in the midline, whereas in organic deficits demarcation is short of the midline.

When deficits are in the lower trunk and legs (Fig 40,B) and are bilateral and almost symmetric, then the lesion probably involves the spinal cord. This is also true of higher deficits if they follow the same basic pattern. Occasionally Guillain-Barré syndrome will produce this pattern. Modalities of sensation may be affected differentially because of the separation of function among the several fasciculi of the cord.

The "stocking-glove" pattern of sensory loss (Fig 40,C) is typical for peripheral neuropathy. Levels should be determined as shown in Figure 39. Sometimes a cerebral or a spinal lesion may cause distal

Fig 40

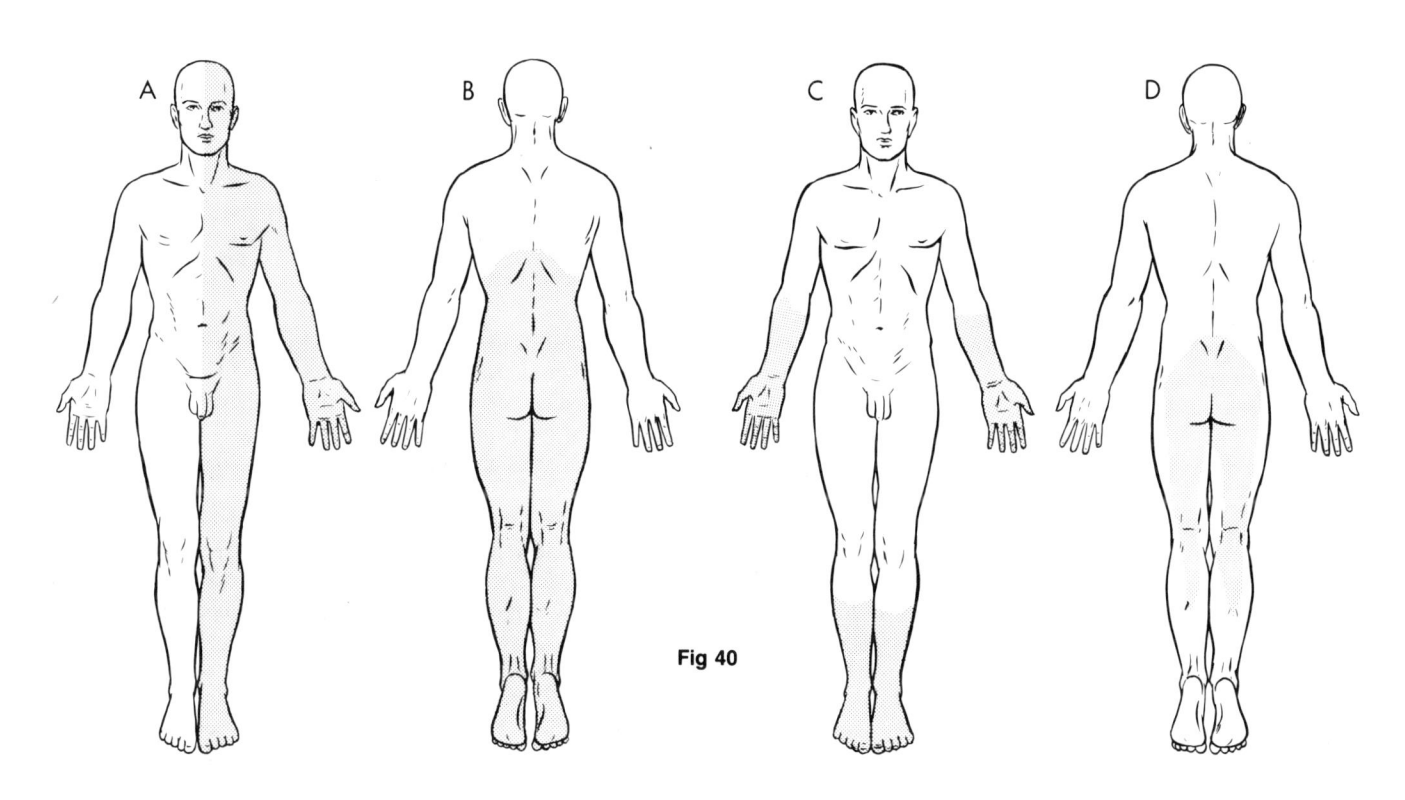

Patterns of Sensory Loss / 61

Fig 41

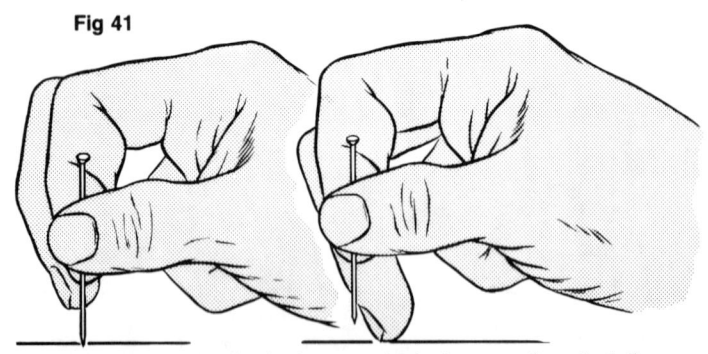

sensory loss, usually of a single extremity in the case of cerebral disease, and often in association with hyperreflexia and the Babinski sign in cases of either cerebral or spinal lesions.

The pattern of sensory loss shown in Figure 40,D is called "saddle-area." This area is the "tail end" of the body and is innervated by the sacral segments of the spinal cord and the sacral roots (p. 69). A lesion producing saddle-area sensory loss will be found in the upper lumbar spinal level if it is due to a lesion of the cord (conus medullaris). The lesion will be at the middle or lower lumbar or upper sacral spinal level if it involves the cauda equina (p. 73). Defective control of the urinary bladder and anal sphincter are regularly associated with this type of sensory deficit. An interesting corollary of the saddle-area pattern is the phenomenon of "sacral sparing," in which this region is relatively spared of sensory loss when lesions are located higher up within the spinal cord.

Lesions in the pons and below in medulla and cord may result in dissociated sensory loss on one or both sides of the body because of different levels of crossing of the sensory pathways. A lesion of the lateral medulla (lateral medullary syndrome, called Wallenberg's syndrome) will cause loss of pain sensation on the ipsilateral side of the face and the opposite side of the body. In this situation, touch is preserved in areas where there is loss of pain perception.

The Brown-Séquard syndrome is due to a lesion involving a lateral half of the cord. The sensory component of the syndrome consists of loss of pain sensation and temperature discrimination contralateral to the lesion, beginning several segments below its level, with position sense lost on the same side as the lesion, below its level.

Since the majority of sensory deficits involve some loss of sensitivity to pain, test this modality first in the adult. Show the patient the common pin to be used and demonstrate on your hand how this stimulus will be applied. Hold the pin so that either your finger or the pinpoint touches the skin. You can thus deliver either a "sharp" or a "dull" stimulus. Do not use an intravenous needle.

Use the pin lightly but consistently, with just enough pressure to elicit a sensation of sharpness and pain. Start on the upper chest, then go to the hands and feet, comparing sensitivity of the two sides of the body, then of distal with proximal areas, and finally of upper with lower aspects of the trunk. If there are differences, ask the patient to report where the sensation of pinprick is normal and where it seems dulled. Go back to the area of reference for reorientation. When sensory loss is partial, consistency will be less because of patchy and incomplete losses. If the patient is inconsistent in responding or does not seem to understand what is sought, resort to irregular alternation of sharp and dull stimuli to note in which areas he is most accurate. Ask him to say "sharp" or "dull" after each stimulus. His response should be immediate. A delayed, perverted, or unpleasant sensation after pinprick usually indicates root or nerve disease but is also found with thalamic lesions (thalamic hyperpathia). Devote the most attention to the hands and feet since differences and deficits will be most intense and easily detected there. The sole of the foot, however, is not a good area to estimate pain loss because of its unusual sensitivity. When pinprick is not felt on the sole, either the part is denervated or the patient has a hysteria of some fortitude.

Pain and temperature sensation are conducted by fibers that, after synapsing, cross in the cord within a few segments upward of their entrance. The secondary neuron ascends in the lateral spinothalamic tract.

Pain and temperature sense are closely associated in the nervous system. Reduction in or loss of either modality has the same meaning, and a deficit in one will usually be accompanied by a deficit in the other. However, some loss of temperature discrimination often precedes unequivocal loss of pain sensation.

Tests for temperature discrimination are done most commonly in cases of suspected thalamic or cord lesions when pain loss is equivocal. At times, pinprick stimulus will elicit dysesthesias, to the confusion of patient and examiner. When this happens, turn to tests of temperature discrimination.

The test shown in Figure 42 is difficult to implement because of the difficulty of maintaining constant temperatures in the test tubes. Obviously the test can be made more sensitive by reducing the difference between the temperatures of the two tubes. Set up the test by putting crushed ice and water in one tube and hot tap water in the other, keeping

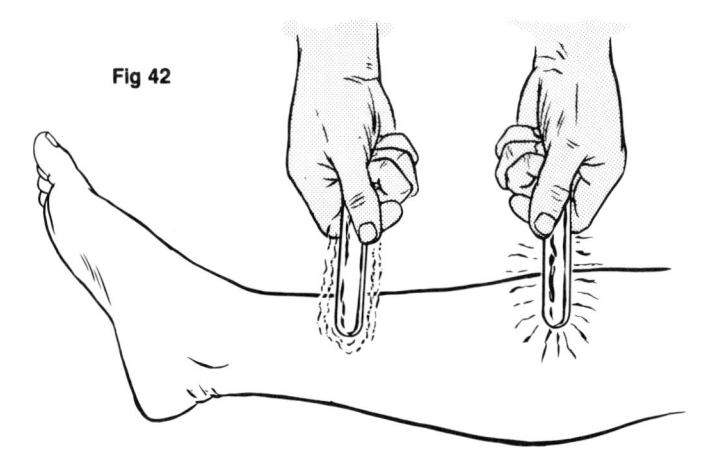

Fig 42

the outside of the tubes dry. Change the water when it approaches room temperature.

Apply the cold and hot tubes in irregular alternation, letting each dwell on the skin long enough to register cold or heat. Start with a normal area of reference and frequently check the ability to sense hot or cold there. Ask the patient to report the sensation. Normally, the patient's reports will show quick discrimination and few mistakes. Compare the two sides and various areas, as indicated, for the ability to discriminate cold from hot, much as one tests for pain. Rough levels or zones of loss should be estimated.

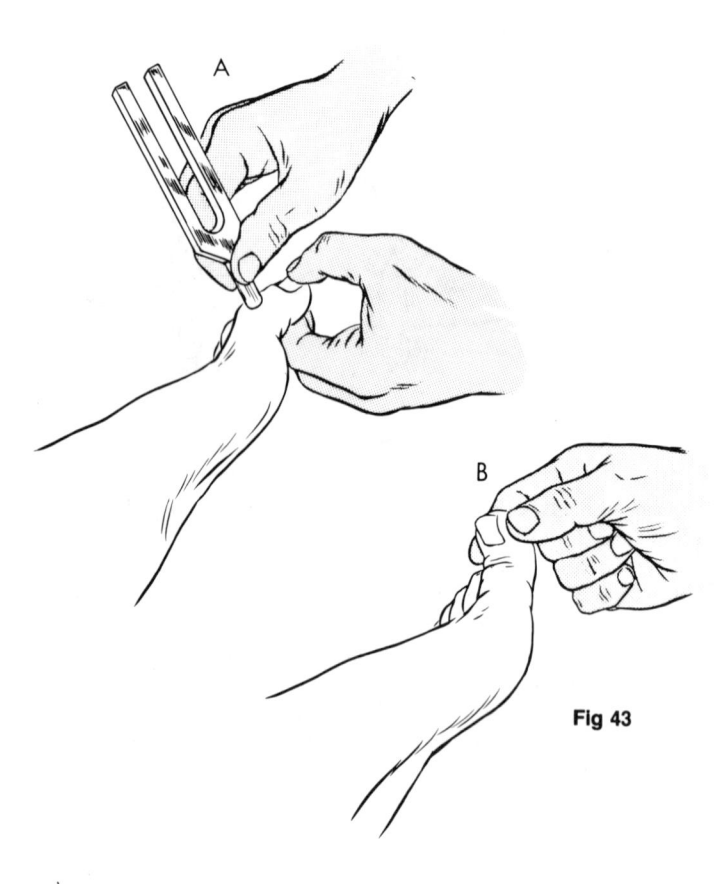

Vibratory sense and position sense are closely allied functions and are diminished or lost when the posterior columns of the cord are diseased, in cases of peripheral neuropathy and lesions of the brain stem and cerebrum. Fibers conducting these modalities do not synapse or cross until they reach the medulla.

Always test first for loss of vibratory sense in the hands and feet and then more proximally when peripheral losses are found. Use a 256-HZ tuning fork. Strike it on some firm but not hard surface and apply the end of the fork firmly to the dorsum of the great toe (Fig 43,A) or to a distal knuckle of a finger. Ask the patient what he feels. Be certain he senses vibration. The fork may be applied to the forehead or sternum if he does not understand what is meant by vibration. Always surreptitiously stop the vibration at some time in the examination to be certain the patient is not reporting only the sensation of pressure. In people over 60, vibratory sensation so tested is often absent in the toes but is never absent on the shin or in the fingers of the healthy person.

When the spinal cord is involved, the level of pallesthesia loss may be discovered by applying the vibrating fork at progressively higher levels, i.e., feet, patella, pelvic brim, and spinous processes of vertebrae, until the vibration is sensed. The test may be refined by holding the fork in position and asking the patient to report when vibration stops. The examiner, feeling the same vibration, will soon learn to judge when normal limits are exceeded. If vibratory sensation is intact in the fingers and toes, there will seldom be loss of position sense as ordinarily measured. Dissociation of these two modalities may occur in lesions of the parietal cortex since preserved cortical function is necessary for proprioception but not for pallesthesia.

Fig 43

To test for position sense, hold the sides of the patient's great toe as shown in Figure 43,B. Have the patient watch while you demonstrate up and down movement. Then ask him to call out "up" or "down" with eyes closed as you move the toe. Normally a few degrees of movement will be sensed and the direction identified. The normal limits are quickly learned. If the initial two or three responses are correct, do not stop here and accept this as evidence of normal position sense. A patient who is guessing will be correct 50% of the time and may well call two or three consecutive movements correctly. Give the patient at least six trials before concluding that position sense is intact. Position sense in the thumb may be tested in a comparable manner.

Always check pallesthesia and position sense carefully when the patient complains of clumsiness of the hands or difficulty in balance or if he demonstrates loss of manual dexterity, unsteady gait, or poor performance on heel-to-knee test or on tandem walking. The differential diagnosis of cerebellar vs. spinal cord, root, and peripheral-nerve disease may rest largely on the demonstration of the presence or absence of disturbed pallesthesia and position sense and their respective distributions.

Testing for touch is done in a manner comparable to testing for pain. A cotton ball is used, with a small piece pulled out as shown in Figure 44 to reduce the area of contact. Apply this to a reference area to acquaint the patient with the sensation. The normal person of any age will be able to sense a wisp of cotton pulled a short distance over the skin anywhere the skin is not calloused. Ask him to close his eyes and say "yes" each time he feels the cotton. Check as before for the patterns of loss that are most common. Compare the regularity of response on the right with that on the left side and on the distal with that on the proximal aspects of the extremities. Then ask the patient if he believes there is any difference in the contrasted areas. Avoid applying the test stimulus with a predictable rhythm lest the patient anticipate that rhythm and respond accordingly. The sensation of touch is relatively enduring, and other losses are apt to be manifested before touch is lost.

Pain and temperature sensation are commonly reduced or absent in the presence of a segmental distribution of syringomyelia or other lesions within the spinal cord. Fibers conducting these modalities have an intramedullary crossing and are preferentially interrupted by such lesions. Touch, however, is often preserved in the same areas by reason of its different pathways, both crossed and uncrossed (pain-touch dissociation).

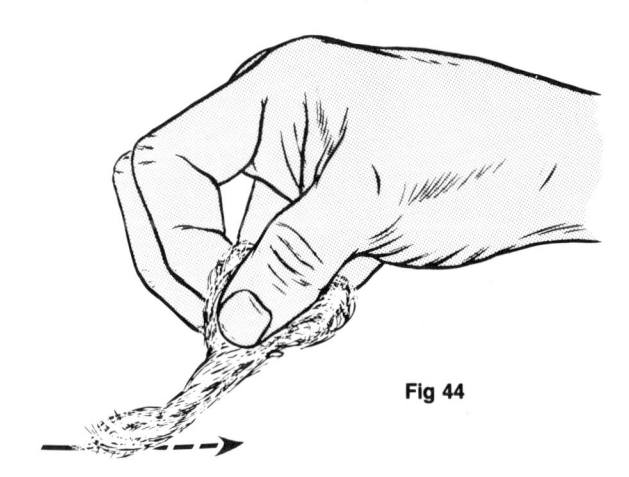

Fig 44

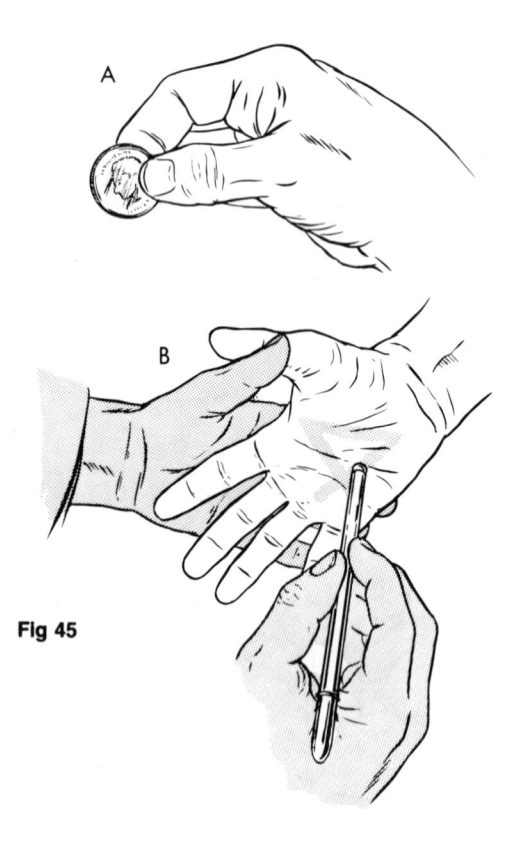

Testing the ability to identify small objects in the hands without visualization is an important part of the sensory examination. Use coins of several denominations, a paper clip, rubber band, small bar of soap, cotton ball, pencil, key, and the like. The normal person will hold the object with the fingertips (Fig 45,A), turn it about, follow its contours, rub and manipulate it in a knowing way, and usually give a correct answer. If the object is handled knowledgeably but not identified or bizarrely misidentified, the integrity of the patient is in question. An exception is the aphasic patient who may not be able to summon the proper name of the object or the patient in whom a lesion has effectively "disconnected" the parietal association areas in the dominant hemisphere from the rest of the brain. The patient with astereognosis does not handle the object well, fumbling it in the palm, trying but failing to grasp it securely with the fingertips, even dropping it. If the patient cannot identify some or all of the objects, the presence of posterior-column disease should be suspected, or, if the patient's difficulty is unilateral and accompanied by little or no other sensory loss, the existence of a parietal lobe disorder is probable.

Graphesthesia refers to the ability to recognize letters or numbers by the feel of them being traced on the skin. Generally this is done on the palm, as shown in Figure 45,B. Make the shape of the numbers as well defined as possible. Before testing with the patient's eyes closed, draw several numbers while his eyes are open to make sure that he understands the test.

Fig 45

This method is used for a more delicate test for sensory loss. It is especially applicable when the presence or absence of sensory loss is important for differential diagnosis, and results of ordinary tests for pain, touch, and pallesthesia are equivocal. Two-point discrimination is commonly determined on fingertips and shins.

For the fingertips, hold two pins as shown in Figure 46,A. Do not stick, but touch simultaneously with the sides of the points. Apply one pin, then two held at a set distance apart, in irregular alternation and ask the patient to report "one" or "two." Normally a distance greater than 5 mm is all that is necessary for the patient to detect that there are two points rather than one. If distances appreciably greater are needed, a sensory defect is suggested. The examiner should measure the distance at which two points can be discriminated from one and thus decide whether normal limits are exceeded. Experience will yield a baseline for future comparison.

A comparable test can be done on the shin using the fingers (Fig 46,B). Two fingers should be sensed if they are over 40 mm apart. Reduction in two-point discrimination is usually accompanied by loss of normal stereognosis and may be based on either central or peripheral sensory loss. When this function is disturbed in the face of relatively preserved superficial and deep sensation, a parietal lobe lesion should be suspected.

Sensory extinction is another finding common in patients with parietal-lobe disease. The technique of double simultaneous stimulation is employed to uncover this abnormality. Any sensory stimulus can be used, but simple touch is usually employed. When the patient's eyes are closed, touch identical parts on each side of his body simultaneously. A patient

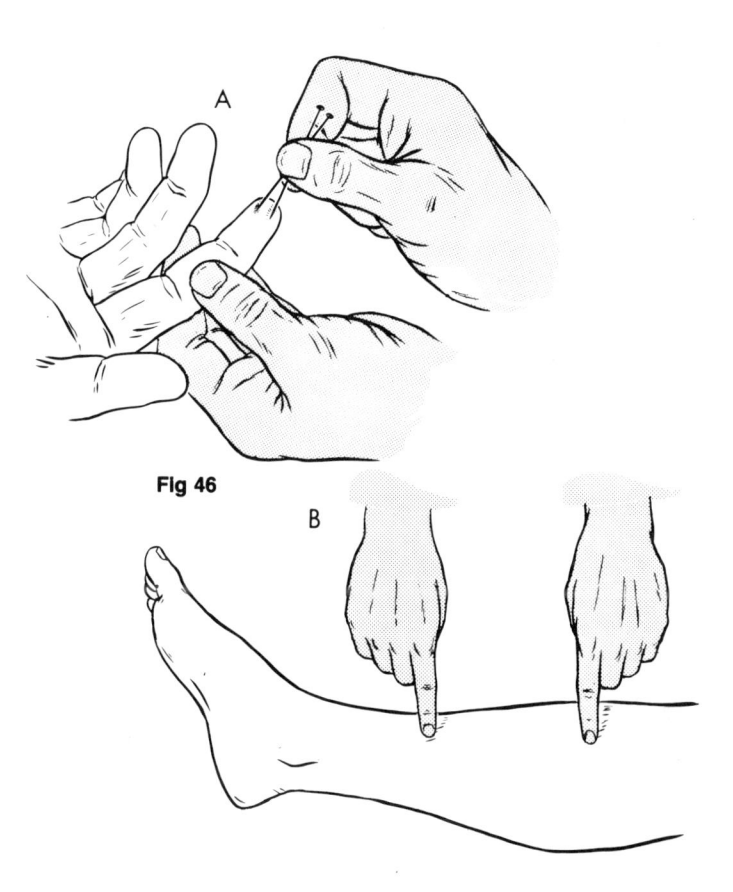

Fig 46

Two-Point Discrimination and Sensory Extinction / **67**

with parietal lobe dysfunction may consistently fail to feel the touch on the side contralateral to the involved hemisphere. When the same part is touched alone it is readily perceived.

The diagrams in Figure 47 depict the distribution of spinal segments and roots. The sensory distribution of several peripheral nerves is shown in a later section.

The anterior neck and upper shoulder are innervated by the cervical plexus, largely C-4, whereas posteriorly the segmental supply follows a regular pattern. The fingers provide a natural division of lower cervical dermatomes C6-8, and their examination allows a more reliable identification of dermatomal involvement than do the arm and forearm. Textbooks give conflicting views in regard to root distribution to the anterior neck and upper chest as well as other areas, but the patterns shown here, drawn in part from Keegan and Garrett, seem most reasonable based on personal experience.

The fifth thoracic (T-5) segment is at nipple level, T-10 at the umbilicus, and T-12 at the groin. The sacral dermatomes innervate the saddle area, and the lower sacral dermatomes take a circumferential distribution about the anus. Examination of the medial thigh is particularly useful in patients with saddle sensory loss because of the apposition of the upper lumbar dermatomes with the S-2 dermatome, between which there is little sensory overlap.

Clinical determination of the level of cord involvement is based on establishing the segmental level at which sensation becomes normal, i.e., from below upward. This level should be established both posteriorly and anteriorly on the trunk so that the diagonal distribution of the dermatomes can be plotted to help establish authenticity of the losses.

Commonly, a cord lesion will be associated with sensory deficits that appear to begin several segments below the lesion. The less severe and less complete the transverse lesion, the less sharp will be the line of demarcation between normal and abnormal sensation and the farther below the lesion will sensory loss be found. As the lesion expands, complete loss of function may take place, and the level of sensory loss will ascend finally to the segment of complete transection.

Herpes zoster is manifested by patchy, painful eruptions that are based on posterior root inflammation and often appear in segmental distribution. One or more roots may be involved, and a striking pattern of root distribution may be evident.

Fig 47

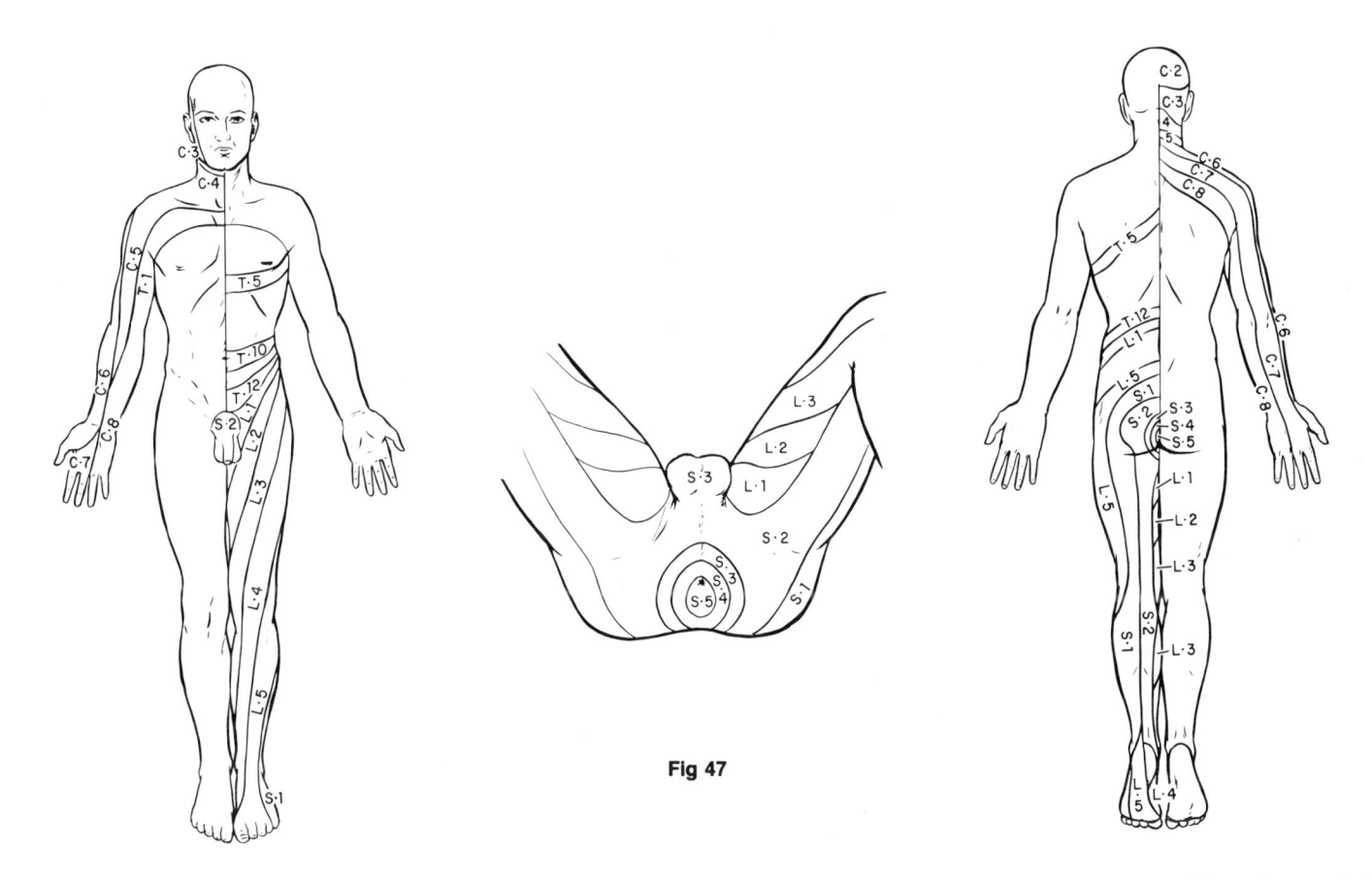

Dermatomes / 69

The diagram in Figure 48 (redrawn from Favill with permission) illustrates the relationship of vertebral levels to cord segments and to spinal roots.

In the cervical region the cord segments approximate the corresponding, numbered vertebrae, and the roots leave the cord at nearly a right angle. The C-1 root has no sensory component. There are eight cervical cord segments and root pairs but only seven vertebrae. The C-8 root exits below the C-7 vertebra, and from that point down, numbered roots leave below the correspondingly numbered vertebrae.

The spinal cord does not lengthen proportionately as the spine grows. In infancy the tip of the spinal cord is at about the L4-5 level but it ascends to the L1-2 level in maturity. For this reason, lumbar puncture may safely be done below the dorsal process of the L-2 vertebra in the adult.

Throughout the thoracic and lumbar regions, the motor and sensory roots are progressively longer as they course from their respective cord segments to their points of exit at the corresponding vertebral levels. Below L-2 this collection of roots is called the cauda equina or "horse's tail."

The relationship of vertebral level to spinal-cord segment is especially important in correlating sites of trauma, radiographic findings (bony erosions, neoplasms, osteomyelitis), and myelographically demonstrated subarachnoid block with clinical findings.

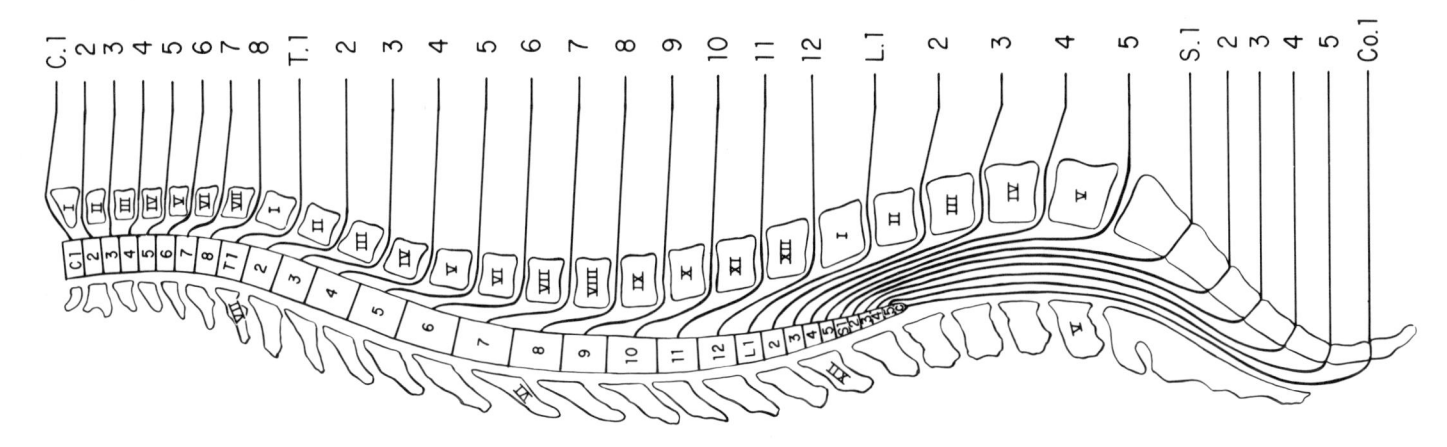

Fig 48

Spine, Spinal Cord, and Roots / 71

The most easily confused relationships of vertebra to cord and to root are shown in the diagram in Figure 49 (redrawn from Favill with permission).

The conus medullaris containing the sacral segments lies at the T-12–L-2 vertebral levels. A spinal fracture causing cord compression or other lesion here will result in saddle-area sensory loss, some weakness in the legs, loss of bowel and bladder control, and loss of potency. Still, the patient may be able to walk fairly well unless the lesion also interrupts the L-1–S-5 roots that traverse this area.

Serious errors may be made in locating a lesion producing saddle-area anesthesia, and bowel and bladder function may be lost if it is not recognized that a lesion in the upper sacral area interrupting the S-1 root and other sacral roots traversing this area may be indistinguishable from a lesion of the conus at the L-1 vertebral level. This knowledge is important for the surgeon. The prognosis for treatment of a lesion that involves only the roots is better than that for a lesion of the cord.

Evaluating such cases is further complicated by the possibility that a lesion such as a tumor at the T-11 vertebral level can cause a combination of lower motor neuron paresis and root compression symptoms from involvement of the L-2 and L-3 cord segments and the T-11–L-3 roots, as well as upper motor neuron paralysis of the cord and its function below this level.

Fig 49

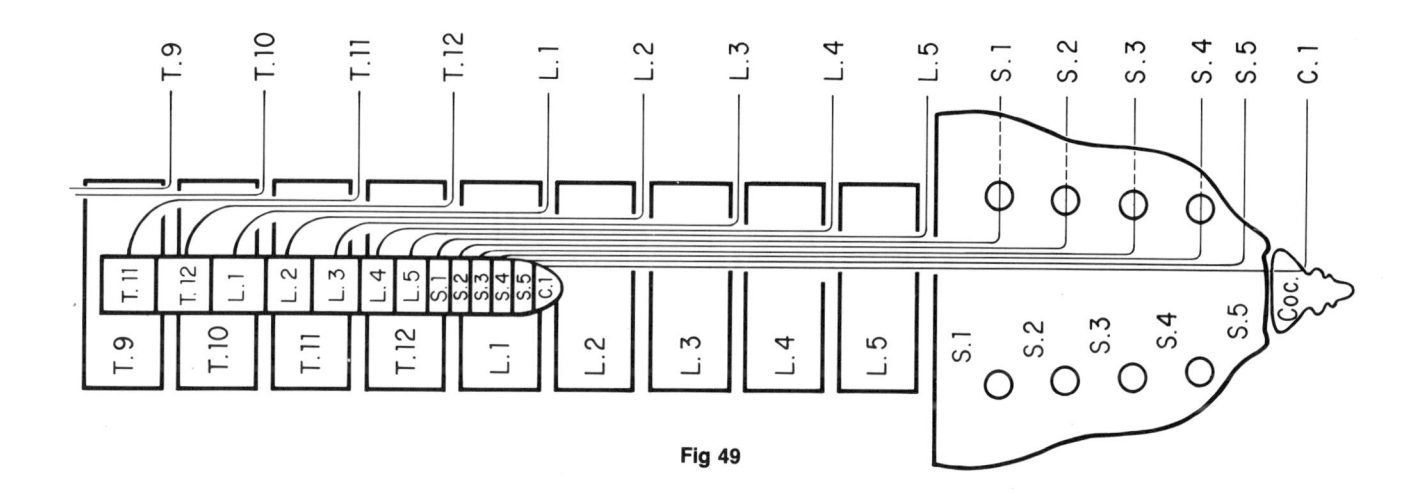

Spine, Conus Medullaris, and Cauda Equina / 73

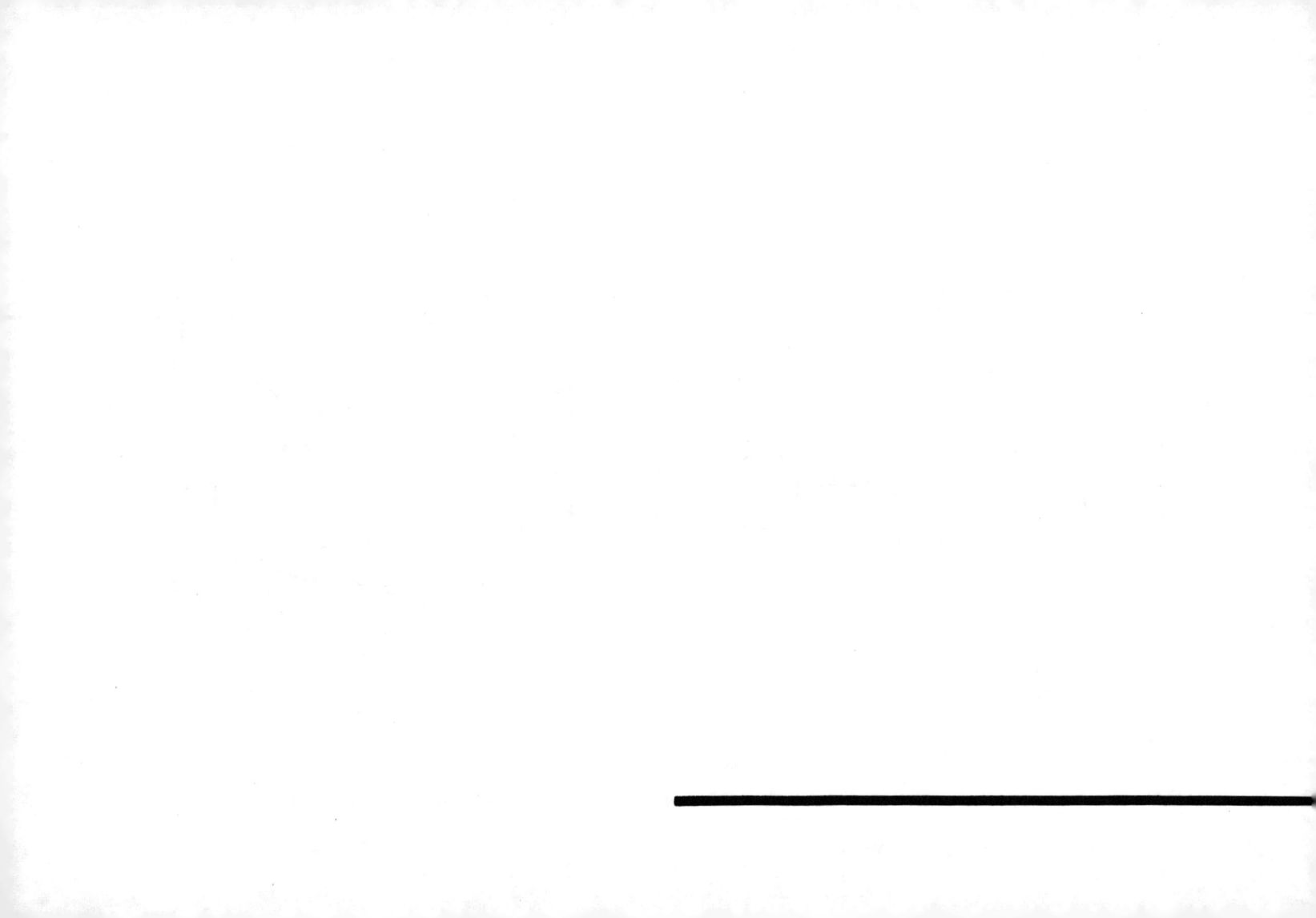

Abnormal Signs and Syndromes—Basis and Interpretation

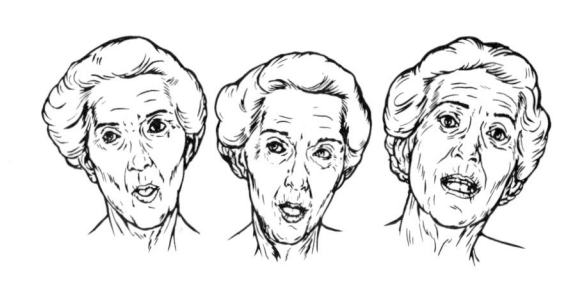

Fig 50

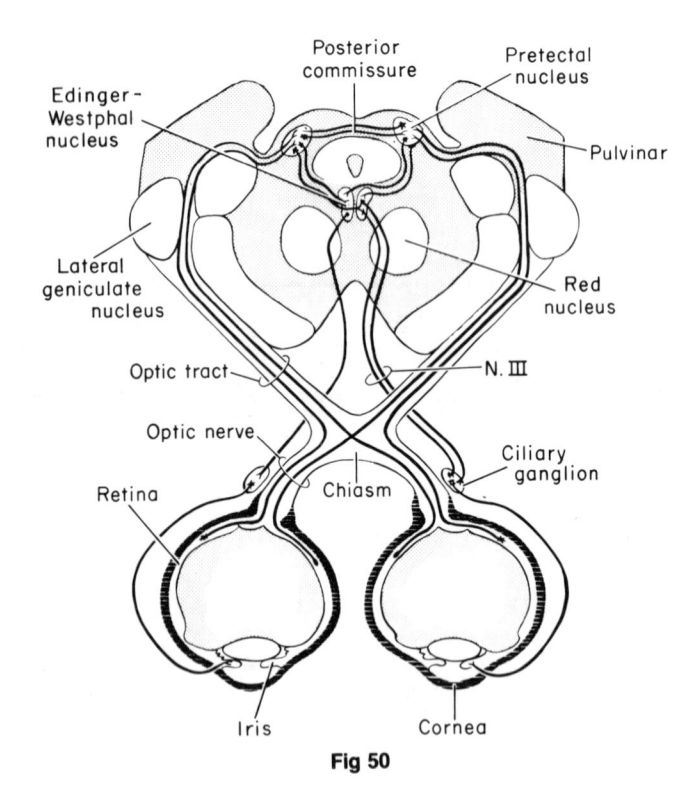

The Cranial Nerves: Their Relationships and Disorders

Fibers carrying impulses resulting from light stimulation of the retina (the afferent side of the reflex arc), both crossed and uncrossed, traverse the optic tract and bypass the lateral geniculate body to synapse in the pretectal region of the midbrain. Here another crossing is made that further ensures that stimulation of one eye will cause the contralateral as well as the stimulated pupil to constrict—the consensual reaction. The pupil of a blind eye will not constrict when its retina is exposed to light, but it will do so when the other, normal eye is stimulated (see Swinging Flashlight Test, p. 80).

The efferent limb of the reflex originates in the Edinger-Westphal nucleus, a part of the third-nerve nucleus. The pupillomotor fibers course with other fibers of the third cranial nerve to synapse again in the *ciliary* ganglion, from which terminal fibers innervate the iris and ciliary body.

Figure 50 was redrawn by permission from Crosby, Humphrey, and Lauer.

Inspect the iris before evaluating the pupillary size and response. Scarring of the iris may distort the pupil and prevent contraction and dilation.

Pupillary signs must be evaluated with due regard to other signs and the state of consciousness (pp. 89, 91, 98). Dilated, nonreactive pupils are most commonly due to local mydriatic drugs. However, such pupils are an ominous sign in the comatose patient, indicating the possibility of irreversible damage to the midbrain. Very small pupils may be due to miotic drugs used for treatment of glaucoma, but they suggest morphine poisoning or pontine hemorrhage if the patient is in a coma. Normal pupils are small in sleep and dilate with arousal. When the pupils are unequal in size (anisocoria), either or both may be abnormal. The larger pupil may react poorly to light as a result of a partial third-nerve paralysis (p. 89), or the smaller pupil may be part of Horner's syndrome (p. 98). When anisocoria is present it is important to examine the pupils in both light and dark. The difference in pupillary size in Horner's syndrome will increase in dark, whereas that due to partial third-nerve paralysis will increase in light.

The Argyll Robertson pupils of tabetic neurosyphilis are small (miotic), irregular, and often unequal in size (Fig 51,A). They react little or not at all to light but constrict promptly when the eyes converge on a near object (Fig 51,B). A similar dissociation between the light reaction and the near response may be seen in patients with diabetes, encephalitis, and midbrain neoplasms.

The pupil of Holmes-Adie syndrome is usually unilateral and is seen preponderantly in young women. The pupil of the affected eye is usually enlarged (Fig 51,C) and reacts slowly if at all to light. Its response to

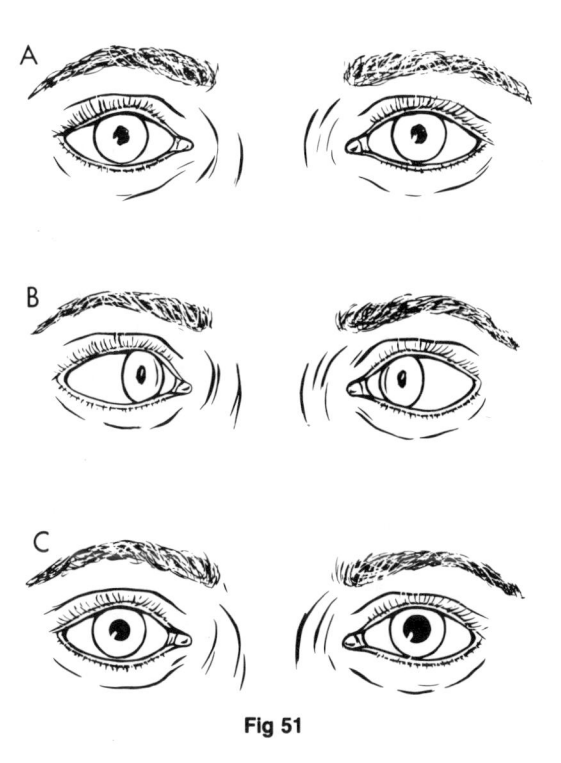

Fig 51

Abnormal Pupillary Signs / 77

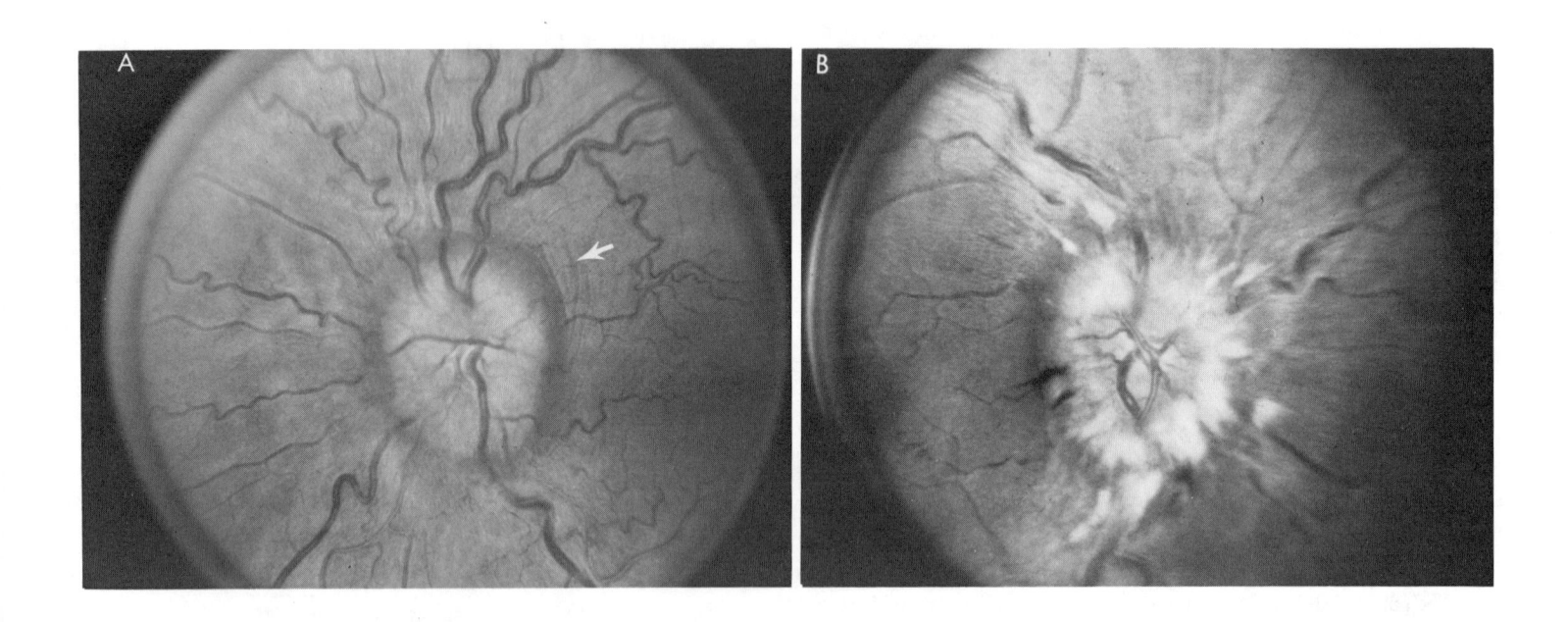

Fig 52

convergence, although slow, is often extensive and its redilation is slow and steady ("tonic pupil"). Conjunctival instillation of 0.125% pilocarpine will cause the tonic pupil to constrict more than its normal fellow. This abnormality seldom signifies a definable disorder but is important because it may be mistaken for a sign of serious disease.

The funduscopic examination is an integral part of the neurologic examination, and papilledema is always sought. Usually papilledema is associated with a history of headache, but sometimes the patient is too confused and forgetful to provide this information. Other symptoms or signs of neurologic disorder also are common. Pseudopapilledema due to anomalies, and drusen (colloid bodies) in and about the nerve head, may make diagnosis difficult, as may changes secondary to hypertension, blood dyscrasias, and vasculitis.

Papilledema is not always symmetrically present. Signs of mild papilledema include congestion, capillary dilation with redness of the disc, engorgement of veins, loss of venous pulsation, and blurring of disc margins, especially at the superior and inferior poles (Fig 52,A). Retinal folds *(arrow)* may also appear. Frequently, a diagnosis cannot be established early and may require repeated examinations every few days.

In more severe papilledema, the normal indentation of the nerve head (optic cup) is lost. Further blurring of the disc margins is evident, with small splinter hemorrhages in radial configuration. Elevation of the disc margins follows, with tortuous and distended overlying vessels. An angry, general hyperemia and multiple hemorrhages are characteristic (Fig 52,B).

As papilledema becomes chronic, gliotic changes obscure details over the nerve head, hemorrhages subside, and vascular distention is less florid. Visual field changes include enlargement of the blind spot and peripheral constriction. Blindness eventually results if intracranial hypertension is not relieved. Subsiding papilledema may reveal some atrophy of the optic disc with diminution of vascularity. Papilledema may arise in hours or days, but it subsides more slowly if pressure is reduced.

Swelling and congestion of the optic disc may be seen in certain primary ocular conditions and are found in cases of vasculitis with ocular involvement. Severe arterial hypertension produces a retinopathy with swelling of the disc, hemorrhages, and exudates. Since neurologic symptoms may also be present, proper interpretation of the retinal changes is quite important. Differentiation is made chiefly by discovering signs of arterial disease such as spasm, arteriovenous crossing phenomena, cotton-wool exudates, and a star figure about the macula. The linear hemorrhages and exudates are not limited to the disc region.

Another problem in differential diagnosis is presented by the swollen nerve head that is secondary to optic neuritis—a common manifestation of multiple sclerosis. Usually the primary complaint is a profound loss of central vision, which usually returns in a few weeks. Some hemorrhages may appear, but vascular engorgement is not ordinarily seen. A principal difference between the nerve-head swelling of intracranial hypertension and that of optic neuritis is that visual loss occurs late in cases of intracranial hypertension but early in optic neuritis. Moreover, papilledema is virtually always bilateral, whereas optic neuritis is usually unilateral. In retrobulbar neuritis there is also substantial central visual loss, but because the lesion is proximal to the optic nerve head there is little evidence of papillitis on ophthalmoscopic examination. Acute ischemic optic neuropathy can produce pale swelling of the optic disc, which may further complicate the task of diagnosis.

Pallor of the optic disc with diminished visual function is evidence of atrophy of the optic nerve. A sharply demarcated, pale disc with fairly normal retinal vessels but a reduction of capillaries over the disc itself, as shown in Figure 53, is typical of "primary optic atrophy." This condition results from damage to the optic nerve or chiasm. The pupillary light reflex is diminished, and vision is either reduced or lost, depending on the severity of the lesion, which cannot always be predicted by the degree of pallor.

Optic atrophy due to retinal artery embolism or thrombosis is associated with attenuated central retinal vessels. That following papilledema is characterized by gliosis and poorly defined disc margins (secondary or postpapilledema optic atrophy). Selective temporal atrophy of the disc may be seen after optic neuritis, but this finding is easily confused with normal variations of the nerve head.

Glaucoma may produce a deep cupping of the nerve head, with atrophy and visual loss. Other retinal findings of neurologic interest include cherry-red macula, arteriovenous angiomas, and pigmentary degeneration (see Bibliography).

The swinging flashlight test uses the direct and consensual pupillary responses to light (p. 76) to detect lesions of the afferent limb of the light reflex (retina and optic nerve). Determine first that the pupillary response to light is present on each side. Inspect the retina, especially the macular area, for primary lesions. Place the patient in a dimly illuminated room and flash a light (the smaller flashlights with concentrated beam are suitable) into one eye, noting the pupillary response. Then swing the light over to the other eye at the same angle and distance. The pupils normally will have dilated slightly in the interim to constrict again as the light is flashed in this eye. When there is an afferent defect on one side, the pupil of that eye will not constrict but will dilate despite the bright light. This apparently paradoxical response is actually a con-

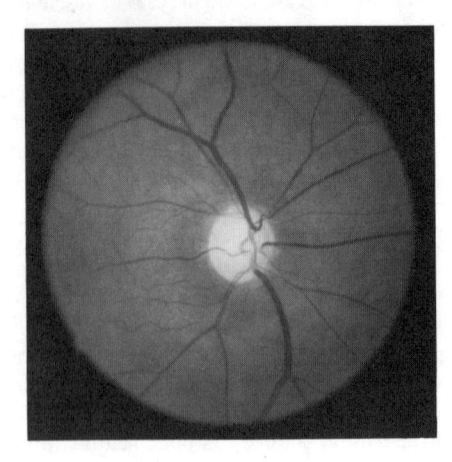

Fig 53

Fig 54

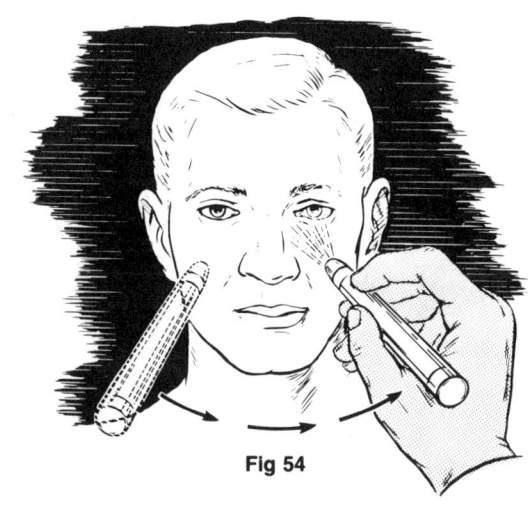

sensual dilation as the light is taken away from the "good eye." (Both pupils are dilating and constricting together.) As the light is shifted to the eye with the optic nerve lesion, the total light stimulus to both eyes is reduced and hence pupillary dilation takes place.

Avoid using the light in a way that may startle the patient and cause a psychosensory dilation, and be sure that the patient looks into the distance, thus avoiding the miosis of the pupillary near reflex.

The result may be positive even when there is no loss of central visual acuity, and the test is especially useful when the retina appears to be normal and optic nerve disease on one side is suspected.

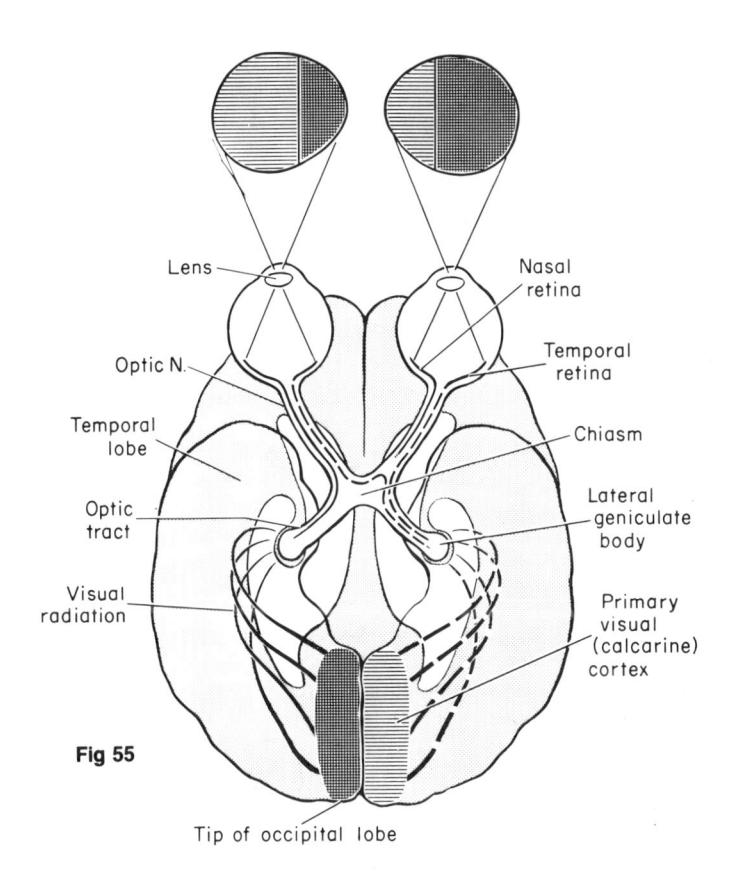

Fig 55

Swinging Flashlight Test/Visual Pathways / 81

Figure 55 is a schematic view of the visual system from the inferior aspect of the brain. This sensory system, including its end organ, extends from the anterior to the posterior aspect of the skull and traverses much of the anteroposterior dimension of the brain. It consists of a three-neuron relay, with the first two neurons in the retina and the third in the lateral geniculate body (a part of the thalamus), which synapses finally with the cells of the primary visual (calcarine) cortex in the occipital lobe.

The lens reverses and inverts the image on the retina. This causes unnecessary confusion to the student and may at first be ignored. The *right side of the brain sees the left half of the field of each eye,* which together compose the left half of the binocular field. Lesions in front of the chiasm will cause loss of vision only in the eye on the affected side. Lesions at the chiasm result in field defects in both eyes, typically involving the *temporal fields* of each eye, but sometimes affecting other portions of the visual field as well. Lesions behind the chiasm (retrochiasmal) cause defects only in the contralateral right or left fields of vision and in the same field of each eye. The loss of vision is *homonymous.*

Occlusion of the central retinal artery results in ischemia of the entire retina and total blindness in the involved eye. Often only the superior or inferior branch of this vessel is occluded, resulting in loss of vision only in the inferior or superior portion of the visual field, respectively (Fig 56, *left*). Such a visual field loss is called an altitudinal hemianopsia and, when unilateral, usually suggests a retinal vascular etiology. Ischemia of the optic disc (ischemic optic neuropathy) can produce a similar pattern

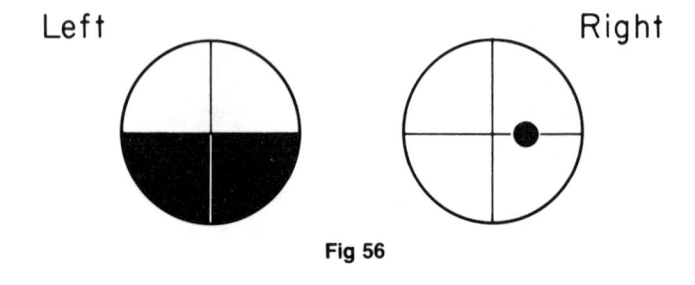

Fig 56

of visual loss. The normal physiologic blind spot is shown in Figure 56 *(right).*

Other abnormalities of the optic nerve or retina may produce islands of visual loss (scotomas) surrounded by areas of normal vision, but these usually are not demonstrated easily on confrontation testing, nor is enlargement of the physiologic blind spot due to papilledema.

In Figure 57,A, transection of the right optic *nerve* results in ipsilateral monocular blindness. Ordinarily any defect in vision that is monocular is attributable to a lesion in the eye, retina, or optic nerve on that side.

A lesion of the right optic *tract* (Fig 57,B) will interrupt uncrossed fibers from the temporal retina (nasal field) of the right eye and crossed fibers from the nasal retina (temporal field) of the opposite eye. Hence, a left homonymous hemianopsia results. A lesion so located is uncommon.

In a chiasmal lesion producing bitemporal hemianopsia (Fig 57,C), crossed fibers from both nasal retinas are interrupted. This is the characteristic pattern of field loss in pituitary tumors that distort the chiasm. When visual field defects are bitemporal in distribution, the lesion is almost always in the chiasm.

Figure 57,D represents a more complex situation. Here the lesion involves both the left optic nerve and the chiasm, producing ipsilateral blindness and interrupting crossing fibers from the nasal retina of the right eye, which causes a temporal field defect in the right eye. The crossing fibers are involved as they loop into the region of the junction between the optic nerve and the chiasm (see also Fig 55). Complex defects can result from small lesions in this area.

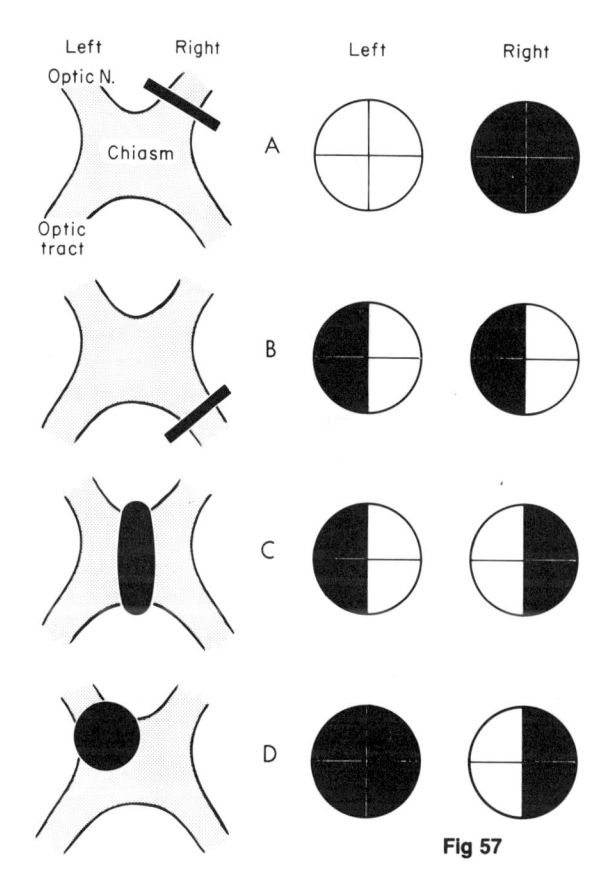

Fig 57

Chiasmic Lesions / Visual Field Defects

In Figure 58 the visual radiations are seen in a schematic lateral projection, and the right side of the brain is shown with the lateral ventricle shaded in.

The optic radiation arising deep from the geniculate body swings forward in the white matter around the ventricle and is dispersed vertically as shown, looping backward to be distributed to the visual cortex of the occipital lobe. Note how far forward the lower fibers of the radiation extend in the temporal lobe (Meyer's loop) and, consequently, how vulnerable they are to temporal lobe lesions.

The upper fibers in the parietal lobe carry impulses from the lower half of the visual field, and the lower fibers coursing through the temporal lobe subserve vision in the upper field of the opposite side. Accordingly, a characteristic of parietal-lobe lesions (Fig 58,A) is a contralateral homonymous, *inferior* quadrantanopsia. Temporal lobe lesions (Fig 58,B) result in a contralateral homonymous, *superior* quadrantanopsia, whereas interruption of the entire radiation (Fig 58,C) causes complete loss of vision on the opposite side, *homonymous hemianopsia*.

As the radiation progresses posteriorly, those fibers representing corresponding retinal areas of the two eyes become more closely associated. Hence, the more posterior the lesion, the more nearly do the visual field defects in the two eyes resemble each other, i.e., the more nearly congruous they are.

Fibers carrying impulses from the peripheral retina and thus representing vision in the peripheral fields are distributed more anteriorly in the visual cortex than are the macular fibers. A large part of the visual cortex, including the tip of the occipital pole, is devoted to central vision.

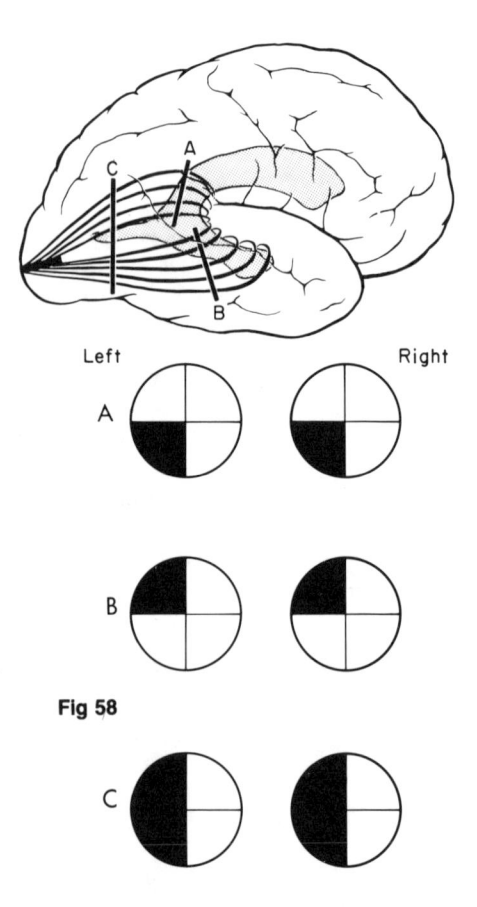

Fig 58

84 / *Lesions of Optic Radiation/Visual Field Defects*

Gaze movements are the normal conjugate movements of the two eyes moving in the same direction. Supranuclear disorders of ocular movement result in limited or absent gaze or forced deviation but usually do not disturb the movement of the eyes in relationship to each other or cause diplopia. Areas in the frontal lobes and posterior hemispheres subserve voluntary lateral gaze, the frontal area governing rapid or saccadic movements to the opposite side, and an area at the juncture of the anterior occipital, superior temporal, and parietal lobes governing slower pursuit movements to the ipsilateral side. In acute destruction of the frontal "eye fields," gaze preponderance is to the side of the lesion. The patient "looks at" his lesion. (The gaze may deviate to the opposite side during a focal or adversive epileptic seizure.) Usually this gaze imbalance is soon compensated. In acute homonymous hemianopsia the patient may only with difficulty gaze in the direction of visual loss or follow an object moved into the hemianoptic region.

Pontine lesions may destroy "centers" that subserve lateral gaze at this lower level. They will paralyze gaze to the same side, and the eyes will deviate to the other side. The patient "looks away" from his lesion. This gaze paralysis tends to persist.

Upward gaze is frequently limited in older people. Vertical gaze paralysis up or down in younger people can be attributed to a midbrain lesion. Upward gaze paresis is supranuclear, leaving the upward gaze reflex (p. 102) intact. The combination of supranuclear gaze paresis, lid retraction, and light-near pupillary reflex dissociaton is called Parinaud's syndrome. This is a classic finding in pinealoma or other neoplasms of the dorsal midbrain region.

Ask the patient to look right and left and up and down, and then ask him to fix his attention on a small object as you move it slowly from one side to the other and vertically. He may be able to follow an object laterally even though he cannot make the same movement voluntarily, if posterior "pursuit" areas are intact but frontal gaze centers are not. An example of paralysis of gaze up is shown in Figure 59. That an effort is being made to look up is established by the elevation of the brows.

In patients with supranuclear gaze palsies (such as lesions of the cerebral hemisphere or upper brain stem), quick, passive movements of the head may result in the eyes deviating to the opposite direction, by this means arriving at a position not voluntarily attainable. If so, lower-level gaze mechanisms and oculomotor apparatus are intact. Eye movements thus induced are called doll's head phenomena (oculocephalogyric

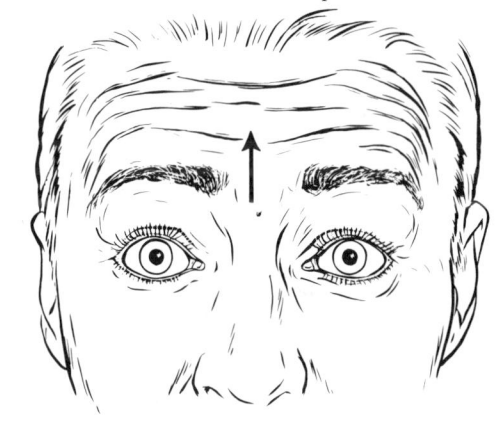

Fig 59

Gaze Paralysis / 85

Fig 60

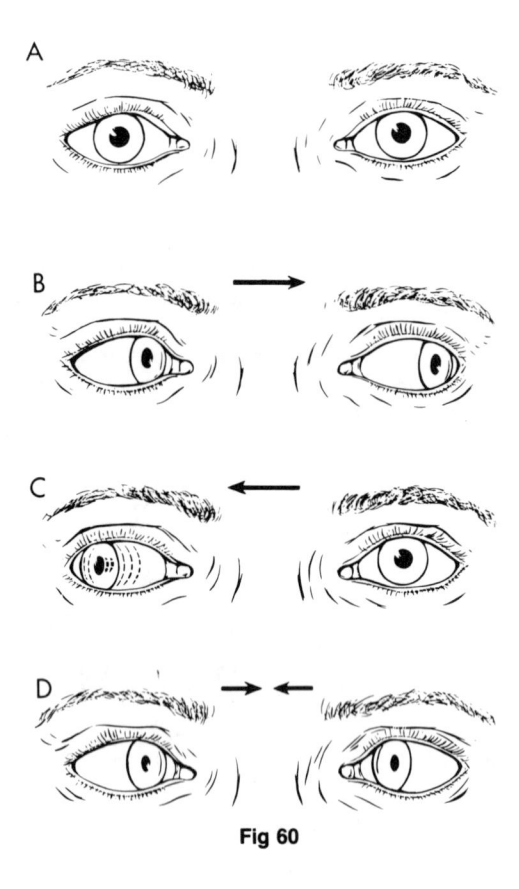

reflex). A gaze paralysis that is due to direct involvement of gaze centers in the brain stem cannot be overcome with this maneuver, nor can the doll's head phenomenon be elicited in patients who are in a state of deep coma, irrespective of the anatomic substrate of the gaze palsy.

Internuclear ophthalmoplegia is not common but has important anatomic and pathologic correlates. A unilateral, left-sided syndrome is displayed. Usually the eyes are straight in forward gaze (Fig 60,A) and diplopia is not constant. On gaze to the left the movement is normal and the eyes are conjugate (Fig 60,B), but on gaze to the right the abducting eye maintains its position poorly, with nystagmus of rapid component in the direction of gaze (Fig 60,C). The adducting eye moves only to the midline or, in milder forms of the syndrome, may move past the midline but noticeably more slowly than the abducting eye. The vertical alignment of the eyes also may be disturbed.

Although these findings are usually sufficient to support a diagnosis of internuclear ophthalmoplegia, the common preservation of adduction for convergence (Fig 60,D, the same movement that is absent in lateral gaze) makes the diagnosis certain. To test lateral gaze for this finding, have the patient fix his eyes on an object at least 5 ft away to avoid convergence that might obscure the difference between the action of the medial rectus muscle in lateral gaze and its action in convergence.

This condition is attributable to a lesion of the medial longitudinal fasciculus (MLF) between the nuclei of the third and sixth cranial nerves. Lateral gaze is integrated by this path, whereas the adduction of convergence is part of a movement pattern using other supranuclear pathways. Thus the paradox results of a muscle paralyzed for one movement but not another.

In young patients, multiple sclerosis is the most common cause of internuclear ophthalmoplegia, particularly when it is bilateral. In older patients it is more likely to be unilateral and due to a small brain-stem infarction.

A related condition is the "1½ syndrome", which is caused by a lesion of the lateral gaze center and the MLF on one side of the pons. Involvement of the gaze center makes gazing to that side impossible, while the MLF lesion prevents adduction of the ipsilateral eye (i.e., the ipsilateral eye cannot move away from the side of involvement). Consequently, all gaze is lost in one direction whereas "half" of gaze is lost in the other.

The upper lid normally covers 1 to 2 mm of the superior margin of the cornea in forward gaze. Drooping (ptosis) of the upper lid is a common abnormality occurring in any of the following conditions:

1. Edema of the lid due to infection, trauma, or venous stasis and drooping due to aging tissues.
2. Congenital ptosis, which may be unilateral or bilateral (Figs 61,A and B), mild or severe.
3. Horner's syndrome (p. 98), in which ptosis is partial, usually unilateral, and accompanied by ipsilateral miosis.
4. Ptosis of third-nerve paresis (p. 89), which may be partial or complete. It is usually accompanied by ipsilateral enlargement of the pupil and diminished reaction to light. Disorders of ocular movement will often be manifest.

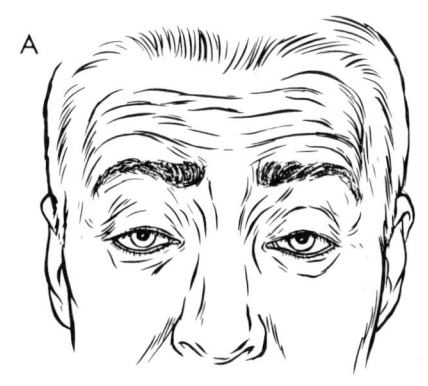

Fig 61

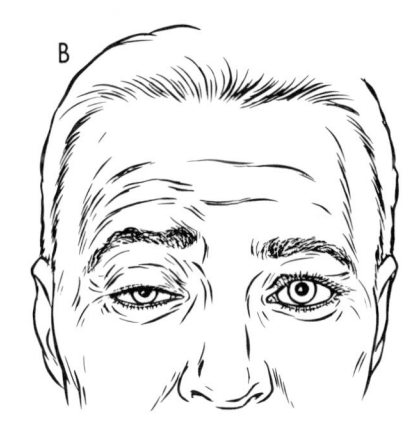

5. Ptosis associated with myopathic disorders (myotonic dystrophy [p. 138]) and with progressive external ophthalmoplegia, which is usually symmetric (Fig 61,A). The pupils will be equal and will constrict to light. Ptosis without anisocoria is likely to be of myopathic origin.

6. Myasthenia gravis. The ptosis is usually partial, asymmetric, and variable. This condition must always be suspected as a cause for ptosis or for external ophthalmoplegia. There are no pupillary changes.

7. Blepharospasm, i.e., involuntary contraction of the orbicularis oculi, which may partially or completely close the eye. When mild it may be mistaken for ptosis, but elevation of the lower lid can be detected and compensatory contraction of the frontalis is not present. Ptosis is sometimes seen in midbrain lesions.

Ptosis of any cause that partially interferes with vision is associated with frontalis contraction, an involuntary effort to maintain elevation of the lid (Figs 61,A and B). Look for ptosis when persistent frontalis contraction is seen.

In Figure 62 the view is caudad, with hemispheres removed. Anatomic landmarks of this region include the optic chiasm, which rises above the sella anteriorly, and the colliculi in the posterior part of the notch. The optic nerves are shown entering the optic foramina. Many syndromes result from disorders in this region.

Aneurysms here are a common cause of paralysis of the third nerve. This area of the midbrain is not only subject to intrinsic pathologic disease but also bears the brunt of damage produced by herniation of the brain. Cerebral masses and extracerebral hematomas may shift the midbrain, impinging the peduncle against the opposite tentorial edge, and thus

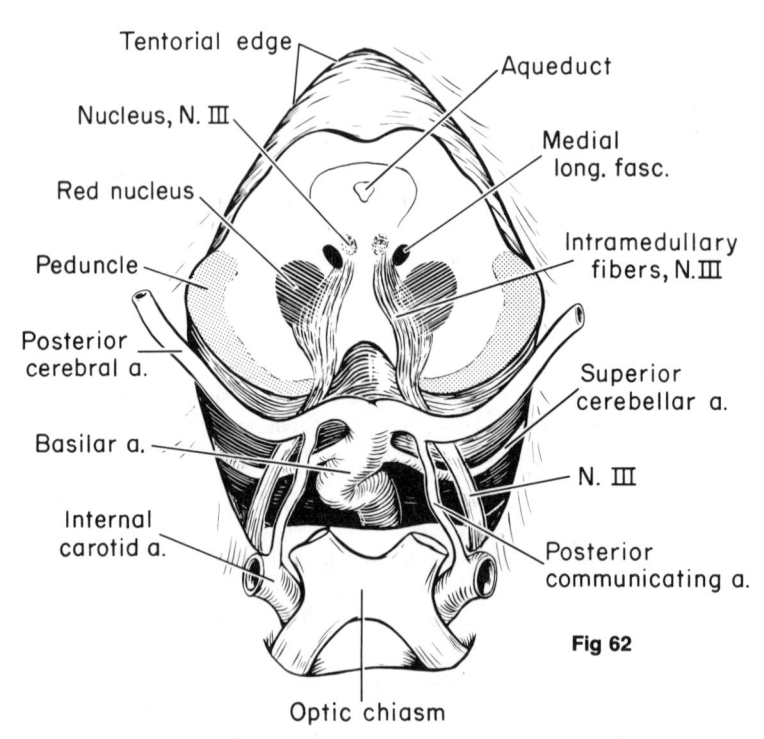

Fig 62

88 / *Tentorial Notch, Midbrain, and Neurovascular Relations*

produce paradoxical ipsilateral hemiparesis. Displacement of the midbrain may impinge the third nerve against the posterior cerebral artery causing paralysis of the nerve (p. 91), one cause of the dilated pupil seen in patients with expanding intracranial masses. Concomitant strangulation of this artery produces infarction in its distribution, which includes the visual cortex. Pressure above may herniate the mesial inferior aspect of the temporal lobe into the tentorial notch, producing serious or fatal embarrassment of midbrain function.

An intrinsic lesion of the midbrain may involve the red nucleus and third-nerve fibers, resulting in paralysis of the nerve and tremor of the opposite arm (Benedikt's syndrome), or it may involve the peduncle and cause ipsilateral third-nerve paralysis and contralateral hemiparesis (Weber's syndrome).

The posterior aspect of the chiasm forms part of the anterior boundary of the third ventricle and does not lie free as shown in Figure 62 for convenience.

The third cranial nerve (oculomotor) innervates the levator palpebrae; the medial, superior, and inferior rectus muscles; and the inferior oblique muscle. In addition, it carries parasympathetic pupillary constrictor fibers (pp. 76, 77). Paralysis of this nerve is caused by pressure from aneurysms of the posterior communicating and internal carotid arteries, by shifts of the midbrain, by tentorial herniation, and by trauma. The nerve may also be affected by meningitis, herpes zoster, syphilis, and cranial neuropathy. Intramedullary syndromes are discussed elsewhere.

Fig 63

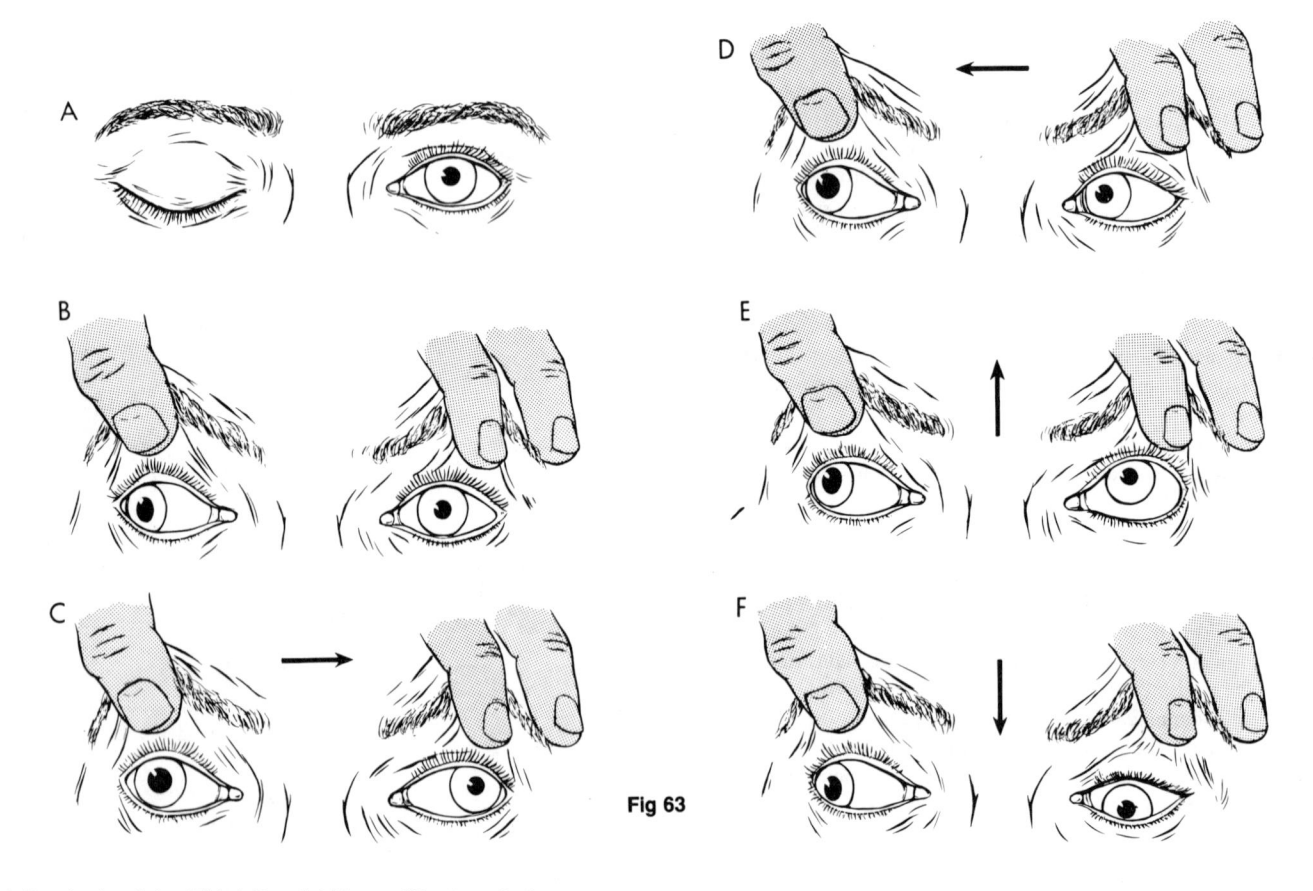

90 / *Paralysis of the Third Cranial Nerve (Oculomotor)*

The findings of total paralysis are shown in Figure 63. Ptosis is complete (Fig 63,A). The pupil is dilated and will not react to light either directly or consensually. The eye is abducted to the outer canthus by action of the unaffected lateral rectus muscle. The appearance on elevation of the lid as shown in Figure 63,B is characteristic of this condition. Some medial movement of the eye is possible because of relaxation of the lateral rectus when the patient looks to the opposite side (Fig 63,C). Virtually no vertical movement can be elicited (Figs 63,E and F).

The fibers subserving pupillary function are located on the outside of the nerve and therefore are very susceptible to extrinsic compression. Accordingly, pressure on the third nerve by an aneurysm may cause pupillary dilation before other signs appear. This is also true of paralysis related to compression of the nerve during tentorial herniation. However, vascular lesions producing ischemia or infarction, as in diabetes, primarily involve the central portion of the nerve and spare the pupillomotor fibers. Thus, the presence of a "pupil-sparing" third-nerve palsy is an extremely important finding in constructing a differential diagnosis. Diplopia appears as soon as any of the muscles attached to globe are weakened. Partial lesions of the nerve may result in confusing signs. Usually partial ptosis and/or abnormalities of pupillary response will be present in third-nerve paresis.

The third nerve is usually involved in its course after exiting the brain stem. Rarely, however, the oculomotor nucleus in the midbrain is the site of pathology. In this case unilateral nuclear involvement results in bilateral weakness of ocular elevation owing to the fact that fibers emanating from the nucleus and destined for the superior rectus muscle decussate and course through the contralateral oculomotor nucleus before joining the nerve.

Regeneration of this nerve with misdirection of peripheral fibers results in anomalous movements. For example, the lid may elevate when the patient attempts to look down or may droop when the eye is abducted.

The fourth cranial nerve (trochlear) innervates the superior oblique muscle. Isolated paralysis of this nerve is uncommon. Its function may be interrupted by trauma, by cranial neuropathy, by aneurysmal pressure in the cavernous sinus, or by inflammatory or neoplastic processes in the superior orbital fissure in company with the third and sixth cranial nerves. The superior oblique muscle deflects the eye down when adducted and rotates it inward when abducted. Its paralysis causes vertical diplopia with a compensatory tilt of the head toward the opposite shoulder. In the presence of third-nerve paralysis, the superior oblique muscle, if active, will rotate the eye inward (intorsion) on looking down. Observation for such torsional movements is made easier by identifying a blood vessel on the sclera and following its position relative to the equator of the globe. In this manner, one may determine whether the fourth nerve is intact in the presence of third-nerve paralysis.

It is important to determine whether the third and fourth cranial nerves are both affected, because involvement of both helps establish the superior orbital fissure, or cavernous sinus, as the most likely location of the causative lesion.

The sixth cranial nerve innervates only the external rectus muscle, which abducts the eye. It has a long course in the subarachnoid space, paralleling the brain stem along the clivus and at the superior border of the petrous portion of the temporal bone, angling sharply forward to traverse the cavernous sinus and then the superior orbital fissure. It is subject to stretching with downward displacement of the brain stem and to vascular compression over the pons. The nerve and its nucleus are compromised in a variety of relatively common disorders—diabetes, trauma, meningitis, Wernicke's syndrome, neoplasia, syphilis, and cranial neuropathy. Abducens palsy, either unilateral or bilateral, in cases of increased intracranial pressure from any cause is relatively common and a notorious false localizing sign.

When paresis is mild the only manifestation may be diplopia on lateral gaze to the side of the weakened external rectus muscle. The image from the paretic eye is displaced to the side of the paresis (uncrossed diplopia). When the nerve is freshly paralyzed, the affected eye is slightly adducted at rest (Fig 64,A). Gaze to the normal side is performed well (Fig 64,B), but as gaze is carried to the midline, diplopia appears; as gaze is directed further toward the affected side, weakness or failure of abduction becomes evident and diplopia increases (Fig 64,C). When paralysis is of long standing, the affected eye deviates further into adduction. This is not true for the peculiar congenital paralysis of abduction, which is based on a different mechanism.

The sixth nerve may also be affected at its nuclear origin or in its intramedullary course. A nuclear lesion is always associated with ipsilateral paralysis of horizontal gaze because of the anatomic proximity of the pontine lateral gaze center; thus, an isolated lateral rectus palsy should never be assigned a nuclear etiology. The anatomic basis for several syndromes that are localized to the region are shown in Figure 64,D. The involvement of the sixth and seventh cranial nerves, the pyramidal tract, the "center for lateral gaze" near the sixth-nerve nucleus, and the cerebellar peduncle in various combinations by lesions, usually vascular, results in several characteristic syndromes. For example, the Millard-Gubler syndrome is characterized by ipsilateral sixth- and seventh-nerve paralysis and contralateral hemiparesis. In the Foville syndrome there are ipsilateral paralysis of the face, paralysis of lateral gaze to the same side, and contralateral hemiplegia. The paralysis of one side of the face and the opposite side of the body is referred to as hemiplegia alternans.

Fig 64

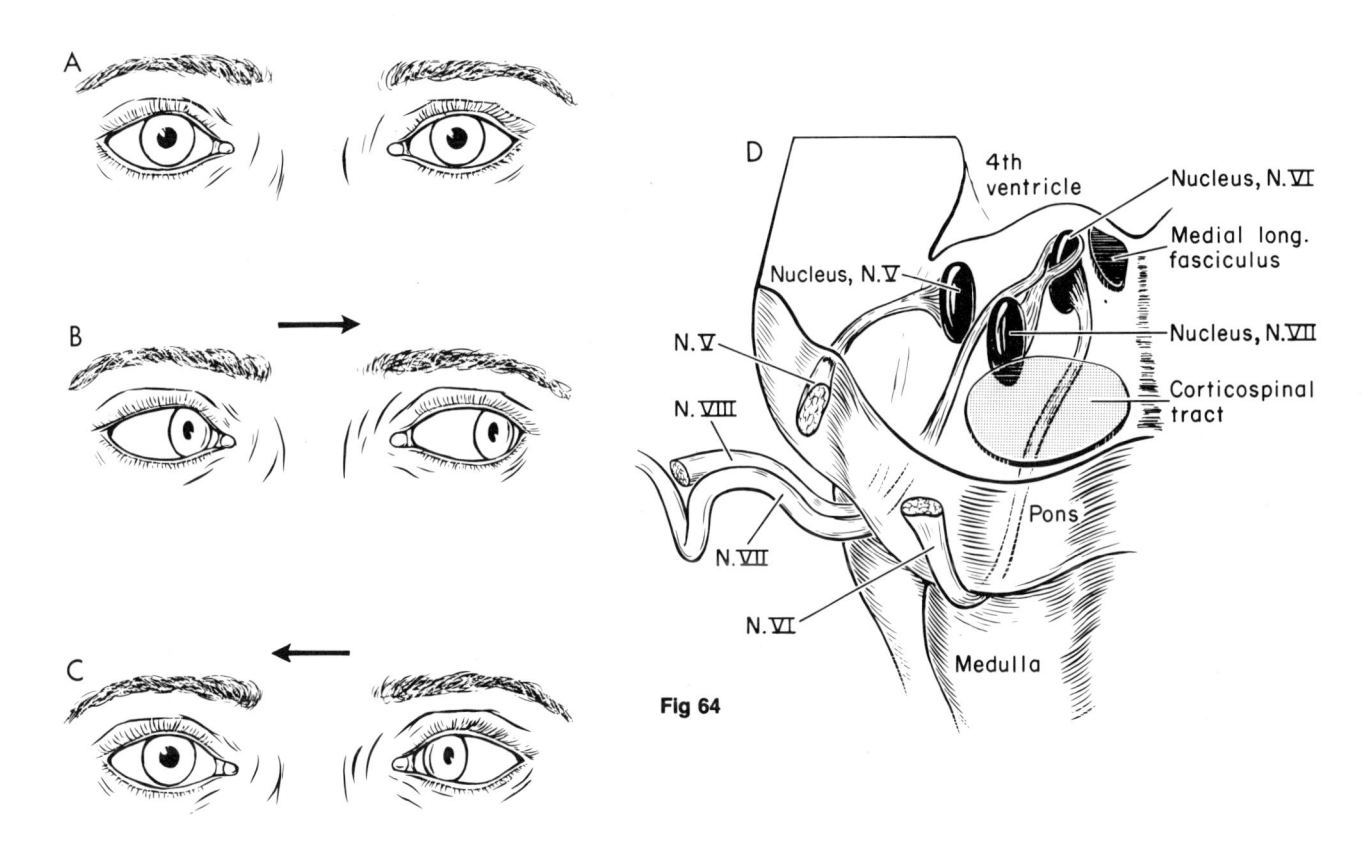

Paralysis of the Sixth Cranial Nerve (Abducens) / 93

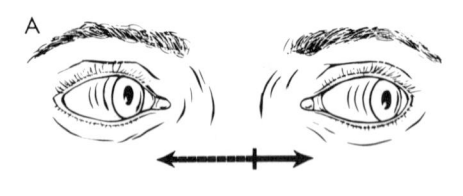

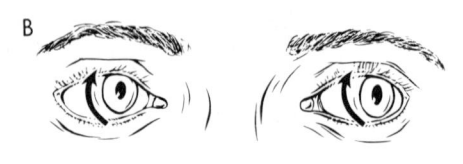

Fig 65

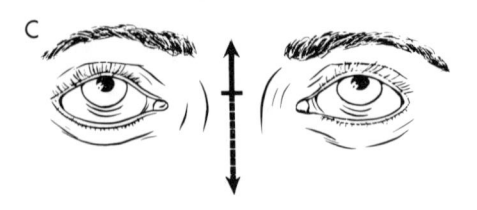

Nystagmus is an oscillatory movement of the eyes of varying amplitude that may be present on forward gaze but usually is found when gaze is directed to either side or vertically (Figs 65,A and C). It should be sought and is usually found during examination for ocular and gaze movements. With some rare exceptions, the movements of the two eyes are similar in amplitude, rate, and direction (p. 86).

Most forms of nystagmus are phasic in that there is a fast movement (jerk) in one direction and a slower movement in the opposite direction. By convention, jerk nystagmus is always described according to the direction of the fast component. In nonphasic (pendular) forms of nystagmus the movements of the eyes are of equal velocity in both directions.

Nystagmus occurs in many normal individuals when the gaze is carried to lateral extremes beyond the normal binocular field. Such physiologic or "end-point" nystagmus, which occurs only with horizontal eye movements, is usually of low amplitude with the fast component in the direction of gaze. It is eliminated when gaze is guided back 10 to 20 degrees toward the midline. Nystagmus of this type has no clinical significance.

When an eye is moved into the range of a weakened muscle, jerking movements will often be seen. The eye intermittently drifts back toward the midline and then jerks back in the direction of gaze as the muscle attempts to hold the eye in position. Any condition that causes weakness of individual eye muscles may result in this form of paretic nystagmus. Since conditions such as ocular mononeuropathy, myasthenia gravis, or ocular myopathy may affect ocular muscles asymmetrically, muscle paretic nystagmus is often asymmetric.

It is convenient to regard most other forms of jerk nystagmus as resulting from an imbalance or weakness of gaze. If gaze to the right is weakened, for example, then on looking to the right there is a tendency

94 / *Nystagmus*

for the eyes to drift slowly to the left, with a subsequent, cortically mediated, corrective jerk to the right. Nystagmus associated with a central lesion involving the vestibular nuclei, the cerebellum, or the brain-stem connections of the vestibular nuclei is usually of this type. In this instance nystagmus is present on both right and left gaze and often on upward gaze, with the fast component in the direction of gaze. Therefore, the direction of the fast component can be in any direction depending on the direction of gaze. The movements are usually of greater amplitude when gaze is directed to the side of the causative lesion. Intoxication with centrally depressant drugs such as phenytoin, barbiturates, or alcohol will result in the same type of nystagmus except that the amplitude is not dependent on the direction of gaze. Patients with toxic or centrally caused nystagmus are usually not aware of movement either of the eyes or of objects in their field of vision but may experience mild vertigo.

Vestibular nystagmus arising from disorders of the end organ is a jerk nystagmus that often has a rotary component (Fig 65,B). If the right vestibular apparatus is suddenly suppressed, as in an attack of Meniere's disease, there will be a slow conjugate movement of the eyes to the right followed by a corrective jerk to the left. It is important to remember that the direction of the jerk in vestibular nystagmus does not change with direction of gaze but rather is always opposite of the suppressed vestibule. The nystagmus is more prominent, however, when gaze is in the same direction as the fast component—in this example, to the left. Unlike central nystagmus, vestibular end-organ nystagmus is often associated with severe vertigo and nausea. Another difference is that visual fixation enhances central nystagmus but suppresses end-organ nystagmus. Accordingly, central nystagmus is best demonstrated by having the patient fixate on the examiner's moving finger, which will accentuate the tendency. Vestibular end-organ nystagmus may be accentuated by techniques that interfere with fixation, such as thick lenses that obscure vision. Finally, central nystagmus is often associated with other brain-stem signs, whereas patients with end-organ vestibular nystagmus commonly have evidence of associated cochlear dysfunction, such as hearing loss or tinnitus.

Optokinetic nystagmus can be induced in a normal subject by moving a series of patterns across his visual field. Fixation of attention on a moving pattern carries the eyes in the direction of movement until visual fixation is broken and the eyes rapidly return to a central position to pick up and follow another pattern. Hence, the nystagmus (fast phase) is opposite in direction to the moving targets. Usually a revolving drum with vertical lines is used. An ordinary tape measure can also be used for this purpose by having the patient read off the numbers as the tape is passed in front of his eyes. In the presence of a parietal-lobe lesion, optokinetic nystagmus may be diminished or eliminated when the targets are moved toward the side of the lesion, i.e., from left to right in a patient with right-hemisphere lesion.

Pendular nystagmus refers to to-and-fro movements of the eyes around a center point, usually near the forward position of the eyes. Movement is of equal velocity and amplitude to either side and has no jerk component unless the gaze is carried to either side when a component may be found in the direction of gaze. This type of nystagmus is characteristic for patients who have from birth suffered a substantial and bilateral loss of visual acuity. It is also called "fixation nystagmus". If pendular nystagmus is acquired rather than congenital, it is likely to be due to multiple sclerosis, or, in older patients, to a brain-stem infarction. In acquired cases, the patient tends to complain of movement of the visual field or blurring of vision corresponding to the movement with reduction in visual acuity (oscillopsia). When amplitude is small, pendular nystagmus may be discovered only on ophthalmoscopic examination. *Congenital latent nystagmus* is made manifest by covering one eye. Then nystagmus of both eyes toward the side of the uncovered eye appears, often reducing visual acuity.

See-saw nystagmus is a condition in which one eye rises and intorts while the other falls and extorts. It is usually seen in patients with bitemporal visual-field loss and large parasellar tumors.

Convergence-retraction nystagmus occurs in conditions that limit upward eye movement, such a pineal tumor (see p. 85). When such movement is attempted, cocontraction of all extraocular muscles occurs instead, with resultant contraction of the globes into the orbits. Since medial rectus contraction is usually stronger than that of the other ocular muscles, concurrent convergence movements follow. When induced by downward-moving optokinetic targets, rhythmic, repetitive convergence-contraction movements result.

Coarse *downbeat* or *upbeat jerk nystagmus* in the primary position, i.e., not evoked by vertical gazes, is always indicative of a central structural disorder. Downbeat nystagmus is usually associated with lesions of the cervicomedullary junction and is accentuated when the patient gazes down or to the right or left. Upbeat nystagmus is most commonly seen accompanying lesions of the medulla or within the fourth ventricule.

Opsoclonus is a rare and striking phenomenon in which there are repetitive, irregular but conjugate, multidirectional jerks of both eyes, giving rise to various colorful descriptive labels such as "dancing eyes." Often it is associated with myoclonus of the limbs and ataxia. It is usually a result of neoplastic, degenerative, or encephalitic involvement of the cerebellum. The movements occur when eyes are in the primary position and are often accentuated by eye movement in any direction.

Although nystagmus is a complex subject, some general rules, although not absolute, can be followed.

1. Pendular nystagmus, when congenital, is almost always of ocular origin and not related to disease of the brain.

2. Nystagmus noted only in the extremes of lateral gaze is not abnormal.

3. Vertical nystagmus, unless associated with sedative drugs, is always indicative of disease of the brain.

4. Nystagmus that does not change direction when gaze changes direction is probably of peripheral vestibular origin.

5. Nystagmus that is associated with severe subjective vertigo is also likely to be of peripheral vestibular origin.

The circuitous route of the sympathetic nervous system in supplying structures to the head is shown in the schematic drawing of Figure 66. The outflow originating in the diencephalon courses downward in ill-defined pathways that are closely associated with the spinothalamic tracts at pontine-medullary levels. There is a synapse in the intermediolateral gray column at C-8 and T-1. The sympathetic nerves emerge from the spinal cord via anterior roots at this level and then contribute to the ascending cervical chain. Fibers mediating tonus of the smooth muscle of the levator mechanism and the pupil ascend into the skull again in the carotid plexus and join the ophthalmic division of the trigeminal nerve before entering the orbit.

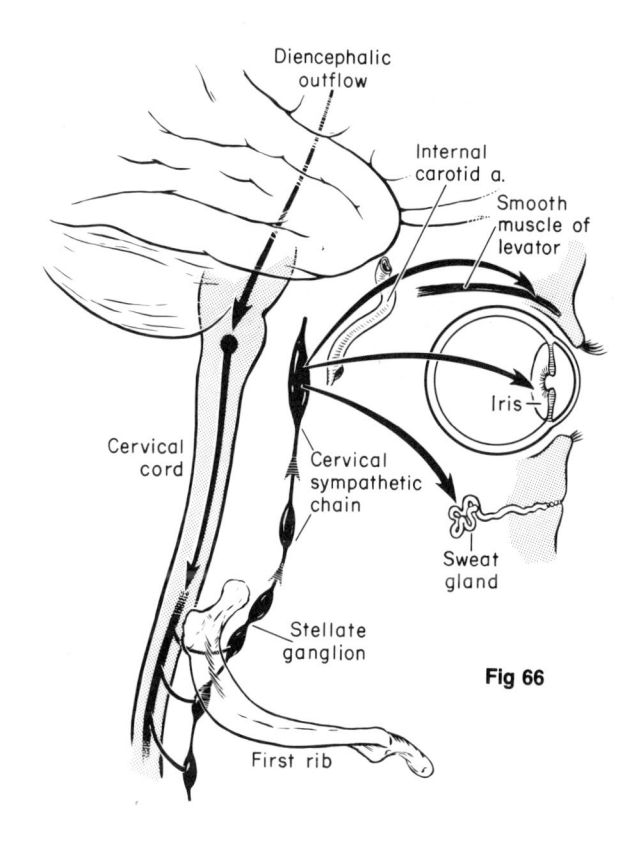

Fig 66

Sympathetic Innervation of the Face and Eye / **97**

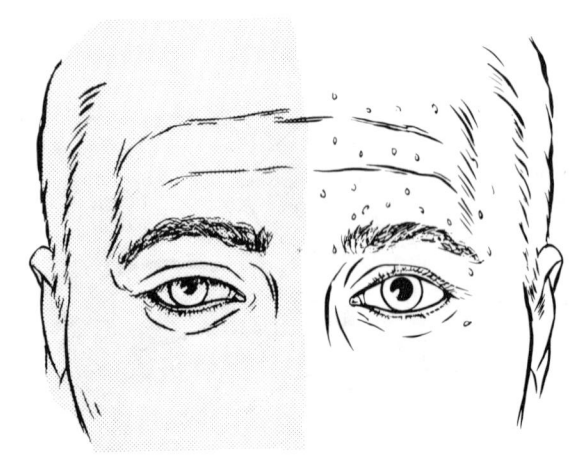

Fig 67

Horner's syndrome, when complete, is characterized by ptosis of the upper lid, miosis, and loss of sweating on the same side of the face. Pupillary reaction to light is normal, but the pupil does not dilate to psychosenory stimuli such as a loud noise. The syndrome may be produced by a central or peripheral lesion and may be partial or complete. The importance of the syndrome derives from the vulnerability of the sympathetic pathways at different points in their long course (see above). Associated signs can help locate the level of a lesion after Horner's syndrome has betrayed the interruption of pathways. When complete, the syndrome is due to a lesion proximal to the superior cervical ganglion. A higher lesion leaves thermoregulatory sweating of the face intact. Lesions at any level may be incomplete.

Pharmacologic tests also can be used to confirm the presence of a lesion in the sympathetic pathway and identify which neuron in the chain is involved. The instillation of cocaine will cause a normal pupil to dilate but has no effect on the pupil in Horner's syndrome, whatever the cause. Having established that Horner's syndrome is present, one can instill a 1% solution of hydroxyamphetamine (Paredrine), which will cause pupillary dilation only if the lesion is proximal to the superior cervical ganglion but not if it is distal to this point, i.e., in the third neuron of the sympathetic chain.

Horner's syndrome may also be congenital or neonatal, in which case there is depigmentation of the iris with a typical blue-gray appearance on the involved side. This is presumably due to the fact that sympathetic innervation is essential to the development of normal iris pigmentation.

Common syndromes and conditions characterized in part by Horner's syndrome include the following:

1. Pontine and medullary infarctions. The syndrome is complete and is ipsilateral to the lesion.
2. Transverse lesions of the cervical cord. These produce bilateral Horner's syndrome as well as sympathectomy of the rest of the body.
3. Infiltrating neoplasms at the apex of the chest—pleural tumors. The noteworthy association of painful and paralytic involvement of the brachial plexus with Horner's syndrome is pathognomonic of such a neoplasm.
4. Traumatic or intrinsic lesions of the common or internal carotid artery in the neck, especially arterial dissection.
5. Miosis and ptosis in the absence of other symptoms. These may be secondary to lesions about the carotid artery in the middle fossa, in the orbital fissure, or within the orbit.

Detection of the presence and nature of facial paresis is a common exercise in neurology. Minor degrees of facial paresis are often apparent when the face is in repose or when the patient changes expression, smiles, or talks. Look especially for asymmetry of the lids in blinking and for asymmetry of the nasolabial folds, bearing in mind that some facial asymmetry is normal. Look for differences in movement of the two sides of the face as the patient executes various expressions on request (p. 28). In very early hemiparesis, weakness of the face may not be discernible (p. 110), and diagnosis may be left in doubt unless disturbed function of the extremities is found.

When weakness of one side of the face is evident, consider whether it is of central or peripheral origin. The distinction can usually be made with a fair degree of certainty. Supranuclear paralysis produces less severe and less complete loss of function than do nuclear and nerve paralysis. The musculature overlying the forehead—the frontalis and corrugator—is almost never involved. Lid closure may be weakened, but less so than in peripheral-nerve paralysis. The lower part of the face is weakened or paralyzed. Movement of the upper part of the face and much of the lid closure function are subject to bilateral cortical influence, whereas movement of the lower area of the face is largely a contralateral cortical function.

Infranuclear lesions commonly resulting from affliction of the seventh nerve within the temporal bone weaken the entire side of the face. Only selective distal lesions of this nerve will paralyze the lower portion of the face while leaving the upper portion functioning normally. Commonly, involvement of the seventh cranial nerve, unless very distal in the facial canal, will be associated with ipsilateral loss of taste. Sagging of the lower lid in cases of lower motor neuron paralysis allows tears to flow onto the face. These signs do not occur in central facial paresis.

Facial reflexes will be reduced or absent. Nuclear and infranuclear paralysis may result from intramedullary lesions that destroy the nuclei or the intramedullary fibers of the nerve before its emergence (p. 92).

In Figure 68,A, the patient is closing his eyes tightly and showing his teeth at the same time. The lids do not close, Bell's phenomenon (p. 102) is seen, and no contraction of musculature of the left side takes place. In Figure 68,B the patient is showing teeth more vigorously; there is some shift of the lower face to the right, and the lower lid on the left is sagging slightly to increase the vertical dimensions of the lid opening. Figures 68,A and B are both typical of Bell's palsy or paralysis of the seventh cranial nerve.

Supranuclear paralysis of moderate degree is seen in Figure 68,C. The forehead is spared, the lid opening is slightly increased, and the lower area of the face is weakened to a lesser degree and is not so hypotonic as in Figures 68,A and B. Facial reflexes in this condition are usually present and often enhanced.

When the facial nerve has been interrupted, recovery is imperfect and characterized by persistent weakness with anomalous movements, presumably due to misdirection of regenerating peripheral fibers. Frequently, twitching about the lips is seen on blinking. Commonly, the nasolabial fold will be more prominent on the side of the old paralysis.

Fig 68

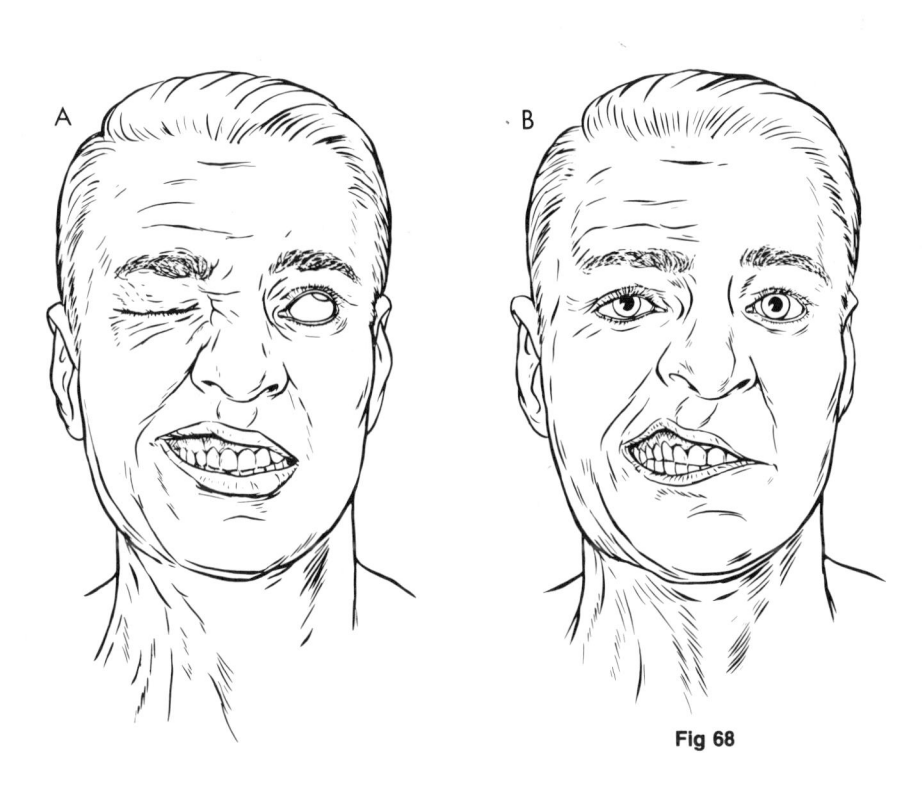

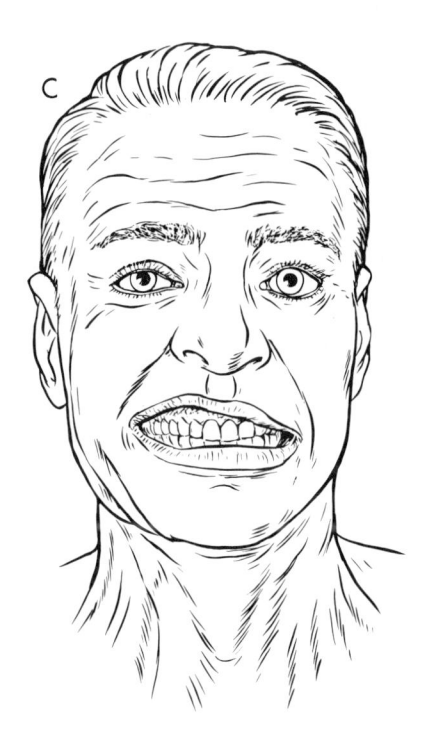

Paralysis of the Face / 101

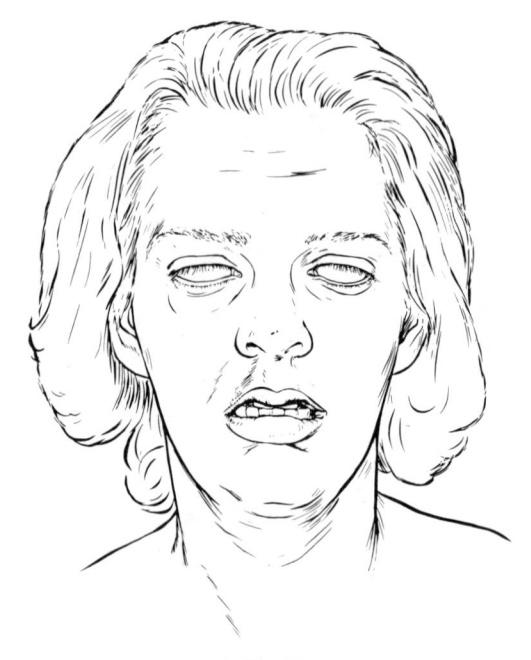

Fig 69

Because the face is symmetric when paralyzed on both sides, bilateral paralysis may be overlooked. Close observation of the face will disclose very incomplete blinking and lack of expressional movements. Attempts to perform various facial movements will betray the presence of paralysis. Bell's phenomenon is usually evident and frequently is seen in blinking.

The face can be paretic on both sides in cases of muscular dystrophy. Acute bilateral peripheral paralysis is usually a part of the polyradicular involvement of the Guillain-Barré syndrome and can be an immediate or delayed complication of basal skull fracture. The facial immobility of bilateral supranuclear paralysis and of Parkinson's disease is described elsewhere (pp. 104 and 114).

Bell's phenomenon is the normal facial-eye synkinesis of upward rotation and slightly outward deviation of the eyes when the lids are closed. One must forcibly hold the lids open to witness this movement except in patients with peripheral facial paralysis. The phenomenon is not always present and is inhibited if the patient fixates on some object. It is based on low-level mechanisms spared in supranuclear paralysis of upward gaze (p. 85). The chief practical application is to seek this automatic rolling up of the eyes on attempted lid closure when paralysis of upward gaze is found or paralysis of ocular muscles is suspected. If Bell's phenomenon is present, the superior rectus-inferior oblique complex is not paralyzed in a lower motor neuron sense.

Taste is mediated from the anterior two thirds of the tongue by the chorda tympani, the fibers of which course with the facial nerve until they branch off within the temporal bone. The glossopharyngeal nerve (ninth cranial nerve) mediates taste function from the posterior third of the tongue. The latter has little clinical significance. Taste is tested chiefly

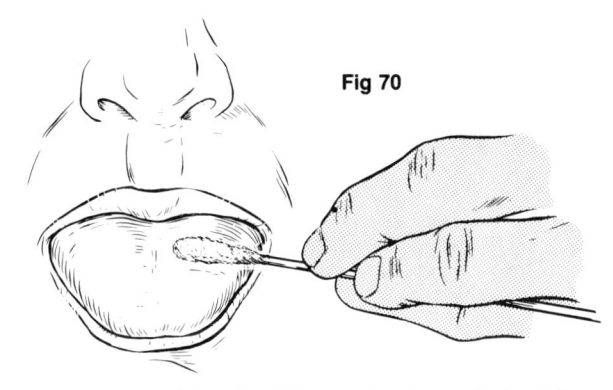

Fig 70

to localize the site of functional interruption in paralysis of the seventh cranial nerve (Bell's palsy). Taste is often inexplicably lost in old age, after head trauma, and in neurosyphilis. The close association of taste and smell, the chemical senses, is such that loss of smell seriously impairs what the patient regards as taste.

Tests for taste are easily done but difficult to evaluate and grade. Test for sweet, sour, salt, and bitter. Use sugar, citric acid, table salt, and quinine. DeJong suggests the use of solutions of 4% glucose, 1% citric acid, 2.5% sodium chloride, and 0.075% quinine hydrochloride.

If these solutions are not at hand, moisten an ordinary cotton applicator and pick up a few crystals or a bit of powder of these substances. Touch to one side of the protruded tongue as shown in Figure 70. Ask the patient not to retract the tongue if possible before identification and to point to one of the words—sweet, sour, salt, or bitter—written on paper as soon as he recognizes the taste. Substances may be alternated, and usually only one side of the tongue should be tested at a time. The patient should thoroughly rinse the mouth with water after each test. Use quinine last.

Pseudobulbar palsy is supranuclear paralysis of the motor functions mediated by the cranial nerves that originate in the "bulb" or brain stem. This includes the 5th, 7th, 9th, 10th, 11th, and 12th nerves. "Pseudobulbar" is used to distinguish the weakness or paralysis from "bulbar" paralysis due to lower motor neuron disease, such as poliomyelitis and neuropathy. The functions involved include breathing, coughing, sneezing, phonation, chewing, swallowing, and facial expression. Patterned expressions of emotion are "released" so that inappropriate crying and laughing, especially crying, are seen.

Commonly, the unilateral "stroke" or paralysis due to infarction of, or hemorrhage into, the corticobulbar pathways will produce some temporary disorders of the functions noted, but these are soon compensated since they are mediated by projections from both hemispheres. However, when disease is bilateral, disabling or fatal disorders of these important functions may occur. Facial expression is diminished; the face becomes blank when it is not contorted in exaggerated emotional responses. The mouth may sag open, and drooling is common. Chewing is slow and incomplete; food cannot be easily moved about in the mouth. The AMR of the tongue is slowed and the tongue may be almost immobile. Swallowing is poorly coordinated, and aspiration pneumonitis is common, especially since coughing is ineffectual. Tube feeding may be necessary. Speech is disturbed, volume is lost, and enunciation is imperfect and slurred. Dysarthria may become so severe that the patient cannot be understood. Poorly coordinated respiratory patterns add to the disability. No muscle atrophy is seen in pure pseudobulbar palsy. The masseter-temporalis stretch reflex (jaw jerk) is increased (p. 28). When spasticity is severe, clonus may be found. Tapping the upper lip (Fig 71,A) will result in a puckering of the lips (Fig 71,B), the snout reflex. Tapping about the forehead may reveal exaggerated muscle responses. The gag reflex remains brisk even though voluntary elevation of the palate may be impossible.

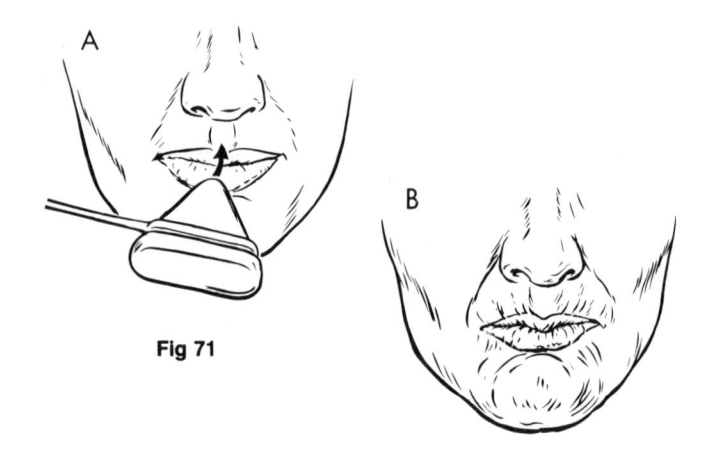

Fig 71

Fig 72

tipped applicator. The musculature will contract on both sides. A unilateral loss of response suggests a sensory lesion of the complex on that side if the palate elevates symmetrically on phonation or contralateral stimulation (p. 32).

Lesions of the tenth cranial nerve (vagus) are manifest largely by hoarseness due to paralysis of a vocal cord. The cough is harsh and loses effectiveness. Laryngoscopic examination is necessary to confirm a suspicion of paralysis. Sometimes acute neuropathy may cause bilateral dysfunction of the vagus nerves and tachycardia results.

Palatal myoclonus is a persistent rhythmic jerking movement of the palate and other nearby musculature. It is associated with lesions (usually an infarction) involving the pathways between the red nucleus, olivary nuclei, and dentate nucleus of the cerebellum.

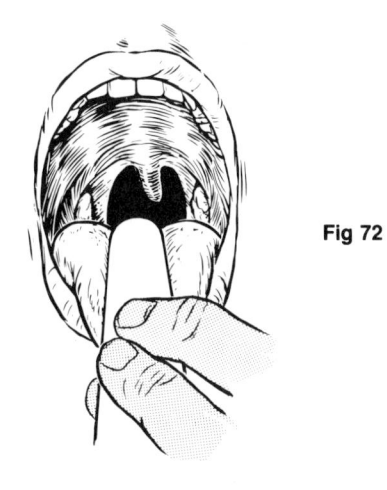

A complex situation exists in amyotrophic lateral sclerosis, in which pseudobulbar palsy may coexist with bulbar palsy resulting from motor neuron loss. Atrophy and fasciculation are seen with the spasticity.

Figure 72 shows paralysis of the right side of the soft palate. The pharyngeal wall is often involved as well. Look closely for a consistent tendency of the soft palate to be pulled to one side (away from the side of paralysis). The musculature involved is innervated by the ninth-tenth cranial nerve complex. Such paresis or paralysis is due to a nuclear or peripheral—not a supranuclear—lesion. Usually some speech change and some difficulty in swallowing are concomitant. The gag reflex can be tested by touching the region of the tonsillar pillars with a cotton-

Fig 73

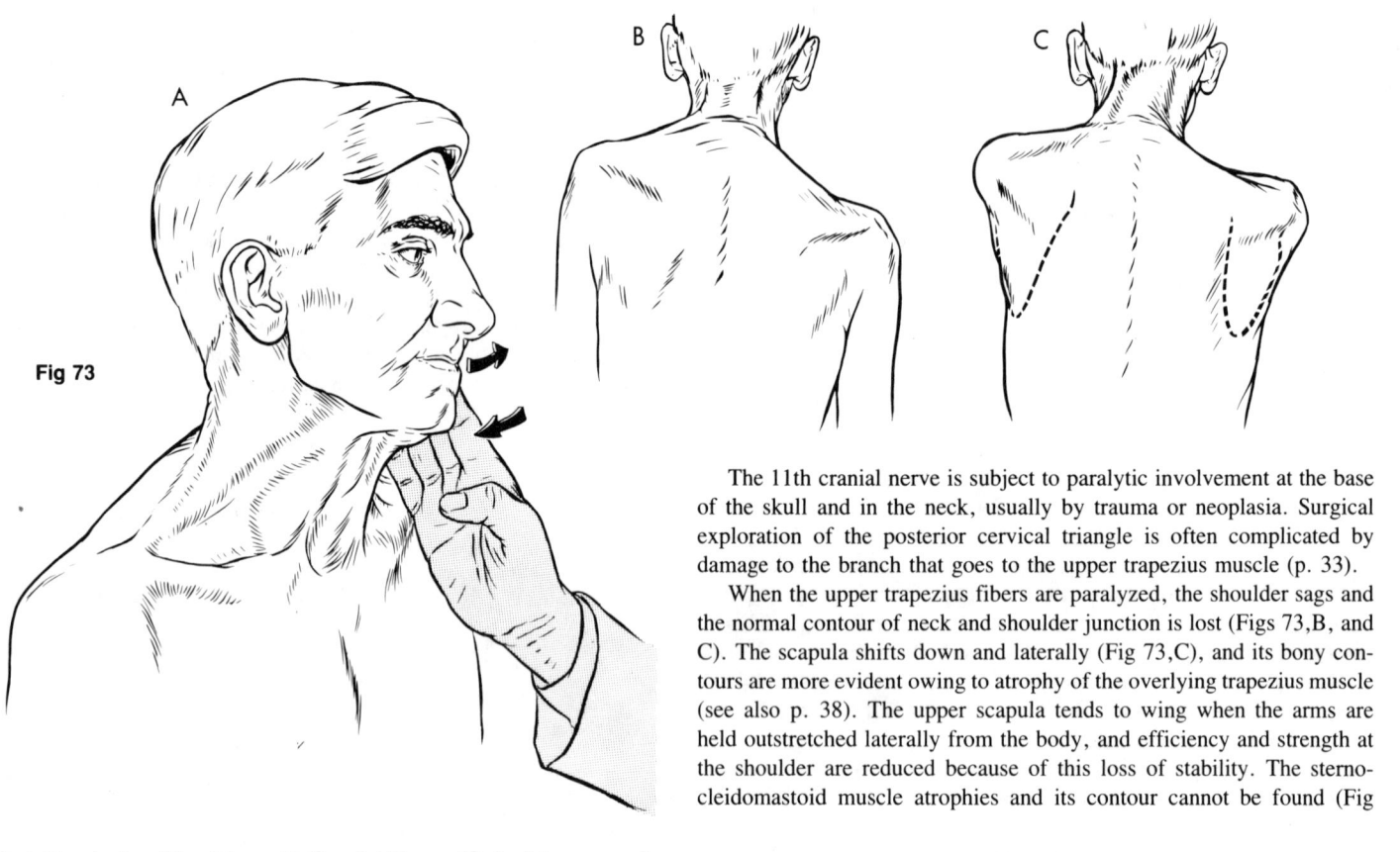

The 11th cranial nerve is subject to paralytic involvement at the base of the skull and in the neck, usually by trauma or neoplasia. Surgical exploration of the posterior cervical triangle is often complicated by damage to the branch that goes to the upper trapezius muscle (p. 33).

When the upper trapezius fibers are paralyzed, the shoulder sags and the normal contour of neck and shoulder junction is lost (Figs 73,B, and C). The scapula shifts down and laterally (Fig 73,C), and its bony contours are more evident owing to atrophy of the overlying trapezius muscle (see also p. 38). The upper scapula tends to wing when the arms are held outstretched laterally from the body, and efficiency and strength at the shoulder are reduced because of this loss of stability. The sternocleidomastoid muscle atrophies and its contour cannot be found (Fig

106 / *Paralysis of the Eleventh Cranial Nerve (Spinal Accessory)*

73,A). Little disability results from this. Atrophy of these and other neck muscles is seen in association with muscular dystrophy and is then usually symmetric. Hemiparesis is often associated with a sagging shoulder and a weakness of musculature, including the sternocleidomastoid muscle, which turns the face toward the side of the paralyzed arm and leg. The sternocleidomastoid muscle, subserving movements to the opposite side, is weakened ipsilateral to the cerebral lesion.

The tongue will *deviate to the side of weakness*, whether the weakness is of supranuclear, nuclear, or infranuclear origin. Inspect the tongue both when it is protruded and when it is lying quietly in the floor of the mouth, where the distinction between normal tremors under tension and abnormal fasciculations present at rest is more easily made.

Atrophy of the tongue is manifest by loss of bulk, corrugations of the edges, and longitudinal furrowing as pictured in Figure 74. Unilateral atrophy of lower motor neuron paralysis is easy to detect (Fig 74,A) and is accompanied by deviation. This condition is usually due to neoplastic or traumatic involvement of the hypoglossal nerve at or below the base of the skull and is seldom due to intramedullary disease.

Bilateral atrophy is shown in Figure 74,B. The tongue protrudes weakly, if at all, and deviation is weak. This condition is most commonly due to motor neuron disease. In both conditions illustrated (Figs 73,A and B) fasciculations are common and are seen as rapidly, irregularly contracting fascicles so that the surface appears in constant motion.

Unilateral supranuclear disease, as in hemiparesis, will produce some dysfunction of the tongue—slowness in motion, clumsiness, or deviation

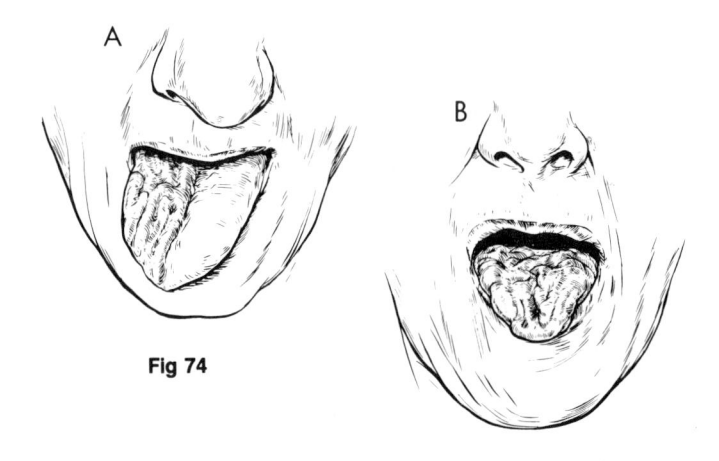

Fig 74

without atrophy—but as with other bulbar functions this is usually compensated in time so that little detectable disability persists. However, bilateral supranuclear disease may seriously limit the extent and rapidity of tongue movement. This is part of the syndrome of pseudobulbar palsy (p. 104) and is associated with difficulties in swallowing and slurred speech (dysarthria). Commonly, the musculature of the pharynx and palate will be similarly involved. In patients with pernicious anemia the mucosa of the tongue is often atrophic and the surface appears smooth and reddened.

"Cerebellar Signs"

This term is often misused to categorize any difficulty in maintaining balance or executing coordinated movement. The cerebellum is an important station for integration of the motor activity of the cortex, basal ganglia, vestibular apparatus, and spinal cord. It has extensive connections via its brachia for both incoming and outgoing signals. Lesions of the sensory end organs and their pathways, which send information to the cerebellum, and lesions of the cerebellum itself or its outflow, especially to the midbrain, may produce "cerebellar signs." For example, ataxia is seen in peripheral neuropathy, in demyelination of the posterior columns, in brain-stem infarcts, and in frontal lobe lesions. Postural disorders result from acute disease or destruction of the vestibular end organ. For these reasons, little use of the term "cerebellar signs" has been made in this book.

Lesions of the midline cerebellum (vermis) cause difficulty in maintaining upright posture, ataxia of gait, and truncal ataxia. Because the same symptoms can result from spinal-cord disease, radiculopathy, and neuropathy, differentiation is necessary, especially by sensory examination (p. xx), since intrinsic lesions of the cerebellum do not produce the type of sensory deficits discernible on ordinary examination. An acute, cerebellar hemispheric lesion produces a tendency to fall to the involved side, with poor application of strength, hypotonia, dysynergia, and reduced AMR of the *ipsilateral* arm and leg. An oscillating tremor may appear on attempted movement; it is accentuated and becomes more coarse as the finger approaches its target (intention tremor). Nystagmus is often present. See the sections on Romberg Test (p. 8), Tandem Walking (p. 9), Hopping (p. 10), Finger-to-Nose Test (p. 36), Heel-to-Knee Test (p. 46), AMR (pp. 44, 46), and Nystagmus (p. 94).

Hemiplegia and Hemiparesis

Hemiplegia or hemiparesis, i.e., paralysis or weakness of one side of the body, is perhaps the most common physical manifestation of disease of the brain, partly because of the vulnerability of the cortex and its radiations to the lesions of vascular disease, either infarction or hemorrhage. Furthermore, contralateral weakness is apt to result from a lesion of a hemisphere even when there is no immediate impingement of the motor cortex and its descending radiations. Hemiparesis that does not involve the face sometimes is seen in association with lower medullary and upper cervical cord lesions.

Acutely acquired hemiplegia is manifested by complete paralysis of arm, leg, and lower portion of the face on one side, with decreased muscular tone. The head and eyes may be deviated to the side of the lesion. The extremities are floppy (flaccid) when moved about by the examiner. The Babinski sign is usually present but the muscle stretch reflexes may be absent, equal to those of the other side, or exaggerated. Later, some proximal movement and strength return, with hyperreflexia. Often the end result is characterized by a severe, spastic hemiparesis (Fig 75). There is residual paresis of the lower face. The upper extremity is useless, shows increased tonus, and is usually held in a flexion posture with the hand flexed, thumb in palm. Some slow, gross movements are possible at the shoulder and elbow, and a little flexion of the fingers may be accomplished. The arm posture is variable, however, depending in part on the involvement of extrapyramidal structures.

Fig 75

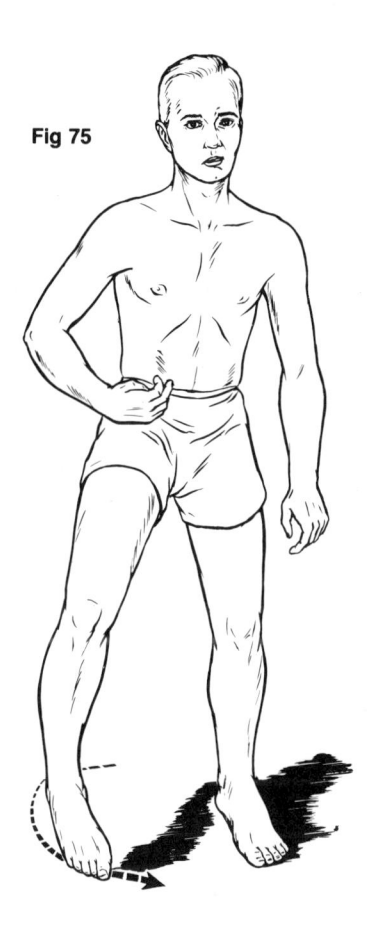

Often the hemiplegic will recover the ability to walk, thanks to strong contraction in antigravity muscles. The paretic leg is moved slowly and in less than the normal range. It is dragged forward, often in circumduction, because the toes of the spastic, dropped foot will not otherwise clear the floor. Flexion at the hip is always weak and the leg cannot be elevated, as in steppage gait due to the footdrop of peripheral origin. There are variations of this pattern. Elderly patients and those who suffer severe hemisensory losses and hemianopsia are more disabled and less apt to learn to walk again.

Early or mild hemiparesis is much less obvious. Discovery of early signs, though sometimes difficult, is of great importance for refined diagnosis. Always be alert for these signs when disease of the brain is suspected. Minor degrees of facial weakness are often best seen in repose and may not be evident on forced expression. Reduced mobility of the lower part of the face is sometimes the first sign of brain dysfunction. Observe especially for slight drooping of the lower lid and of the upper lip, with loss of prominence of the nasolabial fold. Figure 76 depicts the minor nature of the early facial paresis to which one should be sensitive.

The gait may be normal, or the involved leg may be slightly stiff and its normal swing inhibited. While walking, a slightly diminished arm swing on one side is also a sensitive indicator of hemiparesis. Walking on the heels may reveal incomplete dorsiflexion of foot and toes. Hopping will disclose a loss of springiness and coordination; the heel will hit the floor too hard (Fig 77,A). As previously emphasized, hopping is one of the best screening tests to detect early spastic paresis of a leg (p. 10).

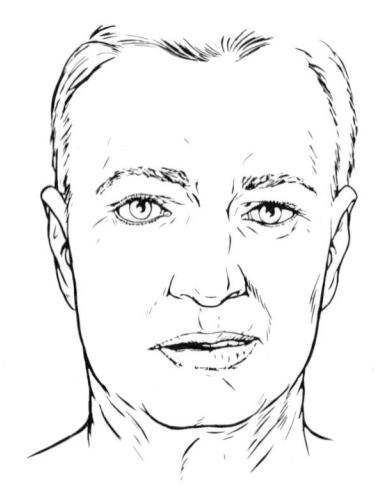

Fig 76

Even before loss of strength is evident, the test of arm posture (p. 36) may reveal a tendency to flexion and droop of the affected arm and hand (Fig 77,B).

Loss of strength is often first evident when the patient holds the arms vertically against resistance (p. 39) or flexes the hip in the sitting position (p. xx), another important screening test. Later, all movements of the arm and leg may be weakened, but extension of the knee and plantar flexion of the foot usually remain strong. The muscle stretch reflexes are usually exaggerated on the hemiparetic side. Alternating motion rate, e.g., rapid finger tapping (Fig 77,C; p. 43), and fine finger movements are reduced early. The Babinski sign (Fig 77,D) lends strong support to a suspicion of dysfunction that may be created by other signs.

The upper and lower extremities may not be affected equally, particularly when the causative lesion primarily involves the cortex. Anterior cerebral artery distribution infarction, for example, predominantly involves the cortical representation area of the contralateral lower extremity and therefore results in a monoplegia with the upper extremity being relatively unaffected. Lesions strategically placed elsewhere in the motor cortex can result in a similar, relatively isolated paralysis of the upper extremity or face. On the other hand, lesions deep in the hemisphere involving the internal capsule are more likely to result in a severe, total hemiplegia, because at this level the outflow of the motor cortex has converged into a more compact bundle.

In most patients with hemiplegia due to vascular or neoplastic causes, a variable degree of sensory dysfunction is also present. The syndrome of pure motor hemiplegia is usually the result of a very small infarction strategically placed in the internal capsule or in the brain-stem pyramidal

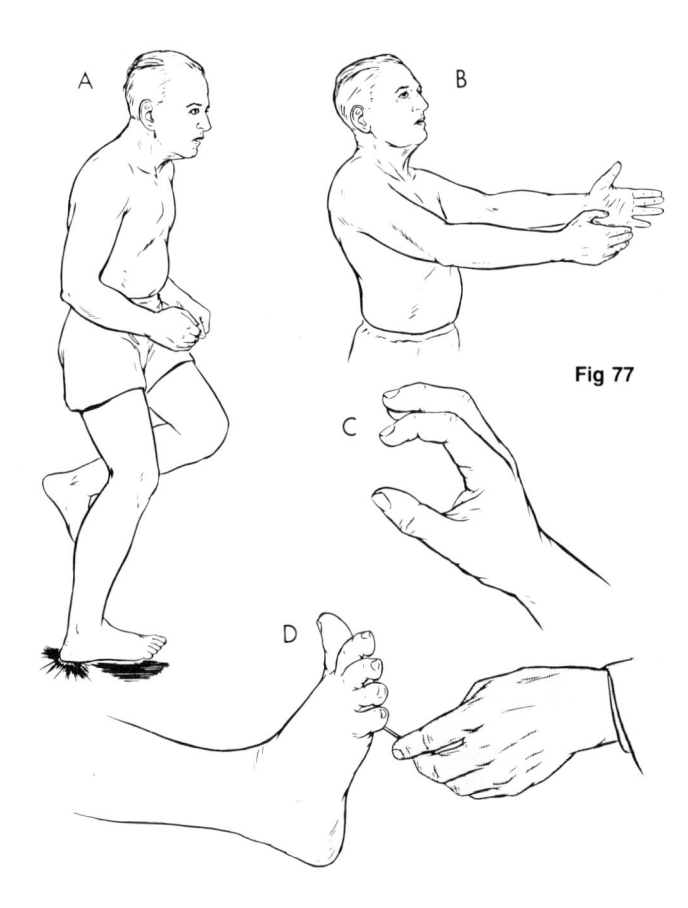

Fig 77

tract. It is typically the result of a lacunar infarction, a lesion usually less than 2 cm in diameter, found in patients with hypertensive disease of the small vessels. A lacunar stroke involving the thalamus can produce the opposite result—a pure hemisensory stroke.

The search for early hemiparesis is to a considerable extent based on the assumption that one side is normal. This is not always true, and bilateral mild hemiparesis may pass unnoticed unless the Babinski sign is present on both sides. Some confusion may arise in distinguishing early hemiparesis from an early unilateral parkinsonian syndrome in which loss of arm swinging and a dragging foot may mimic spastic paresis. The characteristic cogwheel rigidity in parkinsonism and the hyperreflexia and Babinski sign in the spastic state may be helpful in differentiation.

When right-sided weakness is evident, look especially for aphasia (p. 219).

Dyskinesias

Dyskinesia is a general term indicating an involuntary abnormal movement. These movements can be classified into several categories, but the distinction between them is not always entirely clear. With only a few exceptions, dyskinesias tend to worsen with action or with emotional tension and disappear during sleep. Therefore, worsening or improvement under these circumstances should not be taken as evidence that a movement disorder is a hysterical symptom.

Chorea refers to relatively rapid, irregularly recurrent, unpredictable nonrhythmic involuntary movements of the trunk, face, or extremities. This condition is usually caused by an abnormality of the striatum. When chorea predominantly involves proximal muscles, it is often violent and flinging and is then referred to as *ballism*. Ballism is usually caused by abnormalities of the subthalamic nucleus or its connections. It often involves only one side of the body (hemiballism), particularly when caused by an infarction.

Dystonia is a prolonged contraction of agonist and antagonist muscles. When sustained over a long period, a *dystonic posture* results; when more brief and recurrent, *dystonic spasms* are produced. Often, as a patient attempts to oppose dystonia, it is rhythmically interrupted, resulting in a *dystonic tremor*. Examples of dystonia are spasmodic torticollis, a dystonia of the neck, and writer's cramp, a dystonia of the hand and fingers occurring exclusively during the act of writing. Generalized dystonia of the face, trunk, and extremities is seen in conditions such as dystonia musculoram deformans.

Athetosis is related to both dystonia and chorea. It consists of slow, twisting, flowing movements, affecting the distal more than the proximal muscles and resulting in unusual postures. When these movements are very sustained, they resemble dystonia, and when very brief they are similar to chorea, giving rise to the term *choreoathetosis*. Because of this overlap, the term *athetosis* is used increasingly less in favor of chorea or dystonia as the situation demands.

Myoclonus is a term applied to rapid, shocklike jerks of a muscle or part. Myoclonus can occur in diverse conditions, including epilepsy and metabolic encephalopathy, and during normal sleep.

Tremor is an involuntary rhythmic movement of a part. Tremors may appear largely at rest (rest tremors), be manifest on movement (action tremor), or occur on assuming a sustained posture of an extremity (postural tremor). The "pill rolling" tremor of Parkinson's disease is typical of a rest tremor; that occuring with cerebellar disease is an example of action tremor; and essential or familial tremor represents the postural form.

A *tic* is a quick movement that is more complex than myoclonus. Often the movement is repetitive and stereotyped and can be, at least temporarily, voluntarily suppressed. A typical motor tic might consist of eye blinking or touching a specific body part. Tics can also be manifested as vocalizations consisting of stereotyped utterances or throat clearing. In Gilles de la Tourette's syndrome, multiple tics, usually motor and verbal, appear.

Bradykinesia means slowness and poverty of movement, most classically seen in Parkinson's disease. *Hyperkinesia* is a general term referring to any excessive involuntary movement, although the term is also applied to excessive activity of a basically normal pattern as well.

Abnormal dystonic and athetotic movements are seen in children with brain damage of perinatal origin. They are also seen in degenerative diseases of the brain and are usually attributed to disorders of the basal ganglia. Rheumatic fever is occasionally associated with chorea in childhood (Sydenham's chorea), and here the involuntary movements are relatively rapid. Huntington's chorea is characterized by somewhat slower, smoother movements, with contortions of posture, movements of the limbs, and changes of expression. The series of pictures of the head and face in Figure 78,A attempt to show the fleeting changes in posture, the grimacing, and the involuntary tongue movements seen in this disorder. In advanced cases, such movements may continue almost unceasingly

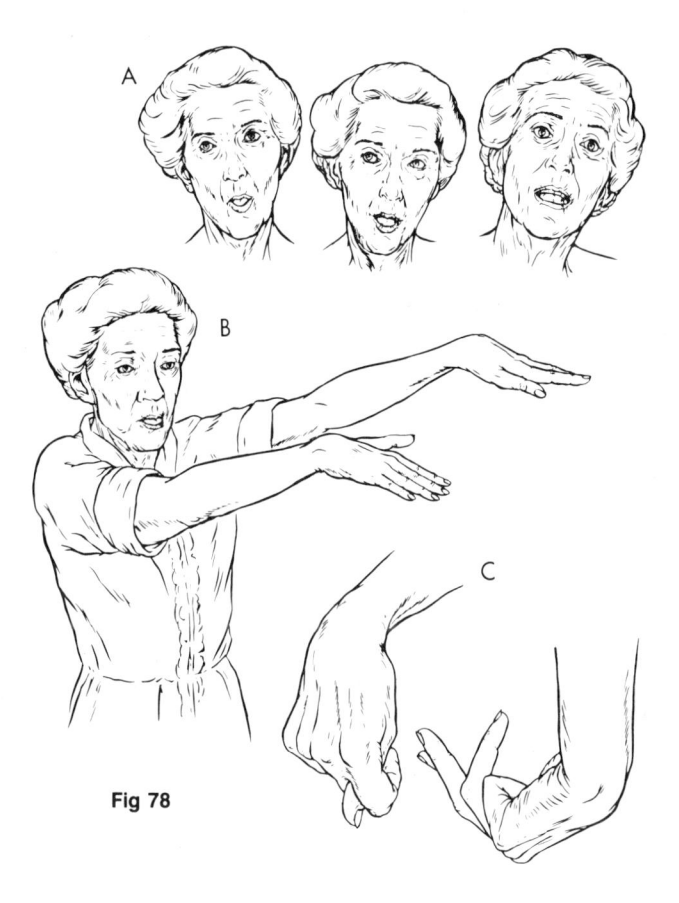

Fig 78

Dyskinesias / **113**

throughout waking hours. Similar movements, especially those involving the face, mouth, and tongue, may appear after chronic phenothiazine, butyrophenone, or metoclopramide administration (tardive dyskinesia) or after treatment with levodopa.

In Figure 78,B the patient cannot maintain normal arm posture. The wrists and hands often assume a peculiar and unnatural forklike configuration. Posture cannot be held and is disturbed by quick drops and deviations, all the while accompanied by grimacing and changes in head and trunk position. Rigidity is variable. Amplitude of movement may be impressive.

Shown in Figure 78,C are two of the many variations in hand posturing common to dystonia. Subtle dystonia of the hands may be aggravated while walking on heels or toes (overflow dystonia). A mild dystonia of the hand, however, can be normal during this maneuver.

One must be attentive to minor shifts in position, such as aborted movement patterns and quick facial grimaces, which may constitute early signs of chorea and related states. When such diseases are advanced, the abnormalities are recognizable at a distance.

Akathisia also can result from administration of a phenothiazine or butyrophenone and is manifested by constant restless movements. The patient generally reports a compelling desire to remain in motion, resulting in constant pacing, shifting of feet, or rocking movements.

Asterixis is seen in patients with metabolic encephalopathy, particularly of hepatic origin. It is characterized by irregular, repetitive loss of tonus, most easily seen in the hyperextended hand, where it results in a flapping tremor.

Parkinson's Disease

Parkinson's disease is a spontaneously occurring condition related to loss of dopamine-producing neurons in the substantia nigra. When a grouping of signs (a syndrome) similar to that occurring in Parkinson's disease is seen in other conditions such as neuroleptic use or after cerebral trauma, the term *parkinsonism* is used. In either true Parkinson's disease or parkinsonism, not all the parts of the syndrome may be found in every patient.

Bradykinesia, a slowness and poverty of movement, is a constant feature and may be so severe that the patient is almost immobilized. Commonly, expressional movements of the face and rate of spontaneous blinking are reduced (masked facies). Speech loses intonation and volume and becomes monotonous. Later, dysarthria may become severe and the patient is understood only with difficulty. Chewing and swallowing may become slow and inefficient. Drooling is common, and aspiration may become a threat.

Slumping of the shoulders and forward stoop (simian posture) are characteristic of parkinsonism. Turning of the head when changing direction of gait and swinging of the arms in walking (associated movements) are reduced or lost. The patient "turns in one piece." Early in the development of the disease asymmetry of involvement is likely, and arm swinging may be reduced on one side only.

A kind of increased tonus called rigidity is present in patients with this disease and can be discovered by first asking the patient to relax an extremity or his neck and then rapidly but gently moving the part. A sense of abnormal resistance punctuated at regular intervals by brief relaxation in tonus gives a ratchety feeling (cogwheel rigidity).

Tremor is common but not universal for the syndrome. The head, hands, arms, legs, and even trunk may be tremorous. Most often the fingers manifest alternating, rhythmic flexion and extension movements with the thumb roughly at right angles to the movement — the pill-rolling tremor. This also may be unilateral early in the disease. Other parts may show tremors of a complex pattern, but these are basically alternating, at a rate of four to six per second. These tremors are present at rest, can be inhibited briefly, and are absent in sleep. It is this tremor, superimposed on the rigidity, that accounts for the cogwheel phenomenon. The tremors of the parkinsonian state often disappear during the course of movement, whereas cerebellar tremors are aggravated during movement.

Shown in Figure 79 is a patient with the expressionless facies typical of parkinsonism. He tends to lean forward in walking, proceeding with a short-stepped, shuffling gait. In some severe cases the forward-leaning posture is so exaggerated that progressively rapid steps are taken in order to "catch up" with the center of gravity (festination). The upper extremities are flexed.

Parkinson's disease appears in middle age. When signs similar to those of Parkinson's disease appear as early as childhood or the teen years, they may represent Wilson's disease instead. In later life, various aspects of parkinsonism may occur secondary to diffuse cerebrovascular disease with multiple small infarctions scattered throughout the brain. Encephalopathic (e.g., due to carbon monoxide poisoning) or drug-induced parkinsonism may be seen at any age.

When severe, the condition is recognizable at a glance. Early signs, however, may easily be missed. Look especially for loss of swinging of an arm, which may be unilateral, slight tremor of a hand, reduced expres-

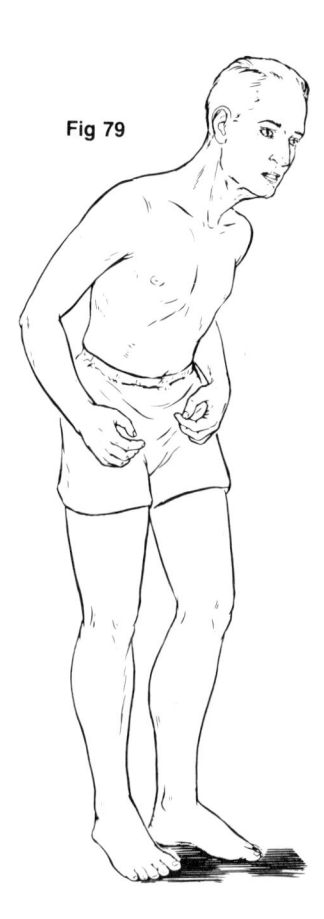

Fig 79

sion, infrequent blinking, slight cogwheeling of the neck, or a "stiff" arm. Change in handwriting with a cramped, tremorous, progressively smaller script is characteristic and usually appears early in the disease.

Sometimes it is difficult to distinguish early hemiparesis from the early and often unilateral manifestations of parkinsonism (p. 112).

Essential tremor is commonly mistaken for parkinsonism. In this condition, also called senile tremor when it occurs in older people, tremor is more prominent during sustained posture than at rest. It is further distinguished from parkinsonism by the lack of associated rigidity or bradykinesia.

Motor Neuron Disease: Amyotrophic Lateral Sclerosis

Motor neuron disease (amyotrophic lateral sclerosis) is a disorder characterized by the signs of progressive motor neuron loss with or without the paresis and spasticity of corticospinal tract degeneration. The disorder may begin in any decade of life but usually is first manifest in early middle age. This is a painless disorder except for muscle cramping. There are no sensory deficits.

Onset is often asymmetric, with wasting of a hand, arm, or shoulder girdle. Fasciculations are common and are often widespread before diffuse atrophy is evident. Weakness is proportionate to atrophy unless the upper motor component is also present, which will cause more severe paresis. The apparent paradox of a hyperactive stretch reflex of a weak, wasted muscle is characteristic of this disorder.

Bulbar involvement may occur early or late and leads to fatal respiratory complications. Bowel and bladder functions become involved late. As the disease progresses, the widespread involvement and lack of sensory signs will establish the diagnosis, but earlier the disease may mimic radiculopathy, neuropathy, or myopathy. Cervical spondylosis with myelopathy or neoplasm of the cervical spinal cord can closely mimic amyotrophic lateral sclerosis because of the concurrent finding of lower motor neuron signs in cervical myotomes and spasticity in all extremities.

Poliomyelitis produces lower motor neuron paralysis acutely. Isolated asymmetric involvement is characteristic, but widespread paralysis also occurs, including bulbar musculature. There are no long-tract signs or sensory losses. Fasciculations may persist for years, and years after the acute paralysis, weakness may begin slowly to progress again.

Fasciculations

Almost any disorder of a motor neuron (cell body or axon) may result in spontaneous, irregular, recurrent contractions of the fascicle of muscle innervated by that neuron. These "fasciculations" are seen as twitching in the muscle not sufficient to move the part. Fasciculations are especially prominent in and characteristic of chronic, progressive motor neuron disease. In this disorder a muscle belly may be constantly agitated by such fascicular contractions, and indeed fasciculations may be found throughout the body. In other neuronal disorders, e.g., peripheral neuropathy, fasciculations are much less evident. Cross-illumination of the muscle surface is best for observation. The muscle must be completely relaxed for valid observation, since fascicular twitching is common in contracting muscles, especially in debilitated patients. It also occurs in otherwise normal people. When infrequent and not accompanied by atrophy, it is not necessarily evidence of progressive disease and should be interpreted with caution.

"Fibrillation" is a term now used only in electromyography. It refers to the low-voltage potentials that result from independent contraction of single, denervated muscle fibers that can be recorded electrically but are not visible on clinical examination (see p. 184).

Spinal Paraplegia

When functional deficits are below a horizontal line at right angles to the spinal neuraxis, suspicion of localized spinal-cord dysfunction is appropriate. However, diffuse cerebral disease, midline cerebellar (vermis) lesions, or a brain tumor affecting both frontal lobes (e.g., falx meningioma) can also produce motor dysfunction or ataxia confined to the lower extremities. Signs of neuropathy or motor neuron disease also can be limited largely to the legs. To complicate evaluation further, multiple focal lesions of the cord such as multiple sclerosis may indicate multiple levels, whereas diffuse tract disease such as posterolateral sclerosis may indicate no clear level.

Single, local, or "transverse" lesions of the cord produce symptoms that are, variously, slow or rapid in onset, partial or complete. Fracture-dislocation of the cervical spine with a crushing injury of the cord is common. A fracture with cord transection at the C-6 level, for example, produces an immediate flaccid paralysis of the trunk and extremities, sparing some shoulder movement and flexion at the elbows. There is complete sensory loss below the C-6 or C-7 dermatome (p. 69). Breathing is diaphragmatic only. The patient is sympathectomized, ileus appears, and the urinary bladder distends. This is "spinal shock." Actually, though blood pressure is often low soon after trauma, perfusion is usually within normal limits. Spinal deformity may be evident. There will be painful limitation of motion and tenderness posteriorly over the fracture.

Later the legs become spastic and are subject to involuntary flexor spasms. Voluntary movement and normal urination are not restored. The sensory level may drop one or two dermatomes. At the level of the lesion, local damage to anterior horn cells and roots results in lower motor neuron signs in one or more segmental areas. This is especially noticeable in forearms and hands. Reflexes in this zone will be reduced or absent, whereas those mediated through intact cord segments further down will be hyperreflexic. Findings are comparable when the lesion is at other levels, but motor neuron components are not easily found when thoracic segments are involved. Beevor's sign may be seen in patients with lower thoracic spinal cord lesions (see p. 57).

Spinal paraplegia of a more slowly developing sort begins with sensory change in the feet and possibly in the perineal region. The legs feel heavy or stiff. Later, weakness of the legs and spastic gait with defective hopping will be seen. Urgency and urinary incontinence appear. The sensory long tracts may be differentially involved, as interpreted from the sensory tests. Levels of deficit slowly rise to the level of the lesion (p. 68). Intramedullary spinal lesions in the thoracic or cervical region may selectively spare sensation in the sacral dermatomes ("sacral sparing").

Segmental symptoms and signs are common, especially when a root or roots are involved, and early radicular symptoms in the upper extremity or intercostal neuralgia may herald an intraspinal lesion that will later give signs of cord embarrassment. Often, local spinal tenderness at the site of the lesion may be found by percussing the spinous processes with a reflex hammer. This is especially true in infectious or neoplastic conditions that also involve the vertebral column. Occasionally, in destructive lesions, local deformity or gibbus will also be present.

Fig 80

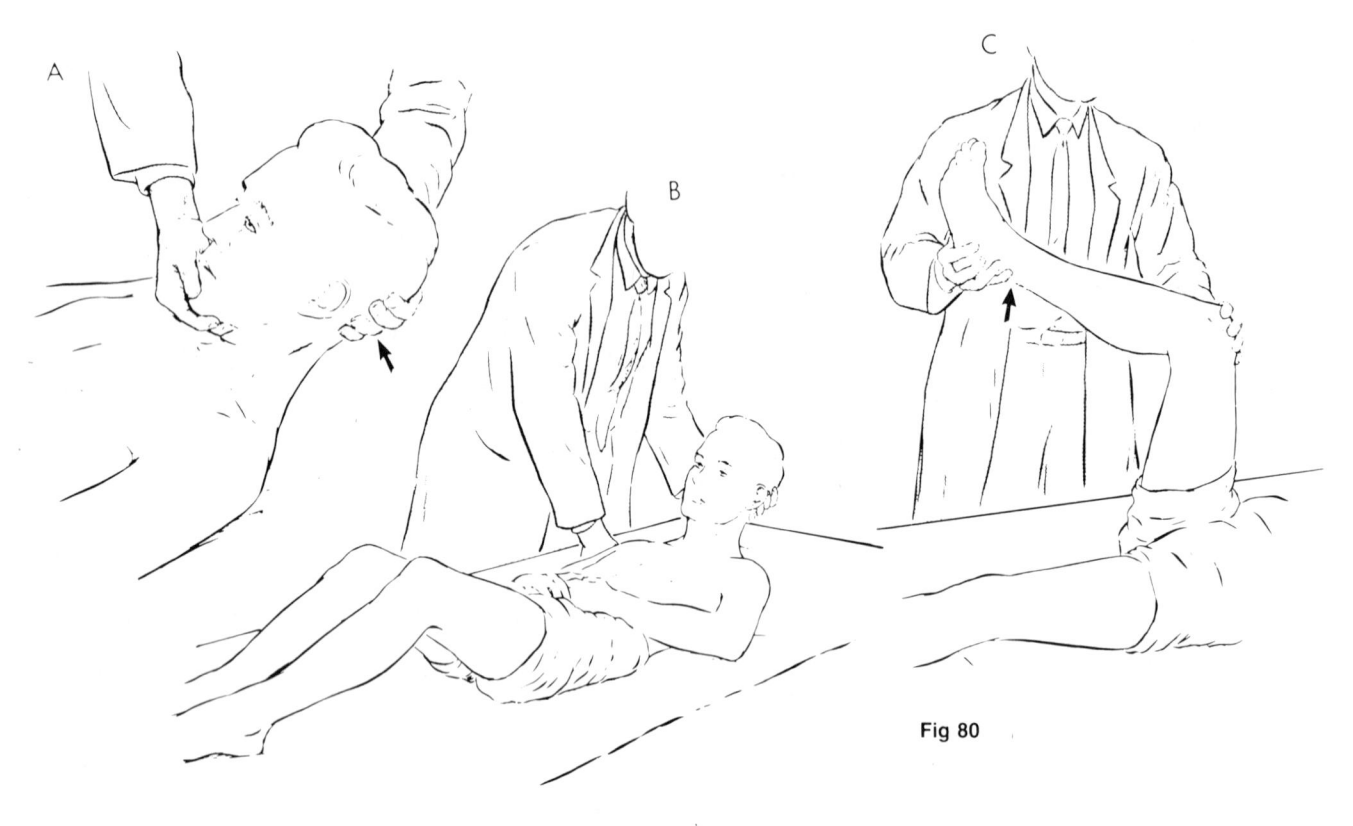

118 / *Signs of Meningeal Irritation*

Signs of Meningeal Irritation

The signs of "meningeal irritation" are probably based on a heightened sensitivity of irritated sensory roots to stretching. Infection in the meninges (meningitis), chemical irritation from injected drugs, subarachnoid hemorrhage, and, infrequently, neoplastic invasion of the meninges and roots are manifested by these signs.

The best sign is the demonstration of stiffness of the neck on flexion. Cradle the head in the hand as shown in Figure 80,A and wait for relaxation of the neck. Then gently flex the neck with chin toward the chest. A boardlike stiffness may be found, and in severe meningitis there may even be a rigid hyperextension of the neck and back. The degree of stiffness is only a rough guide to the severity of meningitis.

Fractures of the neck, paraspinal infection, or acute spinal arthritis may also cause stiffness of the neck. Generally, meningeal irritation does not limit lateral rotation of the neck but degenerative arthritis does; on the other hand, arthritis does not ordinarily cause as much limitation of flexion. The neck may be very stiff in Parkinson's disease, yet continued gentle pressure will result in flexion with little discomfort. The conditions that cause meningeal irritation sufficient to produce a stiff neck are usually accompanied by fever.

The Brudzinski sign (Fig 80,B) is present when flexion of the knees follows an attempt to flex the neck. The Kernig sign is elicited as shown in Figure 80,C. The stretching of lumbar roots consequent to extension of the leg on the thigh produces painful limitation of this movement. Establishing the presence or absence of this sign helps with interpretation of resistance to flexion of the neck when there is a possibility of local disease.

Occasionally, subarachnoid hemorrhage does not produce a stiff neck if it is in an especially early stage or if the patient is moribund.

The signs discussed are not reliable in infants.

Peripheral Neuropathy

One of the simplest and most useful ways to classify peripheral neuropathies is by distribution of involvement. Mononeuropathy refers to dysfunction of a single nerve. Diffuse involvement of peripheral nerves is referred to as polyneuropathy. "Mononeuritis multiplex" means that several nerves are separately involved without general affliction of the entire peripheral nervous system.

Several of the common mononeuropathies have already been described—paralysis of the facial nerve (Bell's palsy), paralysis of the third and the sixth cranial nerves, paralysis of the ninth-tenth cranial nerve complex—and others will be discussed in the section on Paralysis of Peripheral Nerves. The etiology of these apparently spontaneous mononeuropathies is usually vascular occlusive disease, vasculitis, neoplastic infiltration, trauma, or entrapment. Mononeuritis multiplex is often due to infarction of nerve trunks secondary to disseminated vasculitis or diabetic vasculopathy. The onset may be acute and sometimes painful.

Polyneuropathy is one of the most common neurologic disorders and is often overlooked when mild. It may occur as a hereditary condition or as a result of toxic exposure, nutritional deficiencies, autoimmune disease, infection, metabolic disorders, or as a remote effect of cancer. Any combination of motor, sensory, and autonomic dysfunction can be seen among the various polyneuropathies. Because the longest fibers are usually involved first, the initial symptoms often appear in the hands and feet, particularly the feet. For this reason the term "stocking and glove" is often used to describe the sensory loss seen in polyneuropathy. All of the sensory modalities may be involved, as in diabetes, or one may be affected out of proportion to the others, as exemplified by the loss of the pain and temperature sense in hereditary sensory neuropathy. Sensory symptoms may also consist of spontaneous, uncomfortable sensations (paresthesias), usually described by the patient as "pins and needles," or a perversion of sensory stimuli (dysesthesias). In the case of dysesthesias, the patient may find any stimulus, including the touch of clothing or bed sheets, disagreeable. As sensory loss increases, clumsiness of the hands and an uncertain gait appear, particularly when there is involvement of the large myelinated fibers.

In most polyneuropathies, motor involvement is first evident in the form of distal weakness and atrophy corresponding to the early involvement of the distal portions of nerves. An exception is the Guillain-Barré syndrome (acute inflammatory polyradiculopathy), in which the proximal portion of the nerve at the spinal root level is involved early so weakness may be simultaneously evident in proximal and distal muscles.

Since both motor and sensory neurons are usually involved in peripheral neuropathy, diminution or loss of tendon stretch reflexes is an early finding. Again, the distal reflexes, especially the Achilles reflex, are most often affected.

Autonomic denervation will result in orthostatic hypotension, impotence, bladder dysfunction, and loss of sweating. The neuropathies caused by diabetes or amyloidosis have a prominent autonomic component.

Musculature of extremities may be painful when squeezed or slapped, and the skin may be very sensitive to temperature change. The nerve trunks may be tender to pressure. In some neuropathies (leprosy, Charcot-Marie-Tooth disease), nerve trunk enlargement is prominent and can be detected by palpation. Examination of the ulnar nerve at the elbow or of the greater auricular nerve in the posterior neck is useful for this purpose.

Measurement of nerve conduction velocity is the most useful laboratory test to confirm a clinical impression of peripheral neuropathy (see p. 182). Either motor or sensory nerve conduction velocities, or both, may be slowed. Slowing is much more severe in neuropathies involving the myelin sheath, such as the Guillain-Barré syndrome, than in those primarily affecting the axon, as is the case in most toxic neuropathies. When there is a prominent motor component, electromyographic examination of muscle will reveal evidence of denervation.

Root Compression Syndromes

Pain in the segmental distribution of a root is the hallmark of these syndromes. Pain in the spine and restriction of spinal movement are common and are the result of local involvement of sensitive tissues and the root. Herniated disk, metastatic malignancy, a primary neoplasm, recent trauma, or inflammation may be responsible.

Pain radiating down the arm or leg or in intercostal nerve distribution follows the primary anterior division of the nerve and may be localized by the patient anywhere in the distribution of the root. This root pain is characteristically aggravated by spinal movement, by local pressure over the spine, or by straining. Pressure over the muscle in areas of pain usually produces discomfort.

Paresthesias in root distribution are common and are usually experienced distally, in the hand or foot. They may be aggravated or relieved by the same factors that influence the pain, but they tend to be constant.

Weakness and atrophy in the corresponding myotomic distribution result from prolonged or severe root compression, and those stretch reflexes with arcs that are largely or entirely incorporated in the involved root will be diminished or lost.

Suspicion of a single root compression syndrome, then, should be prompted by the combination of a history of pain and the presence of paresthesias in the appropriate distribution of one root only. Findings necessary to confirm the diagnosis are those that relate spinal movement to the radiating pain, that demonstrate muscular weakness and tenderness in the relevant myotome, and that localize sensory and reflex deficits to the dermatome and myotome. The absence of evidence indicating more widespread disease is equally important.

A herniated intervertebral disk generally produces a persistent, unilateral, isolated syndrome. Bilateral and multiple root involvement may be due to extensive degenerative joint disease, but when this is acute or subacute as well as progressive, then metastatic malignancy or inflammation is suggested. Involvement of a single intercostal nerve root (see herpes zoster, p. 68) seldom yields signs. The resulting pain is often mistaken for that of visceral disease.

A root compression syndrome may herald an intraspinal mass that later will impinge on the spinal cord or cauda equina. Always look closely for motor, sensory, and reflex changes below the affected root that may indicate involvement of the cord or cauda equina.

Because herniated intervertebral disk is the most common cause of frank root compression syndromes affecting the extremities, this condition has been selected to illustrate the principles of diagnosis in this book.

Cervical root compression syndromes usually involve one of the three lower cervical roots, C-6, C-7, or C-8. Figure 81,B illustrates the pathologic anatomy of root compression from a common cause, herniated intervertebral disk. Note the possibility for cord compression, particularly if the disk protrusion is more medially placed. Cervical spondylosis is an even more common cause of cervical root impingement. A bulging or partially extruded disk becomes covered with ossified fibrous tissue forming osteophytes or a bony transverse bar capable of compressing nerve roots and/or the cord itself.

Spontaneous pain and tenderness on pressure are typically experienced in the areas marked by the Xs in Figure 81,A. Especially important is localized paraspinal pain and tenderness, which may precede extremital pain and which indicates a focus of disease proximal to the shoulder joint. Often neck movements are restricted because of spinal discomfort. If moderate pressure over the spine enhances pain felt distally in the extremity or if gentle manipulation of the neck reproduces pain felt below the elbow or duplicates paresthesias in the hand, a strong case is made for root impingement from some source.

The next step is to search for evidence of motor and sensory deficit and for reflex loss that, if present, will verify the existence of root or neural compromise and that will help to identify and isolate the site of disease. Check for strength and for muscle atrophy throughout the shoulders, arms, and hands (pp. 38–41). Pain may inhibit maximum exertion. However, range of joint motion, except that of the neck, will not be

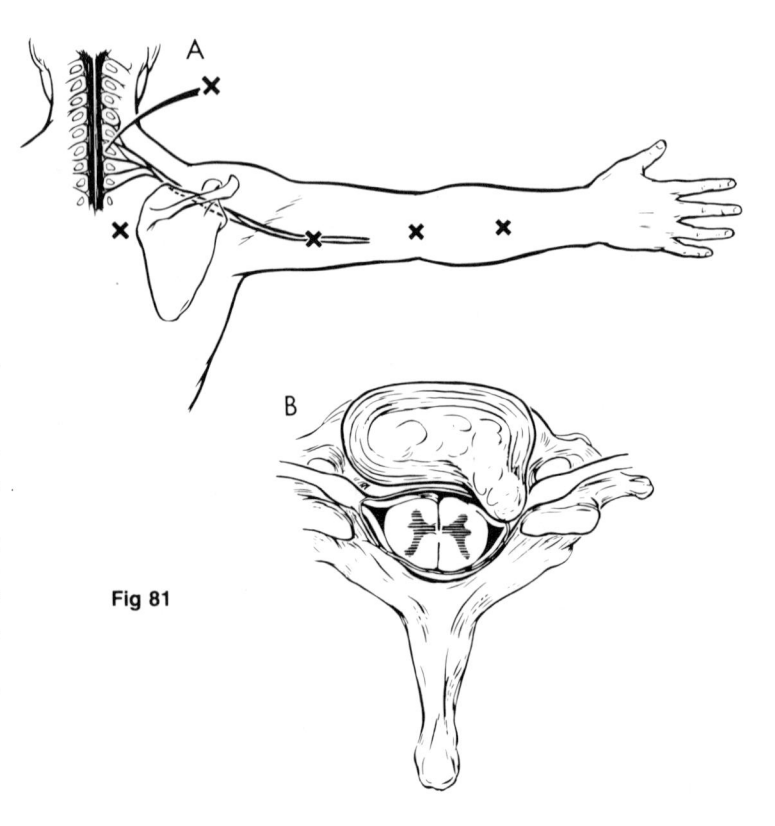

Fig 81

reduced. Watch particularly for painful limitation of shoulder joint movement, which indicates an intrinsic disorder.

Figure 82,A emphasizes the frequent segmental atrophy of the pectoral muscle that results from lower cervical root compression. Figure 82,B shows the test for triceps strength, which is a particularly useful test, since triceps weakness is easily detected and is an early consequence of paresis of lower cervical roots. Strength of dorsiflexion of the wrist (Fig 82,C) should always be checked for the same reasons.

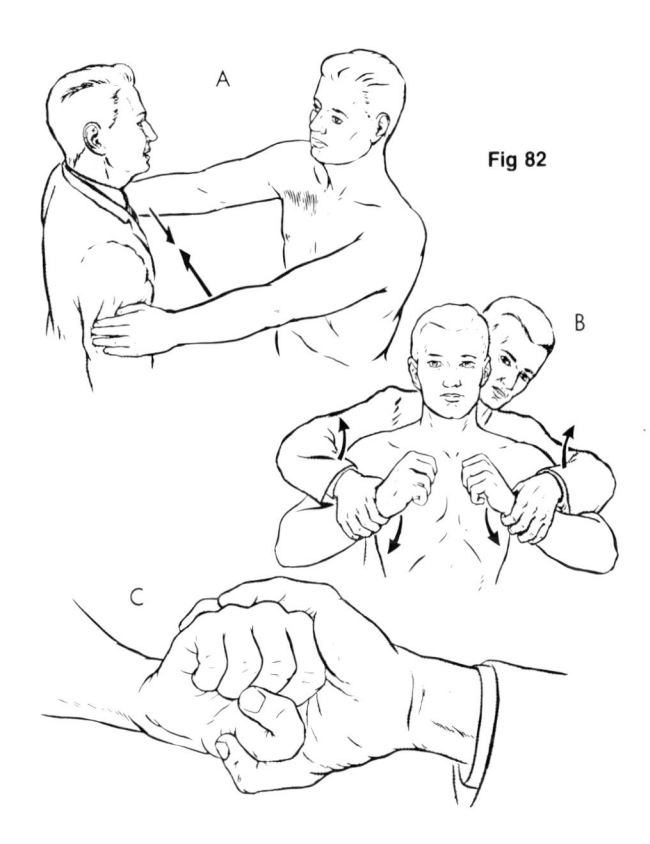

Fig 82

Cervical Root Syndromes / 123

The biceps stretch reflex is mediated chiefly by the C-6 root, so its diminution or loss suggests paresis of that root. The triceps reflex arc employs principally the C-7 root. Thus, some value in localization derives from a differential involvement of these reflexes, and this is relatively common in single-nerve root compression. Figure 83,A depicts the testing procedure previously described (p. 48).

Sensory loss from lower cervical root involvement is most prominent symptomatically and objectively in the digits. The common innervational pattern is shown in Figure 83,B. Variation by one digit is expectable. Test with pin and cotton. Pallesthesia is often diminished or lost in a hypesthetic finger in this condition. The sensory loss is seldom split in one finger, as occurs in ulnar nerve neuropathy (see Fig 90, p. 132). Segmental sensory loss is usually harder to define proximally.

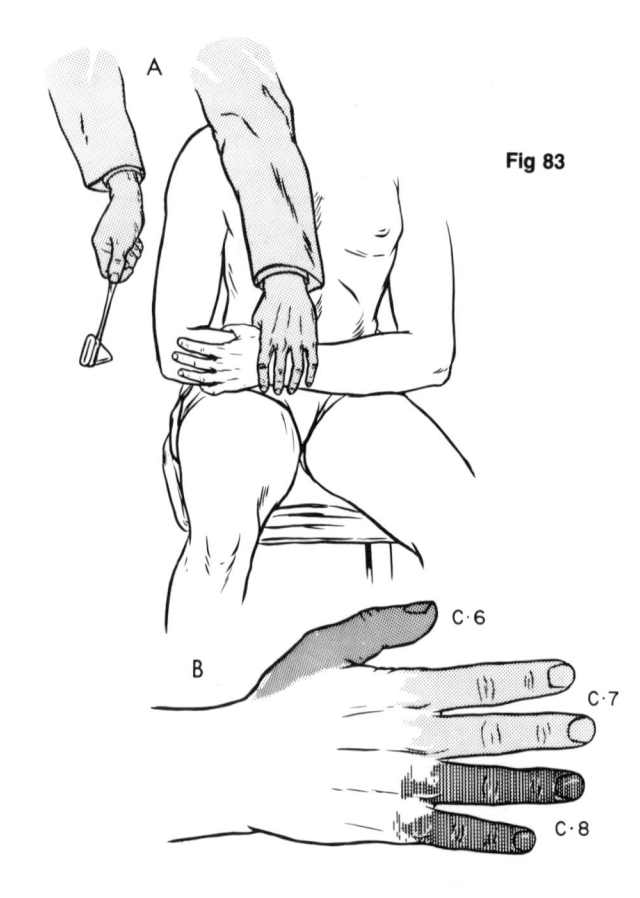

Fig 83

124 / *Cervical Root Syndromes*

Lower lumbar root compression syndromes secondary to degenerating and herniating intervertebral disks produce lower back pain and radiating pain in the buttock, posterior thigh calf, or lateral leg and ankle (sciatica). This is a common affliction, often preceded by months or years of intermittent back pain. A typical posture is shown in Figure 84,A, with deviation and stiffness of the lumbar spine. Common sites of pain and of tenderness on pressure are marked by the Xs. In most cases, the L-4 or L-5 intervertebral disk is involved, causing compression of the L-5 and S-1 nerve roots, respectively (Fig 84,B). The spinal cord does not descend to this level, but a large disk herniation, especially if located centrally, may impinge on other roots of the cauda equina, including those subserving bowel and bladder function.

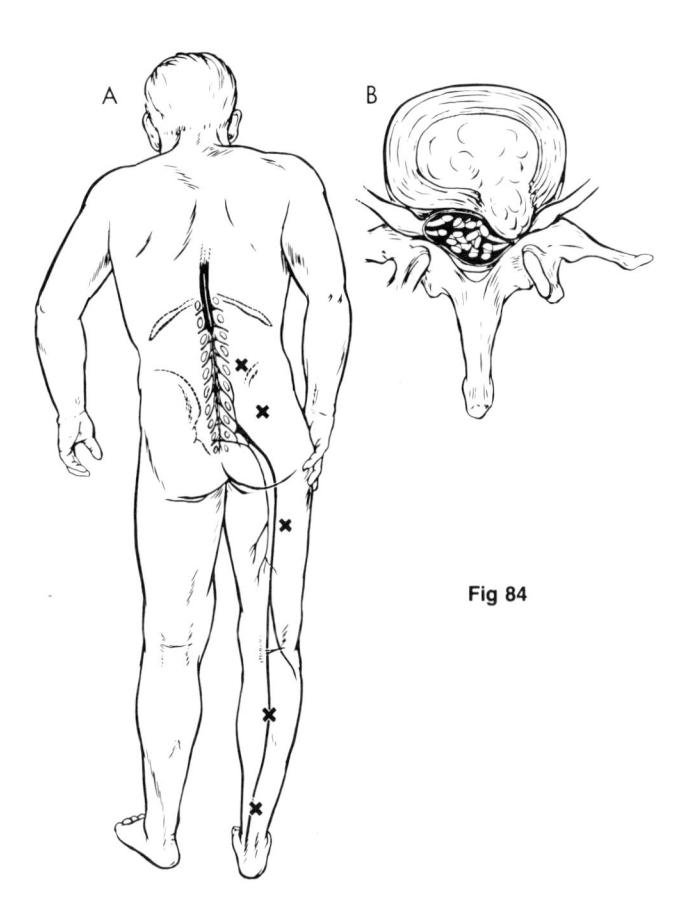

Fig 84

Lumbar Root Syndromes / **125**

In lower lumbar root compression, attempted forward bending is limited by pain and inflexibility of the lumbar spine, and percussion by fist or hammer over the lower lumbar segments, as shown in Figure 85,A, may aggravate pain in the thigh or leg (door-bell sign). The motor deficits ensuing from paresis of these roots are most apparent below the knee. Seldom is weakness of the calf so severe that the patient cannot walk on the toes, but atrophy of the gastrocnemius may be seen, as on the right in Figure 85,B. Heel-walking is especially revealing. Severe footdrop is unlikely, but toe drop is common with some atrophy of the anterior compartment, as seen in the right foot and leg in Figure 85,C. Nevertheless, dorsiflexion of foot and toes should be tested directly as in Figure 86,A (also see p. 44) for minor weakness. The test of straight-leg raising (Fig 86,B) frequently demonstrates marked limitation in range of thigh flexion on the painful side (Lasègue's sign). Squeeze tenderness of the calf is common (Fig 86,C). The ankle jerk reflex (Achilles tendon reflex) is a stretch reflex of the gastrocnemius-soleus. It is commonly diminished or absent in S-1 root impingement but may be normal in L-5 root syndromes. Figure 86,D shows the best method of comparing the two sides when differences in reflex response are important. Typical areas of hypalgesia are shown in Figure 86,E.

Neoplasm or inflammation of the spine or cauda equina may produce a syndrome similar to that produced by compression of the lower lumbar root, as may retroperitoneal tumor and invasive neoplasm in the pelvis. Always do rectal and pelvic examinations when pain is in the distribution of lumbar and sacral roots or the lumbosacral plexus.

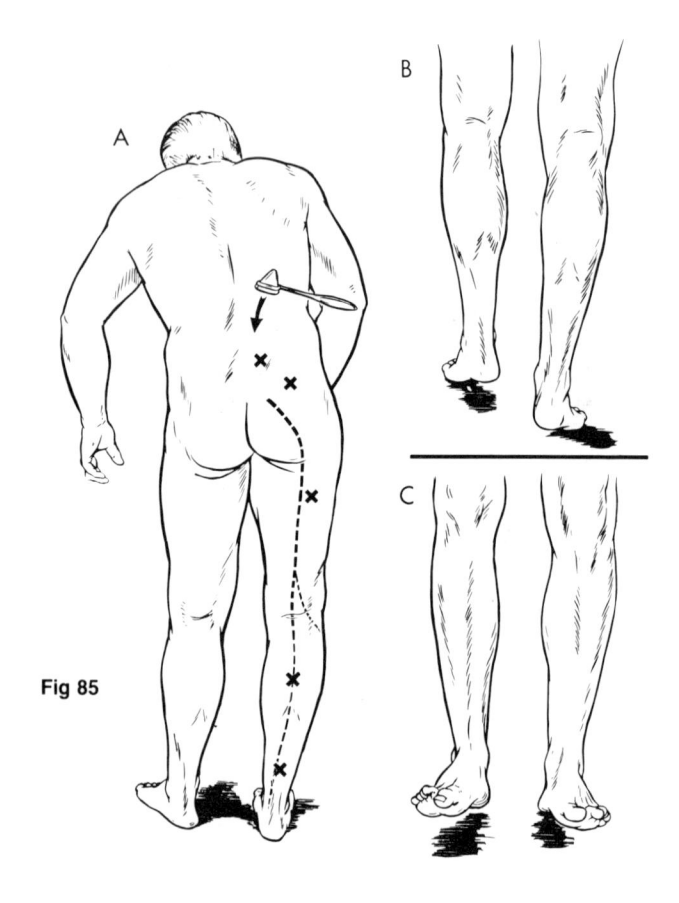

Fig 85

Lumbar Root Syndromes

Fig 86

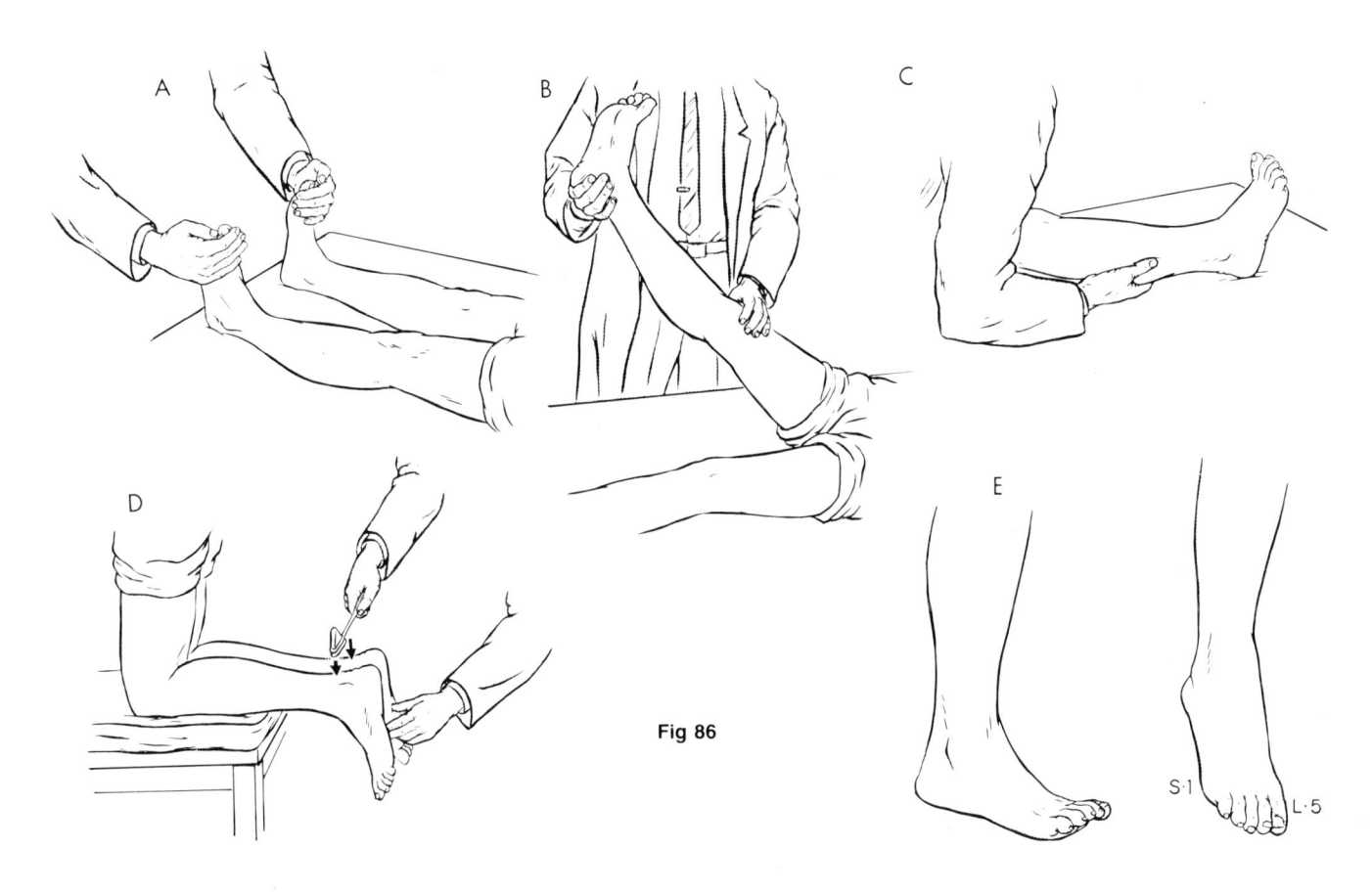

Lumbar Root Syndromes / 127

Paralysis of Peripheral Nerves

Most peripheral nerve lesions are traumatically induced, either acutely by laceration, bruising, or tearing or chronically by repeated minor injury or entrapment at some vulnerable region, often near bone. The functional deficits and tissue changes that result from nerve lesions depend on the site of involvement and the extent and duration of nerve interruption. Injuries of other tissues, bone, muscle, and blood vessels may make neurologic evaluation difficult. Complexity is added if the injury involves more than one nerve or a nerve plexus. Later, imperfect regeneration, secondary contractures, tissue ischemia, and atrophy may complicate evaluation of the degree and nature of peripheral nerve deficits. An additional problem results from anatomic variations in motor and sensory distribution of nerves.

Atrophy of muscle follows soon after interruption of its nerve supply and is usually easily detected when denervation is sufficient to cause weakness. Fasciculations are not common, although they may be seen in any lower motor neuron lesion. Rather minor peripheral nerve lesions reduce or eliminate stretch reflexes since the nerve (e.g., the femoral) may carry both arms of the reflex arc.

Percussion over the course of a nerve is helpful in localizing the site of injury or in following the distal growth of regenerating axons. It may elicit Tinel's sign—tingling paresthesias reported by the patient in the area of normal distal innervation of the nerve being tested, a phenomenon created by heightened sensitivity to mechanical stimuli in portions of the nerve trunk that are undergoing degeneration and/or regeneration.

Since sympathetic fibers course with the peripheral nerves, loss of sweating is a common feature of peripheral nerve paralysis. Dryness and trophic changes in the skin and nails are among the consequences of a complete nerve lesion.

No less important than looking for motor and sensory findings compatible with interruption of a particular peripheral nerve is determining the absence of nearby or general findings that would indicate a more widespread or generalized disorder.

In this section the findings in several common, uncomplicated, peripheral nerve paralyses are described.

The right and left respiratory (*phrenic*) nerves arise from cervical segments C-3, C-4, and C-5 and each innervates its respective hemidiaphragm. Unilateral paralysis may produce no symptoms unless respiration is already compromised from other causes. Bilateral paralysis interferes seriously with depth of respiration, coughing, sneezing, straining, and lifting. Paralysis may result from neuritis, poliomyelitis, trauma, or upper cervical myelopathy. Paralysis may be suspected if the liver fails to descend on deep breathing or if resonance fails to diminish on chest percussion. Fluoroscopy gives the best evidence of diaphragmatic paralysis.

The nerve to the serratus anterior is the *long thoracic nerve* that carries fibers from the C-5, C-6, and C-7 roots, coursing downward on the medial wall of the axilla. Paralysis can be caused by direct trauma but more frequently is a part of brachial neuritis. The nerve may be stretched as a result of a heavy weight on the shoulder, with downward displacement of the brachial plexus. Paralysis of the serratus anterior muscle results in "winging" of the scapula, especially of its lower angle, which is displaced medialward and outward from the chest wall on elevation of the arm or forward thrusting as in Figure 87. The resulting instability weakens the shoulder for these movements. Have the patient extend the straightened arms in front of the body; then press downward on his arm while observing the scapula (p. 39). If the deltoid is also weak, place the patient's palms on a wall and have him push against it to demonstrate weakness of the muscle. See page 106 for scapular displacement caused by trapezius paralysis.

Fig 87

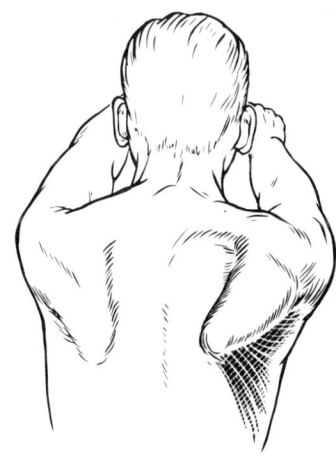

The *axillary* nerve arises from the C-5 and C-6 roots. It partially encircles the upper humerus (Fig 88), where it is prone to trauma from pressure, fracture of the humerus, or shoulder dislocation. It innervates the teres minor and deltoid muscles. Paralysis of the deltoid results in severe reduction of the ability to abduct the arm laterally. The normal, rounded contour of the lateral shoulder is lost as the muscle becomes atrophic. A patch of skin over the upper lateral arm in the region of the insertion of the muscle loses sensation. Sensory examination is valuable when bony or soft tissue trauma prevents study of movement.

The deltoid muscle atrophies quickly in any condition that limits shoulder movement. As the shoulder joint readily becomes fixed and painful from immobility of any cause, it may be difficult to determine whether the muscle atrophy is due to denervation or disuse. Resort to sensory examination and electromyography in difficult cases.

The musculocutaneous nerve innervates the biceps, the coracobrachialis, and the brachialis muscles, which are the principal flexors and supinators of the forearm. It is composed of fibers from the C-5, C-6, and C-7 roots. To test its function, have the patient bend the elbow against resistance while you palpate and inspect the biceps. The biceps stretch reflex is lost in paralysis of this nerve. A sensory component innervates the skin of the anterolateral forearm.

Extension at the elbow is mediated entirely by the *radial* nerve and the triceps muscle. Flexion and supination at the elbow are in part mediated by this nerve through innervation of the brachioradialis muscle. Dorsiflexion of the wrist and fingers, extension of the thumb, and abduction of the thumb in the plane of the palm depend on its innervation of the musculature of the dorsal forearm. This nerve receives fibers from

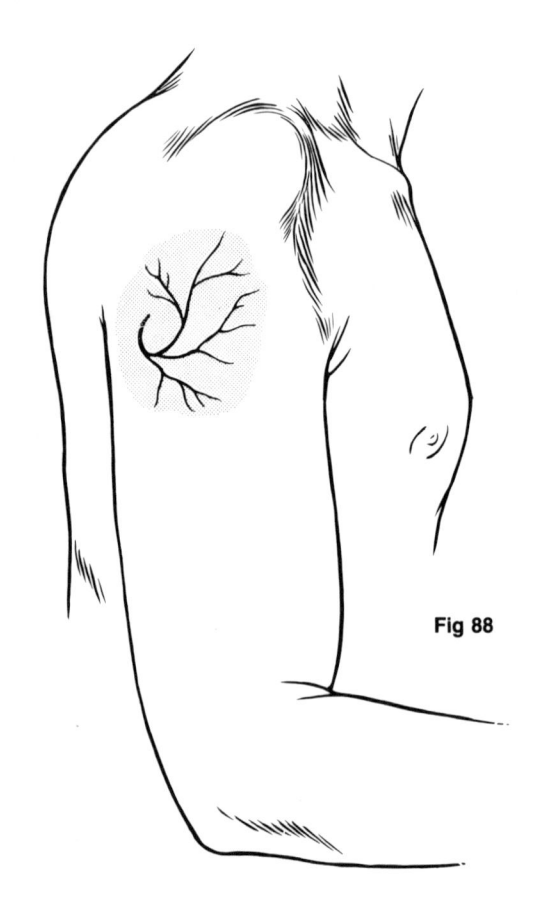

Fig 88

the C-5, C-6, C-7, and C-8 roots, so some loss of function may result from a lesion of any of these roots.

The radial nerve is especially vulnerable where it winds about the humerus. Here it may be injured in fractures of the humerus, in dislocation of the shoulder, by tourniquets and casts, by injections, or by direct trauma. It is classically paralyzed by ischemia from pressure produced when the head is supported on the arm during coma or during a prolonged state of intoxication. The weight of a spouse's head on the arm overnight may have the same result ("honeymoon palsy"). The axilla is another common compression site; in this instance the use of crutches or having fallen asleep with one arm draped over a straight-backed chair ("Saturday night palsy") are the activities responsible. Lead poisoning is another cause of radial nerve palsy.

Functional loss depends on the site of interruption. In a typical injury, extension of the elbow may be strong since most of the triceps innervation is mediated by fibers that enter its upper third. Wrist drop, as shown in Figure 89, is the classic sign of radial nerve paralysis. When loss of function is complete, the wrist cannot be lifted into dorsiflexion, nor can the fingers and thumb. The grip is ineffectual because the wrist cannot be dorsiflexed and stabilized. A penetrating injury of the dorsal forearm may spare branches that mediate dorsiflexion of the wrist but sever the posterior interosseous branch that mediates extension of the thumb and fingers at the metacarpophalangeal joints. Thus a "finger drop" results.

Extension of the distal phalanges, which appears to be absent in wrist drop, will be found to be possible if ulnar and median nerves are intact. Support the wrist by placing the hand palm down on a table top with distal phalanges over the edge so that the metacarpophalangeal joints are stabilized. Then the patient will be able to extend the distal phalanges if

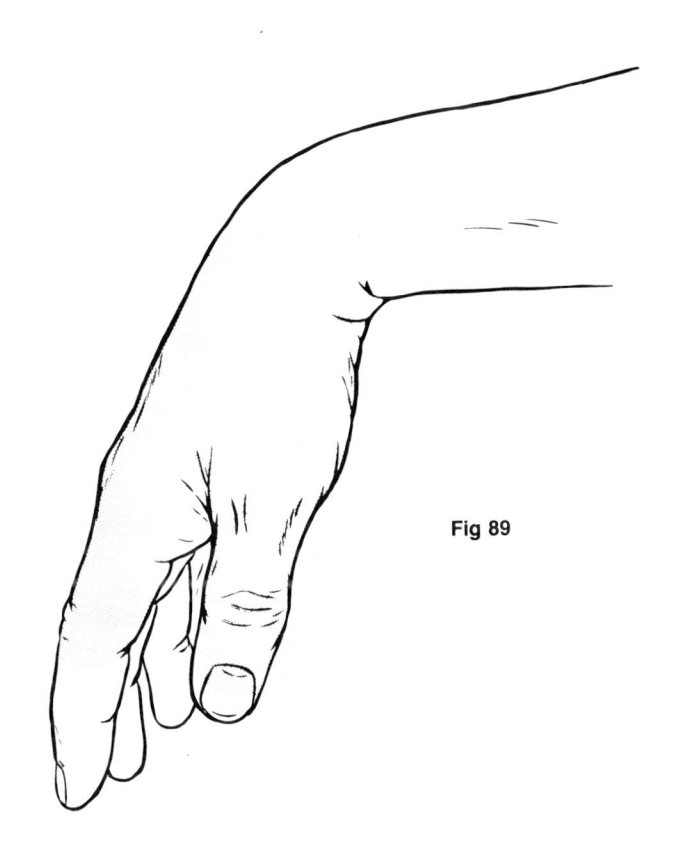

Fig 89

the lumbricales are innervated. This test is occasionally very useful. Abduction and adduction of fingers may falsely seem to be weakened in radial nerve paralysis because these movements are mechanically difficult when the hand is in the wrist drop position. Hold the hand flattened on a tabletop to test these functions.

Sensory loss is variable and may not be as extensive as shown in the figure because of overlap of innervation from adjacent nerves. Test especially in the web area between the thumb and the metacarpal of the second digit.

The *ulnar* nerve carries fibers from the C-8 and T-1 roots. It can be palpated at the elbow where it passes over the medial epicondyle. Functional loss in interruption of this nerve depends on the site of the lesion. Motor fibers first branch off to forearm musculature just above the elbow and then leave the trunk at intervals until the nerve enters the hand to supply the majority of the intrinsic hand muscles. The nerve innervates the flexor carpi ulnaris and the flexor digitorum profundus muscles to the fourth and fifth digits in the forearm. In the hand it innervates the hypothenar musculature, all of the interossei, the two medial lumbricales, the adductor pollicis, and part of the flexor pollicis brevis via its deep palmar branch.

The deformity shown in Figure 90, A and B is typical for paralysis of the ulnar nerve at the elbow. The posture of the fourth and fifth fingers reflects the loss of lumbricales and interosseous muscle function. The grip will be fairly strong, but finger abduction and adduction will be nearly lost. Froment's test is performed by having the patient attempt to hold a piece of paper firmly between the adducted thumb and the radial margin of the forefinger. Because of weakness of the ulnar innervated

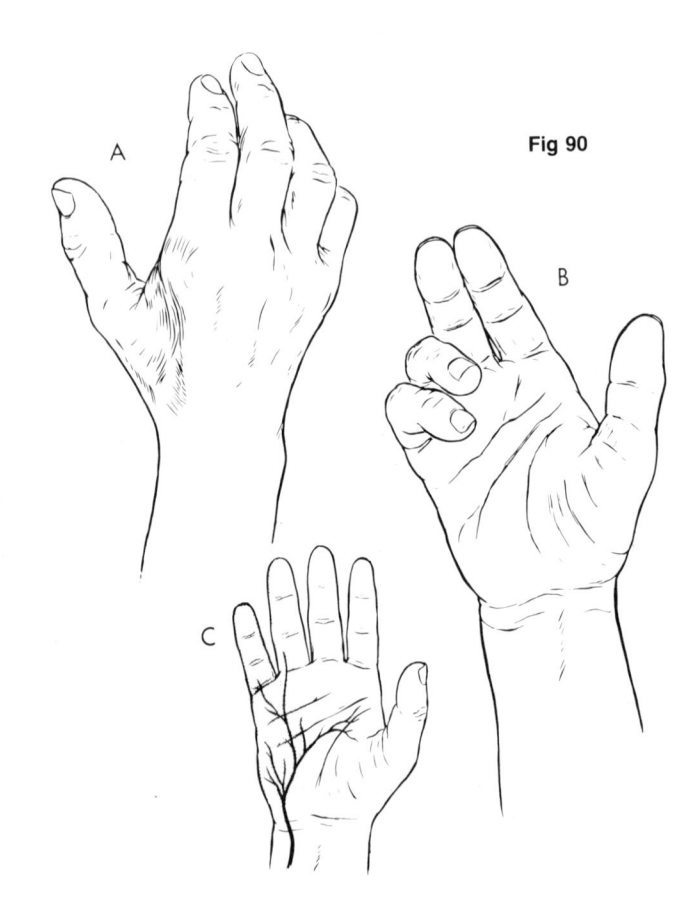

Fig 90

thumb adductor, the patient will compensate by pressing the flexed terminal phalanx of the thumb against the forefinger instead.

Atrophy of the hypothenar eminence and of the interossei, especially the first dorsal interosseus (Fig 90,A), is plainly evident on the dorsum of the hand in patients with ulnar nerve paralysis. Opposition of fifth finger to thumb is lost, and adduction of thumb to second digit is weakened. In cases of early stage or minimal lesions of the ulnar nerve, look closely for atrophy of the first dorsal interosseus and for sensory loss distally in the fifth digit.

The sensory distribution is limited to the ulnar aspect of the hand and with regularity is confined to the ulnar half of the fourth digit. It does not extend above the wrist. When sensory loss is complete, the skin areas shown in Figure 90,C become dry and scaly. The skin and subcutaneous tissue become thin and atrophic and nail changes are seen. Slowly progressive paralysis of the nerve occasionally is seen long after fractures of the elbow or chronic trauma in this region (tardy ulnar palsy). A common cause of paralysis is pressure exerted on the nerve at the elbow in chronically bedridden patients. Habitual or occupational leaning on the elbows has the same result.

If atrophy and weakness of the hand are associated with sensory loss in the forearm or beyond the limits shown here in the hand, look critically for some involvement other than that of the ulnar nerve.

The *median* nerve, carrying fibers from the C-6, C-7, C-8, and T-1 roots, supplies most of the musculature of the anterior forearm and the intrinsic hand muscles not supplied by the ulnar nerve, i.e., the thenar musculature and the lateral two lumbricales.

Interruption of this nerve at the elbow produces weakness of wrist flexion with ulnar deviation, weakness of pronation of forearm, weakness of grip, loss of opposition of the thumb, weakness of thumb abduction perpendicular to the palm, and loss of flexion of the second digit. There is conspicuous atrophy of the thenar eminence with flattening of the palm. Sensory loss involves the palmar surface of the hand and fingers, sparing the ulnar distribution. When complete, the sensory loss is a serious disability. Partial injuries are often painful and paresthetic. Causalgia—pain and sensitivity in the sensory distribution with sympathetic overactivity—may occur.

Most median nerve lesions are traumatic in origin. Tourniquets, casts, and pressure unrelieved during anesthesia or coma may result in paralysis.

Lacerations of the forearm and wrist may damage both median and ulnar nerves. Since the motor functions of the two nerves may overlap considerably, especially in the hand, there is difficulty in evaluating the extent of partial injury of one nerve when the other has been injured. The matter is further complicated by "trick" movements that substitute for lost function.

The carpal tunnel syndrome refers to dysfunction of the median nerve caused by an impingement in its passage under the transverse carpal ligament. Symptoms are paresthesias and pain in the lateral aspect of the hand and the first three digits, with later weakness of the thumb. The syndrome is one of the common nerve entrapments and is seen in conditions such as arthritis or myxedema where there is swelling of the tissues of the wrist, as well as in patients engaging in repetitive flexion and extension of the wrist, such as carpenters. In Figure 91,A the anatomicopathologic features of the syndrome are depicted. Typical selective atrophy of the thenar eminence is shown in Figure 91,B and C; the distribution of sensory loss is also shown in Figure 91,B. Weakness in opposition and in abduction of the thumb above the palm is common.

Forced, sustained extension or flexion of the wrists may produce paresthesias in the sensory distribution shown in the figure (Phalen's sign). Percussion over the carpal ligament may cause similar symptoms (Tinel's sign; see p. 128). Motor and sensory nerve conduction studies are particularly useful in confirming the diagnosis.

Sensory function only is mediated by the lateral femoral cutaneous nerve. It is important to remember that this nerve is not a branch of the femoral nerve and it follows a different peripheral course. Classic entrapment of this nerve where it passes under the inguinal ligament medial

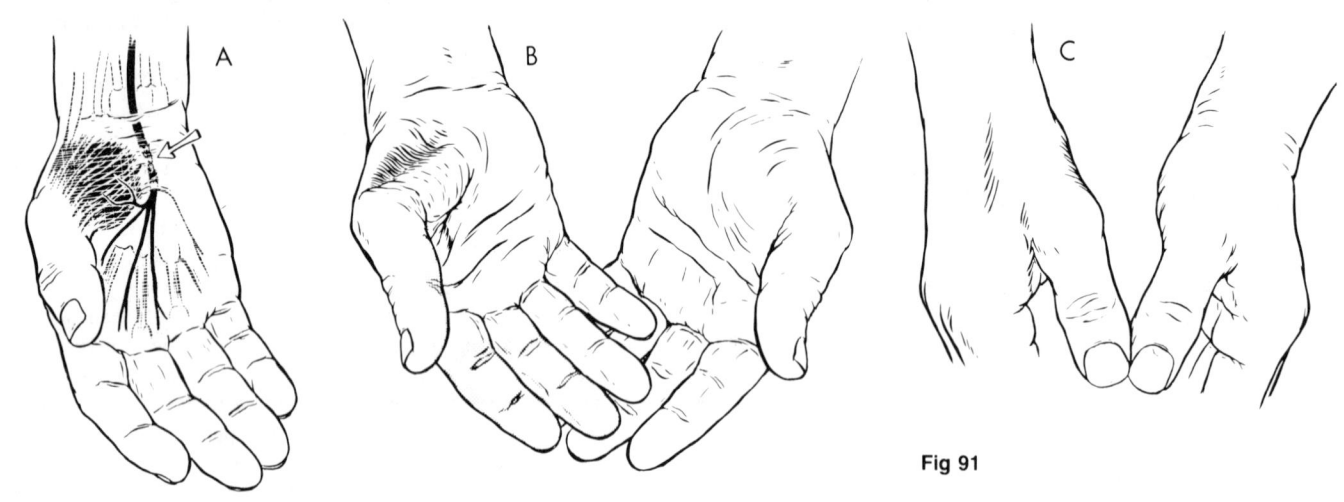

Fig 91

to the anterior superior iliac spine results in a syndrome of dysesthesia and pain along the lateral thigh called *meralgia paresthetica*. Symptoms occur in the area shown in Figure 92. Some sensory loss to pain and touch is typical, often in an area smaller than that shown in the figure. Or the skin may become sensitive to touch and pinching. There is no atrophy and no motor or reflex change. This entity is distinguished by its common occurrence, curability, and tendency to be easily mistaken for symptoms of L-2 and L-3 root compression. It can be initiated by obesity or local trauma from a belt or truss. Like other entrapment syndromes, it seems more apt to occur with metabolic disorders, which may make the peripheral nerves vulnerable to pressure.

The *femoral* nerve arises from the L-1, L-2, L-3, and L-4 spinal roots and innervates the iliopsoas, sartorius, and quadriceps femoris muscles. Proximal lesions result in weakness of thigh flexion or, more prominently, loss of extension at the knee. The nerve can be injured by pelvic fractures, at surgery, and by direct, penetrating wounds. It can be paralyzed by pressure during childbirth, by arterial aneurysms, retroperitoneal hemorrhage, and pelvic neoplasms or abscesses. Probably the most common syndrome involving this nerve is a painful mononeuritis that occurs in diabetes. The quadriceps muscle atrophies quickly, and the knee jerk is lost early. Weakness on stepping up and the inability to rise from a one-legged squat are reliable motor signs of quadriceps paralysis (p. 11), or quadriceps strength may be tested directly (p. 44). Sensory distribution includes the anteromedial thigh and the anteromedial leg to the foot. It is wise to seek signs of more widespread deficits before concluding that this nerve alone is paralyzed, since similar findings may result from a lesion higher in the lumbar plexus.

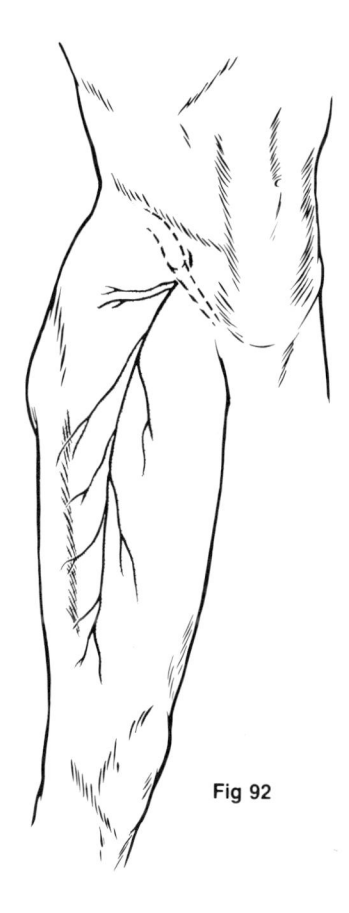

Fig 92

The *sciatic* nerve has two principal divisions, the posterior tibial and the common peroneal. Through the proximal two thirds of the thigh these are usually united into a single trunk. The nerve carries fibers from the L-4, L-5, S-1, and S-2 roots and innervates the hamstring muscles, the adductor magnus, and all the musculature below the knee. Hence, interruption of the nerve will weaken the extension and adduction of the thigh and paralyze flexion of the knee and all movement below the knee. The ankle jerk is lost, and sensory loss involves the lateral aspect of the leg and the lateral dorsum and sole of the foot.

Lesions of the posterior tibial nerve or the posterior tibial portion of the sciatic trunk result in paralysis of the hamstrings (if very high in the thigh) and paralysis of the gastrocnemius and soleus muscles, the long flexors of the toes, and the intrinsic foot muscles. Sensory loss involves much of the sole of the foot, and trophic changes may be prominent. Causalgia may appear.

Sciatic nerve lesions are usually due to fractures of the pelvis, dislocation of the hip, or pelvic neoplasms. One of the all too common causes is medicinal injection, which produces a severe, painful, and compensable neuropathy. Always direct intramuscular injection to the upper outer quadrant of the buttock. "Sciatica" is a term meaning pain in the distribution of this nerve (p. 125).

The *common peroneal* nerve innervates the musculature of the anterior and lateral compartments of the leg via its deep and superficial branches. It receives fibers from the L-4, L-5, S-1, and S-2 roots.

Paralysis of this nerve is common and is often due to trauma in the region of the fibular neck where the nerve is subcutaneous and lies close to bone. It can be easily palpated here. The usual causes of compression include leg crossing, impingement from a cast, or chronic pressure in the immobilized bedridden patient. Interruption of the nerve results in loss of dorsiflexion of ankle and toes (foot drop) and in loss of eversion of the foot. The ankle becomes unstable. There is varying sensory loss along the lateral aspect of the leg and the dorsum of the foot. Atrophy of the tibialis anterior, the extensors of the toes, and the peroneus muscles soon becomes evident, with "sharpening" of the shin from lateral exposure of the tibia.

In walking, the patient lifts the knee to clear the toes from the floor, as depicted in Figure 93. The foot slaps down on the next step. The patient is able to walk on his toes, and the Achilles reflex is preserved. The deep and superficial branches of the nerve may be separately involved, creating partial paralyses. Sensory loss is evident and is most constant over the great toe. Trophic changes in skin and nails are common. When the leg is in a cast, test for dorsiflexion of the great toe and sensory loss on its dorsum.

If there is foot drop with hypotonia and atrophy of muscle but no sensory loss, search for some cause other than peroneal paralysis, e.g., motor neuron disease or myopathy (see also pp. 116, 137–143). Look for weakness in the gastrocnemius and in the hamstrings, which will signify more extensive involvement of the sciatic nerve, plexus, or cauda equina. There is a tendency toward shortening of the gastrocnemius with time, so that eventually the foot cannot be forced into dorsiflexion.

Fig 93

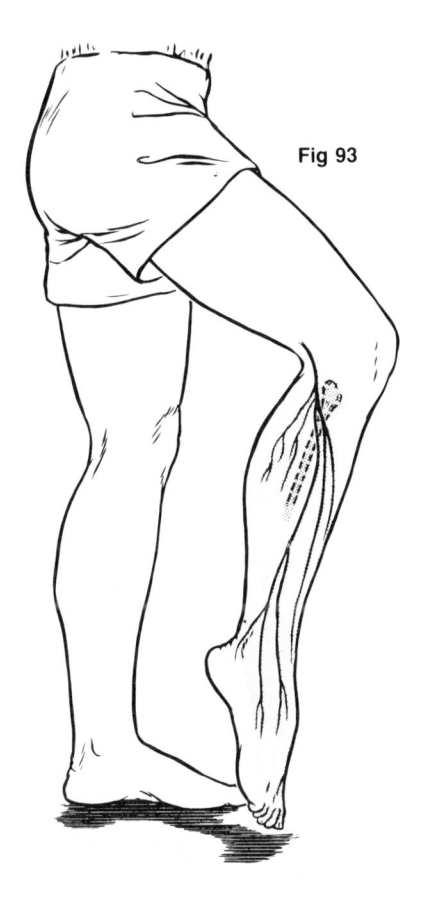

Disorders of Muscle

Primary muscular disease is characterized by progressive loss of strength and muscle tissue without sensory deficit or autonomic dysfunction. There are no reflex changes until the loss of muscle tissue is substantial, when the reflex response will be diminished or lost. Fasciculations are seldom present. Often the musculature of the trunk and girdles is involved early and most severely. However, other patterns of weakness are seen from which some myopathies take their name (e.g., facioscapulohumeral dystrophy, oculopharyngeal dystrophy). Anal and urinary sphincters are spared. The disorders are usually painless unless there is a prominent inflammatory component.

In many varieties of myopathy the distribution of weakened and atrophic muscles is not compatible with the organization of the nervous system. However, this is not always so, and differential diagnosis may be most difficult. Look beyond the positive findings of weakness and wasting for the negative side of the problem, that is, the absence of signs of neurologic disease, central or peripheral.

The subject of muscle disease is complex, and space permits discussion of only a few aspects. Rigid classifications are inappropriate because of wide variations in age at onset, rate of progress, and differential muscle involvement. Duchenne's muscular dystrophy, for example, usually begins early in life, whereas myotonic dystrophy usually does not. Both of these dystrophies are genetically determined. The secondary myopathies, on the other hand, may appear at any age and in several forms and distributions. Thyroid disease, collagen vascular disease, and steroid administration are a few of the conditions that may lead to muscle wasting and weakness. Generally, the involvement is diffuse and symmetric, tending to greater severity in the girdles.

The age at onset, family history, and distribution of weakness provide clues for differentiating the various muscle disorders, a task aided by laboratory studies such as electromyography and muscle biopsy. Muscle biopsy allows identification of abnormal storage products or organelles, enzyme deficiencies, and inflammation. Elevation of serum enzymes, particularly creatine phosphokinase, is a common finding of many disorders of muscle but also is sometimes seen to a lesser degree in cases of neurogenic atrophy. The subject is too complex to permit an exhaustive discussion here. This section will outline the salient features of some common diseases of muscle.

Duchenne's (pseudohypertrophic) dystrophy is a primary, genetic disorder characterized by early weakness and enlargement of the musculature of the calves and (to a lesser extent) the thighs, hips, and shoulders. Onset is in the first 5 years of life, and it occurs almost exclusively in boys. The enlargement of the muscles is due to fibrous and fatty infiltration, and the muscles are weak. On palpation, involved muscles have a firm and rubbery consistency. Figure 94 shows typical gastrocnemius enlargement seen in the Duchenne type of dystrophy of childhood. Later, this enlargement is lost as weakness and death of muscle increase. Weakness of the back, hip girdle, and shoulder girdle is prominent. The patient may not be able to rise from a forward-flexed position without using his hands to assist the movement. If supine, he must roll over and rise on

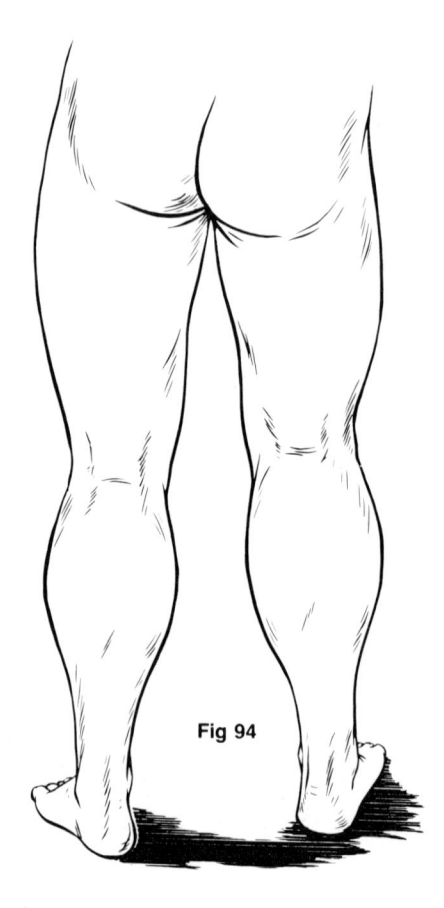

Fig 94

hands and knees and come to an upright position in stages (Gower's sign). An exaggerated lumbar lordosis and kyphoscoliosis ultimately appear, and contractures are common. The patient seldom survives into the third decade. A more slowly progressive form of this disease, with survival into middle adult life, is known as the Becker variant.

Myotonic dystrophy is transmitted in an autosomal dominant pattern. Symptoms usually appear in adulthood, about the third or fourth decades, but may be evident earlier in life. General loss of strength and energy are regularly present, and specific weakness as well as a slowness of grip release may be reported by the patient. It is the weakness, not the myotonia that is disabling.

Electromyography is particularly useful in diagnosing this condition because of the typical "dive bomber" sound recorded during a myotonic discharge of an affected muscle.

Fig 95

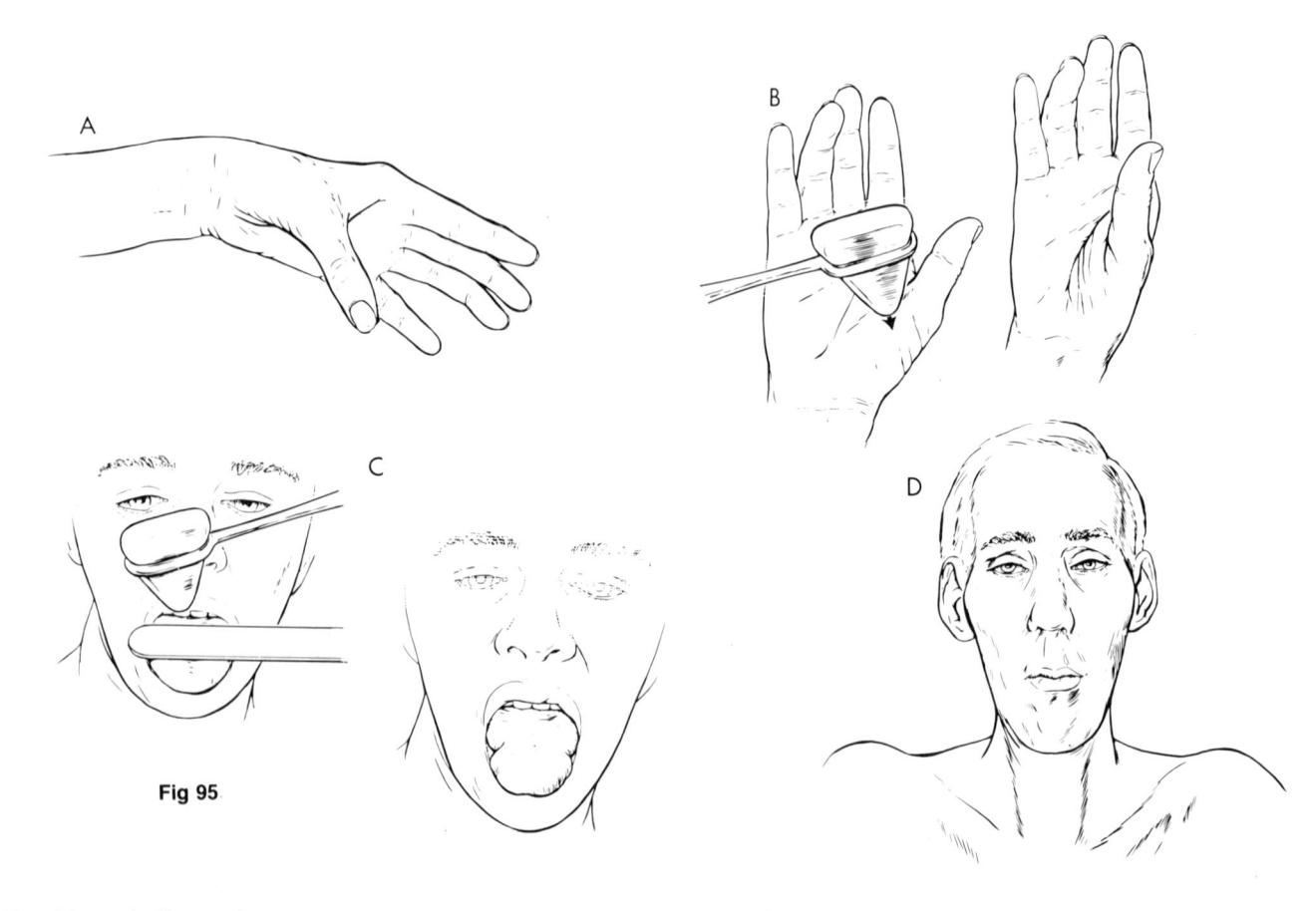

140 / *Myotonic Dystrophy*

In Figure 95,D one sees a typical picture of atrophy of the sternocleidomastoid muscles, the trapezius, and the face. There are ptosis and facial weakness with loss of expression. Atrophy involves both facial and masticatory muscles. The speech is often slurred. An almost regular feature is frontal baldness. Typical also are atrophy of the forearms and hands and atrophy and weakness below the knees with foot drop. No sensory or specific reflex changes are seen. Other features are testicular atrophy, mental dulling, a characteristic cataract, and slowly reactive pupils.

Myotonic features are of special interest and importance in diagnosis but are not usually demonstrable in all muscles. The grip is often weakened. Ask the patient to release his grip quickly. This cannot be done; instead, there is prolonged contraction with posture of the hand as seen in Figure 95,A persisting for some seconds.

The thenar eminence will often demonstrate myotonia. A quick tap on the muscle (Fig 95,B) discharges the muscle membranes, resulting in contraction—a characteristic of normal muscle. However, contraction continues abnormally long, and the thumb adducts into the position shown and remains there for several seconds.

The tongue almost regularly shows myotonia, which is in part responsible for the speech changes and difficulty in swallowing. Hold a tongue blade as shown in Figure 95,C and apply a light, quick tap. This maneuver is a bit painful and should be done with some restraint. Remove the tongue blade at once to witness the peculiar, persisting contraction seen in Figure 95,C. As weakness and atrophy progress, myotonia becomes increasingly difficult to demonstrate.

Myotonia congenita is often manifest early in life and can be inherited in either an autosomal dominant or recessive pattern. The musculature tends to be hypertrophic (not pseudohypertrophic). Congenital myotonia is more generalized and severe than myotonic dystrophy, and strength is usually normal or only minimally diminished. It may be partially incapacitating, and the slowed relaxation especially in cold weather is noteworthy. The same tests used for myotonia are applicable

Facioscapulohumeral dystrophy, transmitted in an autosomal dominant pattern, usually appears in the second decade of life and in either sex. It is slowly progressive, resulting in disability years after onset. Atrophy of the face becomes severe. Facial weakness destroys the ability to whistle, blow up a balloon, or suck through a straw. Eye closure is weak, and there is a weak, horizontal smile. Atrophy and weakness of the shoulder-girdle muscles are prominent. Figure 96 shows prominent loss of arm musculature, with scapular winging and the characteristic upward displacement of the scapulae. Lordosis is exaggerated because of weakness of the back musculature. Ultimately distal limb musculature is involved, most notably the extensors of the wrist and foot.

Limb-girdle dystrophy affects men and women equally and usually appears in the second or third decade. The girdle musculature is most affected. Progression of the disease is slow. There is not complete agreement whether this condition is a distinct entity or represents different myopathies with a predilection for the hip and shoulder musculature.

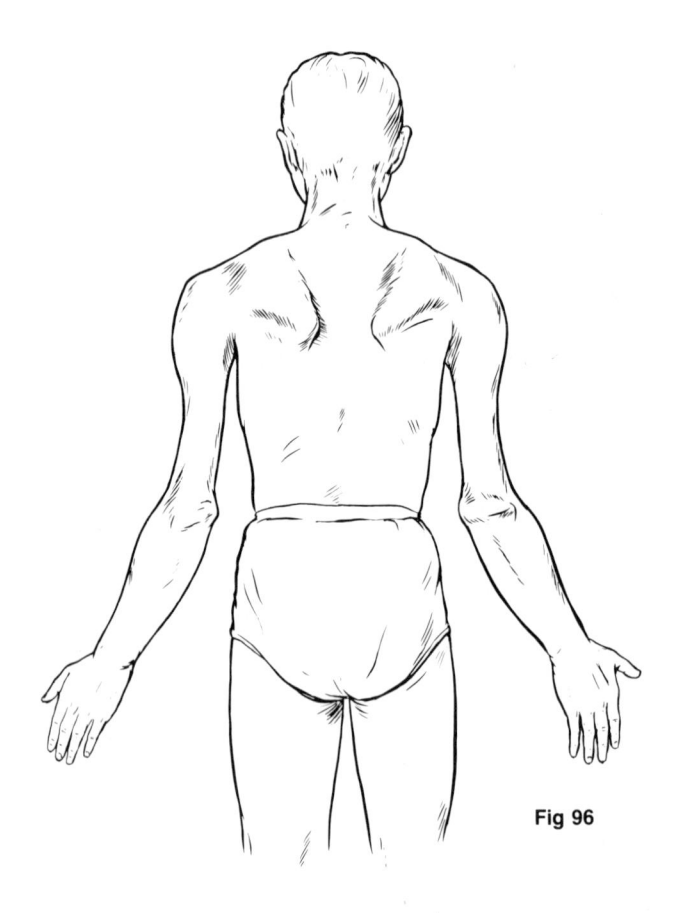

Fig 96

Myoedema is a poorly understood reaction of muscle. It is seen in myxedema but may also be present in chronic debilitating disorders. It can easily be demonstrated on the relaxed triceps but is a general state that can be found widely over the body when present. In testing for the reaction, have the patient stand arms akimbo. Strike the muscle a sharp, quick blow with the hammer at right angles to the muscle fibers. Within 1 or 2 seconds a mounding up is seen, which persists for several more seconds. This localized swelling is parallel to the blow and is not fascicular, as in the contraction of normal myotactic irritability and that of myotonia, which involves contraction of fibers.

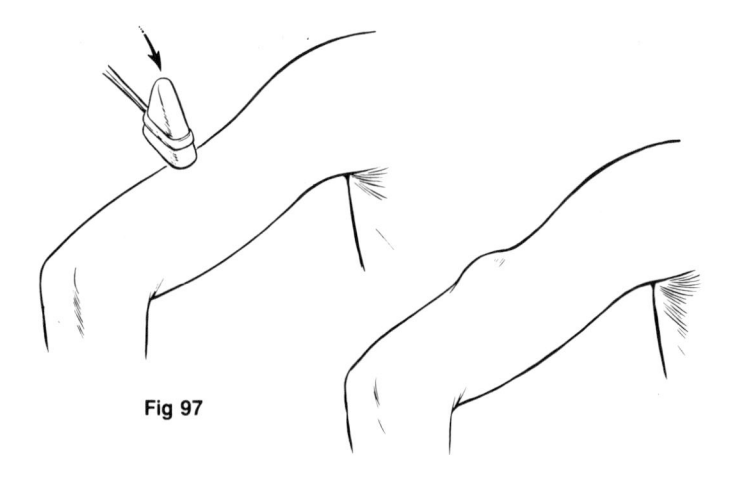

Fig 97

Myoedema / 143

Polymyositis and Dermatomyositis

Inflammation of muscles can result in profound weakness. In polymyositis, muscle alone is involved, whereas in dermatomyositis there is involvement of skin as well. The clinical spectrum in both conditions is wide. Onset can be at any age, although dermatomyositis is most likely to occur during childhood or middle adult life. An acute or subacute course lasting weeks or months is common. Weakness is predominantly proximal at first, and involved muscles may be painful and tender to palpation. Dysphagia is a common complaint, but other bulbar symptoms are uncommon. As the illness progresses, distal limb muscles become involved. The skin rash, when present, simplifies diagnosis. A peculiar purple hue, the so-called heliotrope rash, develops over the upper eyelid. Thickening and erythematous discoloration of the skin over the elbows, knees, and knuckles is common. A deep erythema may develop over the upper anterior thorax.

The association with features of autoimmune disorders such as scleroderma, systemic lupus erythematosis, and rheumatoid arthritis gives strength to the postulation that the inflammation of muscle has a similar etiology. Systemic neoplasm may also be associated, particularly in elderly patients having the typical skin rash. Muscle biopsy demonstrating typical inflammatory changes and electromyography are useful in confirming the diagnosis.

These illnesses follow an either chronic or relapsing course, but complete recovery can occur, especially in childhood.

Myasthenia Gravis

Myasthenia gravis is characterized by weakness and excessive fatigability of muscle. The incidence is highest in young women and elderly men. Dysfunction arises from imperfect neuromuscular transmission owing to an immunologically mediated destruction of acetylcholine receptors at the synaptic site. Involvement is often selective and asymmetric. Weakness of extraocular muscles, with diplopia and ptosis, weakness of bulbar musculature, speech change, and weakness of neck flexion and of shoulder abduction, are the most prevalent manifestations. The degree of paresis varies from day to day in a patient and even during a day. Usually weakness is least noticeable in the morning, progresses during the day with continued activity, and improves to some degree on rest. This pattern is seen in any condition producing muscle weakness but is most conspicuous in myasthenia. some of the findings have been mentioned (pp. 16, 88).

When ptosis is suspected to be due to myasthenia gravis, ask the patient to stare upward strongly for 90 seconds. If the ptosis is myasthenic it will almost always become noticeably worse during this maneuver. Similarly, if the patient is asked to abduct his arms to a horizontal position and maintain that posture for 2 minutes, the arm should droop if myasthenia gravis is present. Repetitive squatting and rising can be used to demonstrate fatigability of the hip-girdle musculature. The grip is evaluated by having the patient repetitively squeeze the examiner's hand. A handgrip ergometer accurately records the change in grip strength, and, slightly less reliably, an ordinary sphygmomanometer can be used by having the patient repetitively squeeze the inflated bladder while the ascent of the mercury column is recorded. Voice fatigue can be provoked by having the patient count to 100.

Commonly, anticholinesterase drugs are administered to help confirm the presence of myasthenia gravis, since resultant objective improvement in the patient's condition is excellent confirmation of the diagnosis. It must be kept in mind, however, that other neuromuscular disorders, including amyotrophic lateral sclerosis, primary myopathies, and polymyositis, may have symptoms similar to those of myasthenia gravis that may be minimally, but never substantially, improved by anticholinesterase drugs.

Before pharmacologic testing is undertaken, establish clearly the features to be observed for functional change. Typically these will be a droopy eyelid, extraocular muscle paresis, vital capacity, a weak face, or a weak neck. Ask a friendly but skeptical colleague to join you in observations. Tell the patient you are going to give him an injection to see its effect on the weakness. If possible, have an assistant draw up two syringes: one containing 1 ml of normal saline solution and the other 1 ml (10 mg) of edrophonium chloride (Tensilon). The test can now be performed in double-blind fashion with the examiners having the responsibility of determining whether the contents of one syringe unequivocally produce more improvement in the targeted function than the contents of the other. Through an established intravenous line, inject 0.2 ml from the first syringe. If there is no untoward reaction or unequivocal improvement in 2 minutes, the remaining 0.8 ml should be administered. After 5 minutes the process is repeated with the contents of the second syringe. Tensilon can be expected to begin to act within 30 to 60 seconds and last for 1 to 5 minutes, rarely slightly longer. Test strength at once and observe critically for improvement of function at 30-second intervals after each injection. A Polaroid photograph showing facial appearance and ptosis before and after each injection is helpful in capturing very transient improvement and providing a permanent, undisputable record of the test results, particularly when positive. A syringe containing 0.4 mg of atropine should always be available as an antidote for severe muscarinic side effects such as bradycardia and hypotension, nausea, and severe abdominal cramps.

When the result of a Tensilon test is equivocal, a similar test can be performed administering 0.04 mg/kg or up to 2 mg of neostigmine methylsulfate intramuscularly. Give 0.4 mg of atropine sulfate intramuscularly at the same time to prevent muscarinic side effects. Test in a comparable fashion, waiting 30 to 60 minutes for maximum effect. When positive, the benefits of the medication will last for 60 to 120 minutes, allowing more time for observation. This is particularly useful in ocular myasthenia, or when limb weakness is being tested.

Fig 98

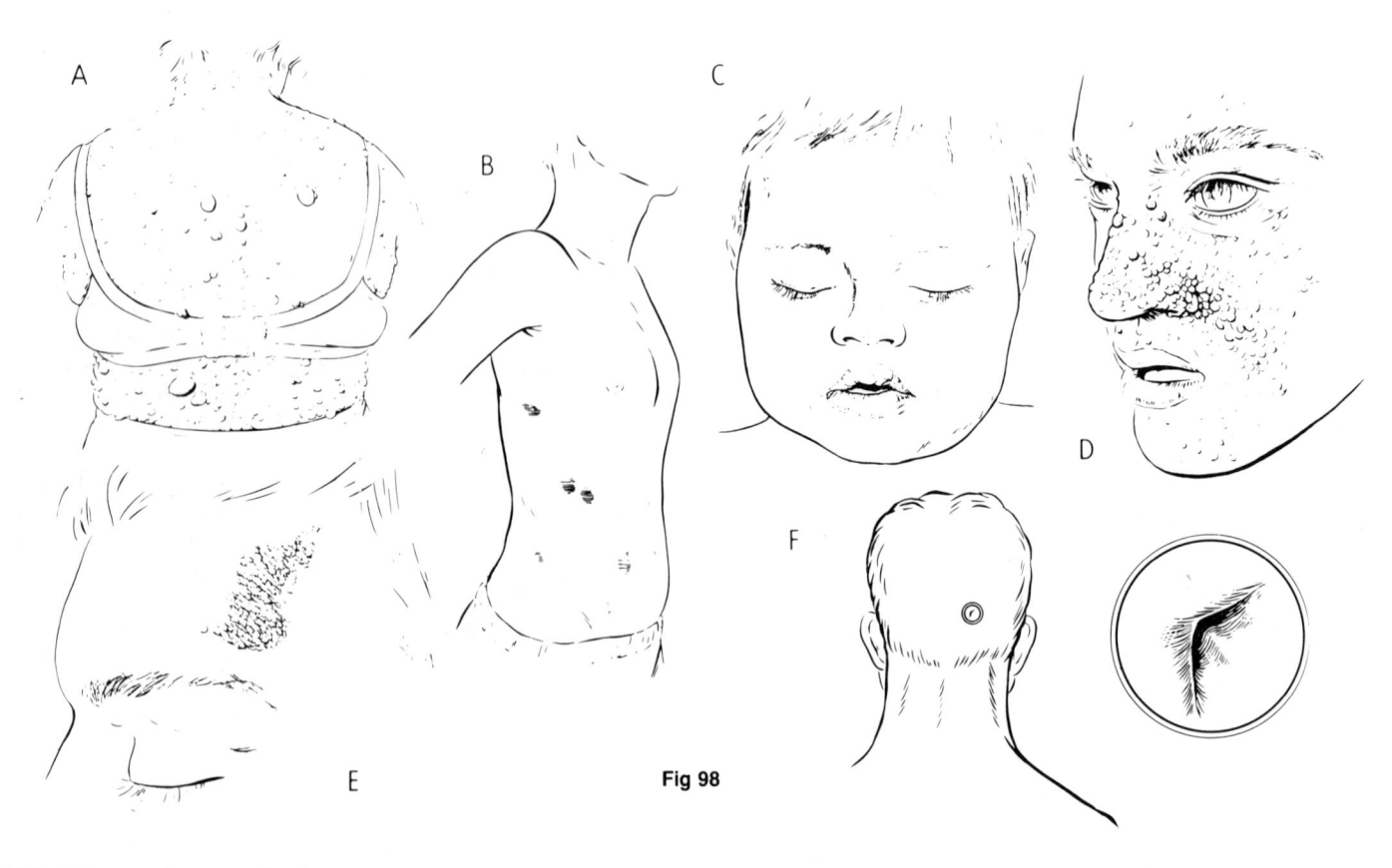

146 / *Neurocutaneous Syndromes*

Neurocutaneous Syndromes

The skin and the nervous system both originate from the embryonic ectodermal layer and are sometimes affected by the same congenital disorder. The cutaneous manifestation may betray the presence and nature of its neurologic counterpart. Some forms of neurocutaneous syndromes can be recognized in infants, but some forms may not be detectable until the patient is an adult.

In neurofibromatosis (von Recklinghausen's disease) subcutaneous fibromas or neurofibromas are widely distributed over the body (Fig 98,A). Café au lait spots (Fig 98,B), so named for their coffee-colored appearance, are also typical of this condition, especially when they are larger than 1.5 cm and multiple. Neurologic symptoms derive from associated tumors of the nervous system involving the brain or the peripheral, spinal, or cranial nerves. The auditory nerve is a particularly common site, and in patients with bilateral acoustic nerve tumors neurofibromatosis is likely. A variety of tumors of the nervous system other than neurofibromas can accompany this condition.

In encephalotrigeminal angiomatosis (Sturge-Weber syndrome), a port-wine-colored nevus covers the distribution of one or more divisions of the trigeminal nerve on one side of the face. The ophthalmic division is most commonly involved (Figure 98,C) and when so situated may be accompanied by an angioma of the meninges and cortex of the posterior hemisphere ipsilateral to the facial nevus. Convulsions and mental retardation are common, and there may be a contralateral hemiparesis. The intracranial angioma is calcified and can be seen on roentgenograms of the skull as a series of linear calcifications conforming to the surface convolutions of the brain and resembling "tram tracks."

Tuberous sclerosis has several characteristic cutaneous manifestations. Most typical and most easily observed are adenoma sebaceum—a collection of small, pink papules located over the bridge of the nose and the malar area (Fig 98,D), which, when mild, may be mistaken for ordinary acne. Shagreen patches (Fig 98,E) are slightly raised, flesh-colored areas with a coarse, leathery surface. Depigmented spots can also result from tuberous sclerosis. The pathologic basis of this disorder is that the brain contains multiple nodules (tubers) that are most abundant in the cortex and around the perimeter of the lateral ventricles. They consist of giant neurons and abnormal-appearing glial cells, the latter of which may undergo neoplastic transformation and form the nidus of a brain tumor. Seizures and mental retardation are the usual neurologic accompaniments. This condition notoriously appears in partial forms, so that one or more features may be mild or entirely absent. Genetic counseling is warranted in these cases.

Neurofibromatosis and tuberous sclerosis are inherited in an autosomal dominant pattern, whereas the Sturge-Weber syndrome appears sporadically.

Other facets of the cutaneous examination may also provide clues to the neurologic diagnosis. A noticeably smaller thumb or thumbnail on one side or a shorter and smaller extremity suggests that a functionally impaired extremity is part of a congenital hemiparesis. These findings in the adult may obviate the need for extensive diagnostic studies searching for a new or active lesion. A cutaneous angioma over the spine should raise the suspicion of an underlying intraspinal angioma at the same spinal level. Failure of the embryonic neural ectoderm to separate from skin ectoderm may result in a dermal sinus. A narrow channel leads from the surface of the skin, where it appears as a small dimple or depression

(Fig 98,F) to the dura or beyond, thereby creating a potential source of recurrent meningitis. An occipital or lumbosacral location is most common for these lesions but they may be seen at any point along the spinal axis.

Neurologic Disorders of Urinary Control

Five types of neurologic disorders of urination and urinary bladder control are generally recognized.

The centrally uninhibited bladder functions well in respect to emptying; but urgency, frequency, and incontinence are common. This type of disorder occurs especially in elderly people and is attributed to diffuse brain disease with resultant inadequate control over the primitive micturition reflex. It is often confused with the symptoms of prostatism.

The sensory paralytic bladder results from peripheral or radicular sensory denervation. The bladder becomes atonic, loses the feeling of distention or the elicitation of reflex emptying, and gradually retains a significant amount of residual urine. This condition occurs in tabes dorsalis, diabetic neuropathy, and the combined-system disease of pernicious anemia.

The motor paralytic bladder is also atonic but is due to neuronal loss in the S2-4 segments or their axons in the parasympathetic outflow. Poliomyelitis and trauma to the conus medullaris may produce this syndrome.

The automatic reflex bladder is a consequence of spinal-cord disease above the S-2 level (e.g., trauma, compression, multiple sclerosis) in which local reflex arcs are intact. The sensation of fullness is impaired or lost. Frequency, urgency, incontinence, incomplete emptying, and the inability to void are the usual symptoms. Though micturition may be possible with incomplete cord lesions, urinary tract damage may still result from ureteral reflux or infected residual urine.

The autonomous bladder has no neural connection on either side of the reflex arc and functions imperfectly on a myogenic basis. An atonic bladder with secondary overflow incontinence and impaired drainage of the upper urinary tract is characteristic.

Bladder function is studied by cystometry, i.e., plotting intravesical pressure against volume. The ability to sense fullness and hot and cold is assessed, and the intravesical pressure produced by voluntary contraction of the detrusor mechanism is noted. Catheterization after voiding to measure the amount of residual urine is a common and valuable procedure, which may be expected to yield abnormal amounts (over 50 ml) in any of the conditions described except the centrally uninhibited bladder. Persistent and substantial amounts of residual urine may require drainage by an indwelling catheter or a suprapubic cystostomy. In some patients external bladder compression (Credé's maneuver) or intermittent self-catheterization is more effective.

Rectal and Pelvic Examinations

From the standpoint of the neurologic examination there are several indications for, and possible findings of, rectal examination. Attention is indicated whenever there is pain in the back, pain in the perineal region, or complaints of poor bowel or urinary control, which suggest a disorder in the distribution of the lumbosacral plexus, and, of course, whenever a search for a source of metastatic malignant neoplasm is in order. Pain may be related to prostatic, cervical, or rectal carcinoma, whereas sphincteric weakness may indicate denervation, either proximal or distal.

The musculature of the anal sphincter, normally at rest, contracts on intention and with coughing and straining. The sphincter is 1 to 2 cm thick as palpated by gloved finger. With finger inserted, ask the patient to cough or voluntarily to contract the sphincter to estimate its responsiveness and strength. Bowel control may be satisfactory with a relatively lax sphincter, but if this muscle contracts poorly, a disorder of urinary control may be suspected to have a neurologic basis. (Previous surgical procedures may weaken the sphincter.) While investigating this region, use a common pin to check sensation around the anus on both sides. The area is supplied by the lower sacral segments, which are also concerned with urinary control and sexual function (p. 69). The skin here is ordinarily quite sensitive. Scratch the skin about 2 cm laterally from the anus with the head of the pin. In most normal people, the external anal sphincter and the skin overlying it will pucker, demonstrating an intact local arc. This response is sometimes referred to as the "anal wink."

The pelvic examination is especially important in investigating syndromes of lower-back pain and leg pain with peripheral neural involvement, because of the propensity of pelvic malignant neoplasms to involve the lumbosacral plexus. Palpation of the pelvic walls may reveal induration or a neoplasm involving nerve trunks. Keep in mind, however, that the plexus or nerve may be abnormally sensitive to pressure when the pathologic involvement is proximal to the area of investigation.

Disturbances of Consciousness

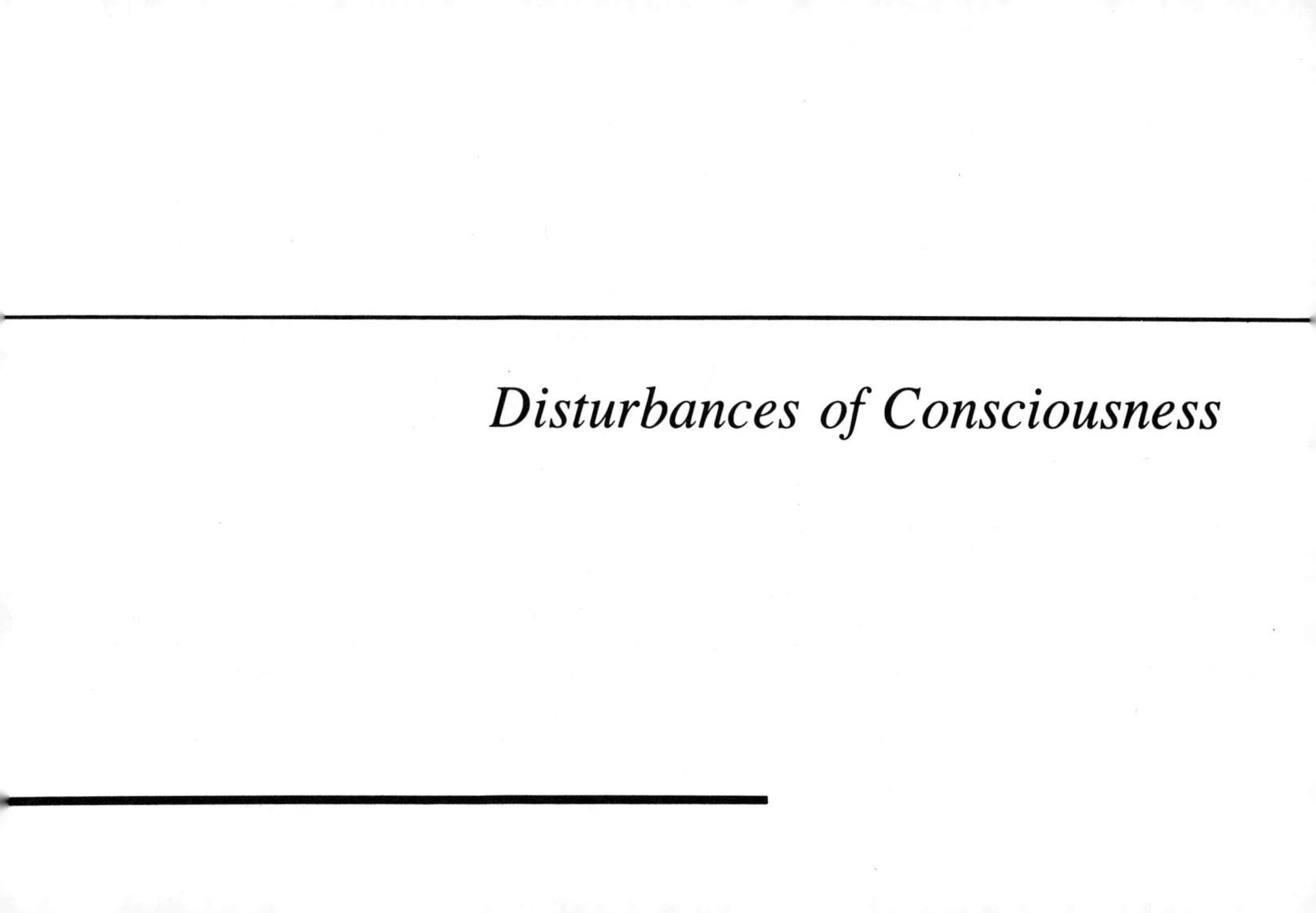

Examination of the Patient in Coma

Whenever cooperation of the patient is reduced by confusion, stupor, or coma, the information that can be gained from the neurologic examination is proportionately less. The approach to such patients therefore depends in part on the interpretation of clues found in the available history and in the examination.

When it has been determined that the comatose patient does not require immediate care for obstructed airway, shock, or hemorrhage, the diagnostic assessment should begin with a pertinent history. Information must be sought from relatives, friends, witnesses, police, and ambulance attendants. If such people are not available, the patient's name and address can be obtained from his billfold and used to contact relatives or to check hospital records. Look for bracelets and medallions identifying disease. Information about medications taken (particularly those with sedative properties) and about previously known illnesses (e.g., diabetes, hypertension, alcoholism, or depression with suicidal tendencies) can provide clues to the cause of coma. One should ask if the patient has had neurologic complaints such as headache, confusion, diplopia, or focal weakness in the hours, days, or weeks prior to the onset of coma.

The waking state demands an intact cortex of at least one cerebral hemisphere interacting with a normally functioning reticular activating system of the upper brain stem. Since it is critically important to determine whether the cerebral hemispheres or the brain stem, or both, are malfunctioning, the examiner should try to identify which one or combination of these anatomic pillars of wakefulness is involved. In the alert patient, localizing brain dysfunction depends on the patient's capability to demonstrate, on command, his strength, coordination, and ability to perceive sensory stimuli. In the comatose patient, localization of brain dysfunction depends instead on careful observation of posture, respiratory pattern, pupillary size and reactivity, ocular position and motility, and spontaneous or reflex motor activity. Depending on the part of the brain involved, each of these functions may be altered in various ways. Specific combinations of dysfunction are characteristic of disease at each level of the brain.

Observing the posture of the patient's trunk, extremities, head, and neck provides much information. An extremity that rests in an awkward or seemingly uncomfortable position, such as over the bedrail, is likely paretic. A lower extremity that is flaccid and externally rotated is probably paralyzed. These observations are less valid in a very deeply comatose patient, whose extremities will rest in whatever position they are placed.

The face may exhibit a flattened nasolabial fold or puffing out of the cheek on one side during respiration, either of which suggests facial weakness. Decorticate and decerebrate posture are both indicative of significant brain dysfunction and are easily recognized. Decorticate posture is typically associated with a lesion involving the pyramidal system above the level of the midbrain and includes flexion at the elbow and wrist with adduction of the upper arm against the thorax and extension and internal rotation of the lower extremities. Decerebrate rigidity implies a lesion involving the upper brain stem between the midbrain and midpontine level. When fully developed it consists of hyperextension of the neck, arching of the back, extension, pronation, and adduction of the arms, and extension of the legs. Although this finding usually implies anatomic disruption of the upper brain stem, metabolic encephalopathy occasionally involves this region and produces typical decerebrate posturing. If not present spontaneously, either of these two abnormal postures can often be provoked by a noxious stimulus such as vigorous sternal pressure.

The rate, rhythm, and depth of respiration may also provide a clue to the locus of the lesion. Cheyne-Stokes respiration consists of alternate hyperpnea and apnea and is commonly attributed to bilateral cerebral dysfunction, either structural or metabolic. Regular, sustained, deep, and rapid breathing may result from many diverse conditions, but in the comatose patient it can be due to dysfunction of the lower midbrain or upper pons, in which case it is termed central neurogenic hyperventilation. Ataxic breathing is an irregular pattern and rhythm of both deep and shallow breaths, which suggest direct involvement of the medullary respiratory centers.

A bright light is needed to accurately determine pupillary activity because the reactive excursion, particularly in very small pupils, may be minimal and easily overlooked. A unilaterally dilated and fixed pupil implies compression of the third nerve, commonly as a result of temporal lobe herniation. Bilaterally fixed but midsize pupils are found in midbrain compression or destruction most commonly associated with transtentorial herniation in patients with increased intracranial pressure. Pontine lesions often produce pinpoint pupils that can be demonstrated to be minimally reactive if examined with a bright light and a magnifying lens. In metabolic or drug-induced coma, the pupils, although sometimes small, are almost always clearly reactive, despite evidence of severe brain-stem dysfunction. Exceptions to this general rule are the metabolic comas associated with atropine or glutethimide intoxication or narcotic overdose.

Ocular position and motility are among the most useful guides to the site of brain dysfunction in the comatose patient. It is worthwhile as a first step in examination to lift the eyelids gently and observe the position of the eyes at rest. Slight ocular divergence is common and does not suggest a lesion at any specific locus. If both eyes are consistently and conjugately deviated to one side, however, it is likely that there is involvement of horizontal gaze mechanisms in either the frontal lobe on the side to which gaze is directed or in the pons on the opposite side. Downward deviation of the eyes results from dysfunction of the pretectal region of the midbrain, usually as a result of thalamic hemorrhage but occasionally resulting from metabolic encephalopathy. "Skew deviation" refers to a vertical disparity of eye position and suggests a pontine lesion, particularly on the side of the inferiorly deviated eye.

Although the unconscious patient cannot cooperate by volitionally moving his eyes, his range of ocular movement usually can be tested nevertheless. In light coma there may be spontaneous, random roving eye movements in the horizontal plane that prove the intactness of the third and sixth cranial nerves bilaterally and of the horizontal gaze centers in the pons. If horizontal eye movements are not present spontaneously, they may be induced by employing the oculocephalic and oculovestibular reflexes. To elicit the oculocephalic reflex, briskly rotate the head first to one side, then the other. Never perform this in a patient with possible cervical spine injury. In the fully awake patient the eyes move in the same direction as the head, but with depressed consciousness the eyes move conjugately in the opposite direction. This movement is the result of a reflex mediated through the brain stem, and its intactness means there is normal function of the third and sixth cranial nerves and their brain-stem connections. Similarly, brisk movement of the head up and down can be used to test for elevation and depression of the eyes. The oculovestibular reflex (see p. 152) is brought into play by positioning the patient's head 30 degrees above the horizontal axis and instilling 10 to 20 ml of icy water into the external auditory canal and against the intact tympanic membrane. In the unconscious patient with normal brain-stem function, the eyes deviate conjugately toward the side of stimulation. In deep coma, both the oculovestibular and the oculocephalic reflexes may be lost, even though the brain stem remains structurally intact.

Gross movements of the limbs should be assessed first by observing whether there is more spontaneous movement on the one side than the other. Withdrawal movements or more complex defensive movements can be provoked by a stimulus such as a pinprick on the sole of the foot. The vigor and appropriateness of the responses on the two sides can then be compared. When there is no spontaneous motor activity, lift the patient's arms above the bed and allow them to drop. A paralyzed limb will drop free and limp. The innervated extremity will fall with some braking action.

Cerebellar function is difficult to assess, but occasionally an intention tremor can be detected as a limb is moved in a defensive manner toward the face. The sensory examination is ordinarily limited to noting whether or not the patient responds to painful stimuli and, if so, the relative vigor of the response to stimulation of various parts of the body. More discriminating sensory testing is usually impossible. The reflexes are examined in a comatose patient just as they are in an awake patient. Asymmetric hyperreflexia usually indicates a lesion of the contralateral hemisphere; a unilateral Babinski sign has the same significance. The interpretation of bilateral Babinski signs is more difficult because in the unconscious patient this finding may be present in the absence of structural disease of the pyramidal system.

Other clues to the cause of coma may be found in the general examination. Lacerations of the face or scalp or a palpable skull depression suggest trauma as the cause of unconsciousness. Look for an ecchymosis behind the ear (Battle's sign); (see p. 15) or cerebrospinal fluid leaking from the nose or ear either of which implies a basilar skull fracture. Careful examination of the skin may help elucidate the cause of coma. A petechial rash raises the possibility of meningococcal meningitis or a thrombocytopenic condition. A red hue to the skin is seen in carbon monoxide poisoning. Jaundice of the skin or sclera should alert one to the possibility of hepatic encephalopathy, whereas dry, coarse skin, particularly when associated with hypothermia, suggests myxedema coma.

Nuchal rigidity (see p. 119) is evidence of either central nervous system infection or hemorrhage. In either condition, however, nuchal rigidity may be delayed 12 to 24 hours after onset, although typically it occurs within 3 to 4 hours. In deeply comatose and flaccid patients, the absence of nuchal rigidity does not rule out hemorrhage or infection. Carefully examine the tongue and buccal mucosa for lacerations or contusions that may have occurred during a seizure. Prolonged unconsciousness occurring after a generalized convulsion (which may have been unwitnessed) is not uncommon and accounts for a significant number of admissions to the emergency room. Fecal or urinary incontinence, though less specific, could indicate the same possibility.

Two conditions in which the patient appears unresponsive but is not truly comatose deserve special mention—psychogenic unresponsiveness and the "locked-in" syndrome. Psychogenic unresponsiveness should be suspected in patients with a history of personality disorder, histrionic behavior, or recent emotional turmoil. Frequently, the coma begins immediately after an emotionally charged incident such as a family quarrel. Although this background is fertile ground for psychogenic unresponsiveness, the diagnosis should not be made until all reasonable metabolic or structural causes of coma have been excluded and special consideration has been given to the possibility of a suicide attempt. On formal testing these patients are typically diffusely flaccid, although when they think they are not under direct observation, purposeful activity such as shifting position, scratching, or rearranging bedsheets may be observed. Focal or lateralized paralysis is seldom present, and the pupils are equal and normally reactive. The oculovestibular test is useful for determining whether the patient's coma is psychogenic, because ice-water irrigation of the external auditory canal produces nystagmus in the awake patient only. Hence, the patient who is flaccid, apparently incapable of volitional motor activity, and unresponsive to all stimuli, but who exhibits nystagmus after ice-water stimulation, is probably not suffering from an organic condition. The catatonic schizophrenic may appear to be in coma. Sometimes this state is betrayed by a peculiar tendency to support the limbs in any posture they are placed for long periods.

The "locked-in" syndrome is caused by a lesion, usually an infarction, in the base of the pons. Descending motor fibers to the lower brain stem and spinal cord are interrupted so that phonation, horizontal eye movements, and movement of all extremities and the face are impossible. Since the reticular formation of the upper brain stem is spared, the patient, although unable to speak or move, remains fully awake. Because the midbrain is uninvolved, the patient retains the ability to move his eyes in the vertical plane and open his lids; in this way he can communicate with the examiner and demonstrate his alertness. It should be remembered that such patients can hear and understand and should be regarded as awake.

Seizures

A generalized tonic-clonic (grand mal) seizure is followed by some degree of confusion and blunting of responsiveness. If several seizures have occurred in close succession, stupor may persist for many hours. The diagnostic problems thus presented are aggravated if emergency administration of an anticonvulsant drug with sedative properties is required.

An accurate assessment of the basic neurologic status of a patient cannot be made in the postictal period, but the observation of focal deficits during this time may be of considerable value in localizing the lesion responsible for the seizure. The clinical features of the seizure itself, particularly the nature of its onset, are also important in this assessment. A physician who by chance has an opportunity to witness a seizure is obligated to make note of the initial manifestations of the episode and the progression of events that follow. Often, the diagnosis of an episodic disorder of consciousness and the clinical localization of the lesion responsible derive mostly from an accurate record of an intelligently observed attack. Obviously, then, it is imperative to have some knowledge of the characteristic features of each of the several types of seizures.

The terminology used to label seizure types has evolved from purely clinical descriptive terms, such as grand mal, petit mal, or psychomotor, to a newer, internationally accepted classification that takes account of the EEG features, anatomic substrates, and clinical features of each

TABLE 1.
Classification of Seizures

I. Partial seizures (seizures beginning locally)
  A. Simple partial seizures (consciousness not impaired)
    1. With motor signs
    2. With somatosensory or special sensory symptoms
    3. With autonomic signs, such as flushing, sweating, pupillary dilatation
    4. With psychic symptoms such as déjà vu, fear, anger, illusions, distortion of time (these are more commonly associated with impairment of consciousness)
  B. Complex partial seizures (with impairment of consciousness)
    1. Simple partial onset (see I.A.) followed by impairment in consciousness
    2. Impairment of consciousness at onset
      a. With impairment of consciousness only
      b. With automatisms
  C. Partial seizures that secondarily become generalized
II. Generalized seizures (first clinical symptoms indicate bilateral, nonfocal onset
  A. Absence
  B. Myoclonic
  C. Clonic
  D. Tonic
  E. Tonic-clonic
  F. Atonic

seizure type. Using this classification, seizures can be divided into two broad groups—generalized and partial—each of which has several subcategories. Generalized seizures are clinically and electroencephalographically symmetric, whereas partial seizures are focal in onset. To circumvent the confusion generated by this changing terminology, it is wise to be aware of both the new and the old nomenclatures. A simplified version of the international classification of the epilepsies is given in Table 1. Although there is not exact equivalency between the older clinical terminology and the newer international categories, both terms will be used where possible.

A generalized tonic-clonic seizure (grand mal) may start with a cry and fall, then generalized stiffening in extension and temporary respiratory arrest (tonic phase). This is followed by violent, rhythmic jerking of the extremities and by stertorous, partially obstructed breathing (clonic phase). Occasionally, seizures are purely tonic or clonic. Finally, relaxation with random, infrequent jerks signals the end of the seizure. The tongue may have been bitten and injuries suffered in falling. Urinary incontinence is frequent. Pupillary dilation or Babinski signs are common immediately after a generalized tonoclonic seizure but are usually transient and seldom indicative of new structural brain lesions. The patient will remain drowsy or stuporous for minutes to hours and then awaken with a headache and muscular aches and pains, in most cases lacking recall of the seizure or its onset. Persistent back pain suggests compression fracture of a vertebra.

Generalized seizures of the absence type (petit mal) occur almost exclusively in children and rarely after the age of 30. An *absence* attack (pronounced "ob-sahnz" as in French) typically consists of a brief (several seconds) lapse of consciousness with interruption of activity and associated staring, followed immediately by a return to normal function. Often there is associated minor, symmetrically clonic movement of the eyelids or fingers at the same three-per-second rate that typifies the EEG discharge recorded during these attacks. The seizure may be so brief as to go unnoticed by others. Slightly longer episodes are sometimes mistakenly considered by parents or school teachers to represent daydreaming or inattentiveness.

In an atonic seizure, postural tone of a part or the entire body is lost, but consciousness is retained.

Partial seizures have their origin in a discrete area of the brain. Simple partial seizures with motor symptomatology (focal motor seizures) originate in the motor cortex of one hemisphere. There may be localized jerking on one side of the face or one arm or leg. Sometimes the convulsive movements spread up one side from leg to arm to face (jacksonian march). Not infrequently, there is forced turning of the head and eye away from the hemisphere harboring the epileptogenic focus. There is little or no alteration in consciousness unless a generalized seizure is triggered. Postictal paralysis of the involved limbs is common, and if the seizure originated in the speech area of the dominant hemisphere, aphasia may also occur. The finding of asymmetric paralysis after an apparent generalized motor seizure suggests that the episode began focally before becoming generalized.

Simple partial seizures with somatosensory symptomatology (focal sensory seizures) originate from a seizure focus in the primary somatosensory cortex of one hemisphere. They are characterized by an unusual spontaneous sensation involving part of one side of the body and often spreading to involve other parts on the same side as the seizure discharge spreads over the sensory cortex. Usually the abnormal sensation is described as a tingling, crawling, or numbness. Any part of the body may be affected initially, but the hand and the perioral region and lips are most often involved. As in focal motor seizures, consciousness is not altered unless there is progression to a generalized seizure.

Complex partial seizures (psychomotor or temporal-lobe seizure) commonly originate from a focus in one temporal lobe. The aura preceding the episode sometimes provides a valuable clue to the precise location of the seizure discharge within the temporal lobe. For example, the aura may consist of a hallucination of an unpleasant odor such as burning rubber or vomitus. The so-called uncinate aura suggests that the initial seizure discharge arose in the medial temporal lobe, an area that subserves olfaction. The partial complex seizure itself consists of an alteration, but not complete loss, of consciousness typically lasting several minutes but occasionally longer. During this time the patient may appear confused, exhibit a blank or distant stare, and swallow repetitively or smack his lips. Sometimes there is purposeless motor activity such as fumbling with clothing or other objects (automatisms). Behavior that is more complex but inappropriate to the situation is also possible. The patient may, for example, clear the dishes off the dinner table even though the meal has not yet begun. A sensation of unusual familiarity (*déjà vu*) or strangeness (*jamais vu*), which represent cognitive symptoms, often accompanies or precedes these attacks. Visual hallucinations or distortions (psychosensory symptoms) can also occur, as can a feeling of intense fear or sadness (affective symptoms). Afterward, the aura may be remembered, but there is imperfect recall of whatever automatic behavior may have occurred. Psychotic, antisocial, or histrionic behavior is sometimes mistakenly diagnosed as a complex partial seizure. Aggressive behavior is uncommon during these convulsive episodes unless the patient is restrained or his automatic activity interfered with. Be circumspect about a diagnosis of partial complex seizures when the patient's behavior, although extreme, is entirely appropriate to the situation.

The manifestations of convulsive disorders are endless in variety. With special attention to both historical and observed evidence of premonitory symptoms as well as to aura and early features of the attack itself, the anatomic location of the epileptogenic focus can often be discerned. The EEG is useful to corroborate one's clinical impression (see p. 176).

Neurologic Evaluation of the Infant

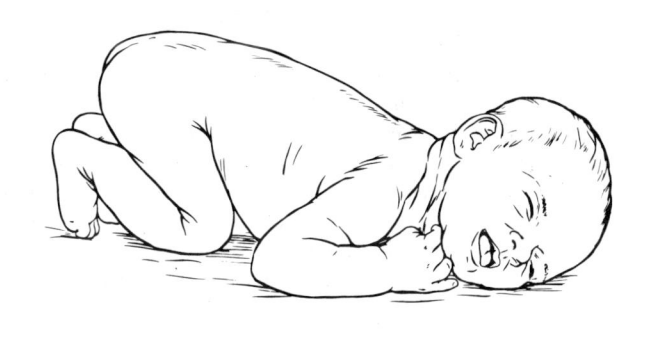

Neurologic Examination of the Infant

Specific neurologic abnormalities helpful in locating lesions are found far less frequently in the infant than in the adult. Much of the nervous system is not functionally effective in infancy, and one deals largely with gross responses and attributes of lower levels of organization. However, function is rapidly acquired and elaborated. The child of 1 year is decidedly more aware of events in his environment than the infant of 1 month. By the age of 2 years the child is capable of quite complex behavior, including verbal comprehension and expression.

Knowledge of normal developmental landmarks is crucial for assessment of the state of nervous system function at various ages in infancy. Motor skills are generally achieved in a rather constant sequence during the first 2 years of life. It is the appearance of these capabilities at the proper time that constitutes evidence of nervous system integrity. However, other factors unrelated to brain disease can also hinder the orderly appearance of the developmental milestones. Maternal or sensory deprivation may result in serious deficits in the child's motor and speech development. Infants with very low birth weight develop more slowly than full-term infants during the first year. Serious generalized disease or recurrent infections may also retard development during the first year even though there is no significant nervous system disorder. This section is designed as a reference for the findings appropriate on examination at birth, 6 weeks, 6 months, 9 months, and 1 year of age.

The prenatal and perinatal history must be obtained because difficulties during that period often predispose the infant to neurologic abnormalities. Maternal illness, use of drugs, exposure to toxins, or trauma during pregnancy are important information, as is the duration of pregnancy and maternal age at the time of conception. The details of labor and delivery are important, particularly complications such as placenta previa, abruptio placentae, premature rupture of membranes, prolonged labor, and precipitous or traumatic delivery. Inquire specifically about perinatal cyanosis, apnea, or the need for resuscitation. If the details of birth and delivery are not known to the parents, the days or weeks of age at which the infant was discharged from the hospital can be a useful guide to the general state of neonatal health.

The neurologic examination of the infant must be done in a less systematized fashion than that of the adult. Much information can be obtained at the outset by a few moments of observation of the baby, whether he is asleep or awake. Observation of the waking infant provides information in many areas, including symmetry of limb movements, organization of ocular movements, and the degree of interest in and awareness of the surrounding environment. Make note of the vigor and persistence of the infant's cry, the ability to suck, the muscle tone on passive movement, and certain reflexes (p. 163). Garments must be removed from the infant for effective observation or examination. Be careful to void chilling the infant, especially the premature infant.

Physical findings vary from hour to hour depending on the child's feeding schedule and the degree of alertness. For example, immediately after a feeding, neonatal reflexes tend to be less distinct and muscle tone may seem diminished compared with the findings just before feeding time. Regardless of the age of the infant, a cardinal rule is that those aspects of the examination that require restraint or discomfort should be left until last. The screaming infant is difficult to assess and will require reevaluation when both patient and physician are more composed.

Elicitation of the Moro reflex should be part of the examination of any infant. It is normally present from birth until age 3 to 4 months. The intensity of the response gradually abates in the normal infant. If it persists after 4 months of age in a full-term infant, neurologic disease should be suspected. In a child more than 6 months of age it almost always indicates a significant cerebral disorder.

Even more important than persistence of the reflex too far in life is its absence in the first few weeks of life. Deeply sedated infants or in those who have suffered a severe cerebral insult prenatally or during birth generally lack the Moro reflex. If the reflex is present, then disappears, the infant may have kernicterus. Absence of the response in the neonate does not necessarily indicate brain disease, and it may be difficult to elicit in premature babies. Birth injury to the upper cervial cord, advanced anterior horn-cell disease, and severe myopathy are unusual causes of a suppressed or absent reflex.

Persistent asymmetry of the response suggests hemiparesis, injury to the brachial plexus, or fracture of the clavicle or humerus.

Among the several methods for evoking the Moro reflex, that pictured in Figure 99 is perhaps safest and most reliable. The infant is held supine (Fig 99,A) and the head is gently but abruptly allowed to drop in partial hyperextension. Overextension of the neck must be prevented or spinal-cord injury could result. In response, the arms briskly abduct and extend while the hands open, the legs flex slightly, and the hips abduct to a lesser degree than the arms (Fig 99,B). The arms then return forward in a clasping fashion over the body. This response is generally regarded as a mass reflex that occurs when normal reticular and brain-stem mechanisms are not yet under significant inhibitory control from higher centers.

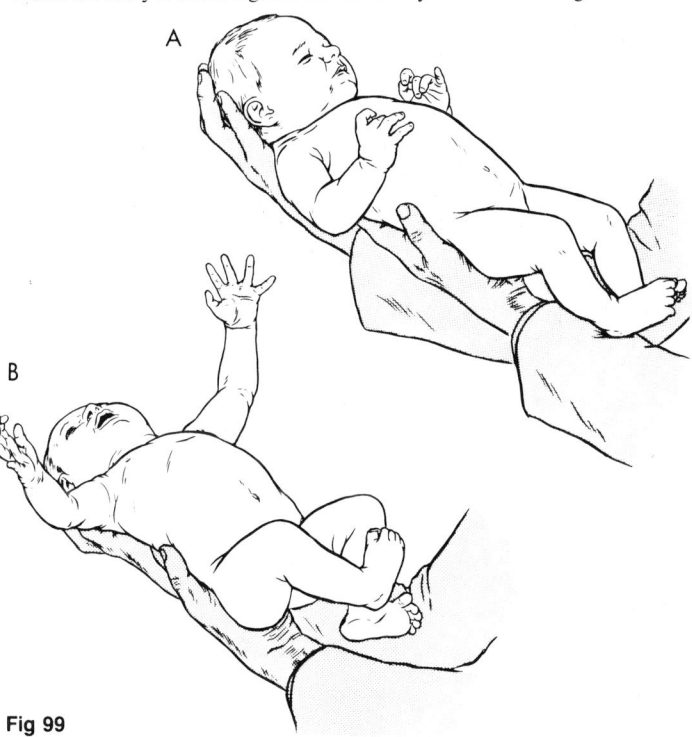

Fig 99

The full-term, healthy newborn infant assumes during sleep a posture of semiflexion of all limbs with the thighs tucked under the lower abdomen as shown in Figure 100.

Rooting and sucking reflexes are active, moreso if the child has not been recently fed, since these reflexes are geared to the nutritional needs of the infant. The rooting reflex can be prompted by gently rubbing the infant's cheek, which should cause him to deviate his mouth to that side. His ability to suck and swallow is best evaluated by observing him at feeding time. Persistence of rooting and sucking reflexes beyond the fourth month suggests bilateral brain dysfunction.

The infant at birth blinks in response to bright light, and the pupils constrict immediately. Conjugate ocular movements develop rapidly after birth, although the eyes may not be able to follow objects for the first few weeks.

The newborn infant's hands are in the fisted position during much of the waking period. The hands tend to open after 4 weeks of age. Persistence of a fisted posture of one hand after 2 months of age may be an early manifestation of a developing spastic hemiparesis. A grasp reflex is symmetrically present at birth and persists for 2 or 3 months. To elicit it, stimulate the ulnar side of the child's palm with your finger. The response should be a forceful grasp of your finger. Persistence of the grasp relex in the full-term infant beyond 4 months of age is evidence of cerebral dysfunction.

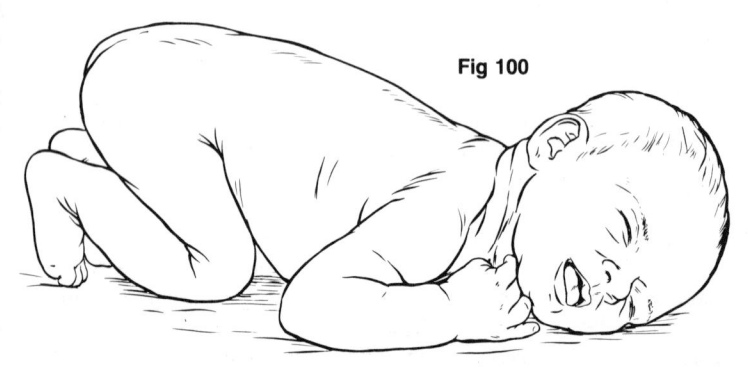

Fig 100

The tonic neck reflex is elicitied by rotating the head of the supine infant to one side. A normal response consists of extension of the extremities on the side to which the head has been turned and flexion at the elbow and knee on the opposite side. The resultant posture has been likened to a fencer's stance. The reflex can often, but not invariably, be elicited in the normal infant between the ages of 1 and 5 months, but then is only partially developed and easily overcome. A tonic neck reflex that cannot be overcome or that persists in an infant beyond 6 months of age suggests an abnormality in the motor system.

The normal, waking newborn infant will engage in reflex stepping movements if placed in a suitable position, as shown in Figure 101. As the child is supported in an upright position, the bottom of one of his feet should come into firm contact with the examining table. This neonatal reflex, lasting for 3 to 4 weeks, provides evidence of neurologic integrity.

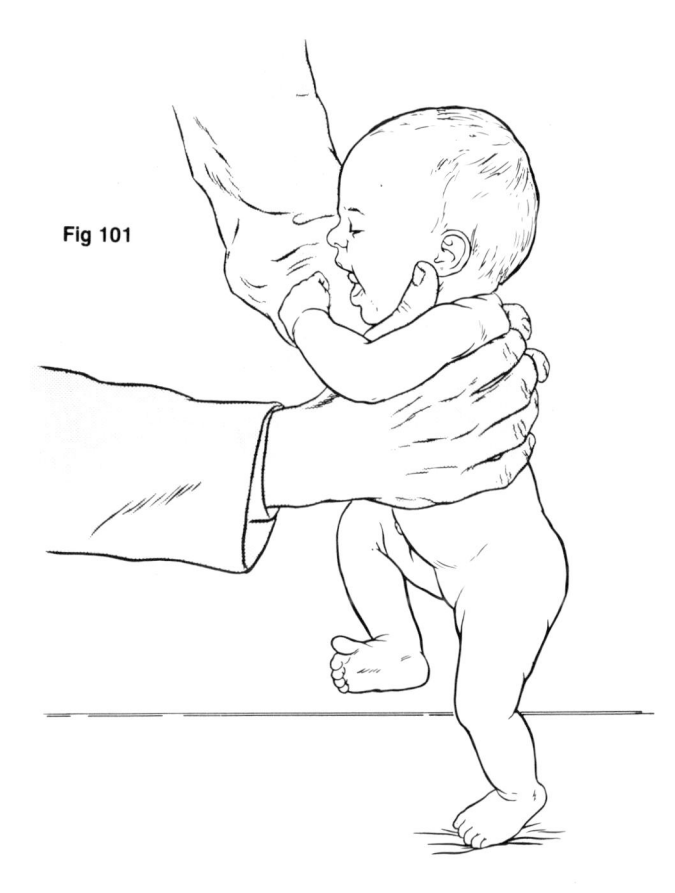

Fig 101

A

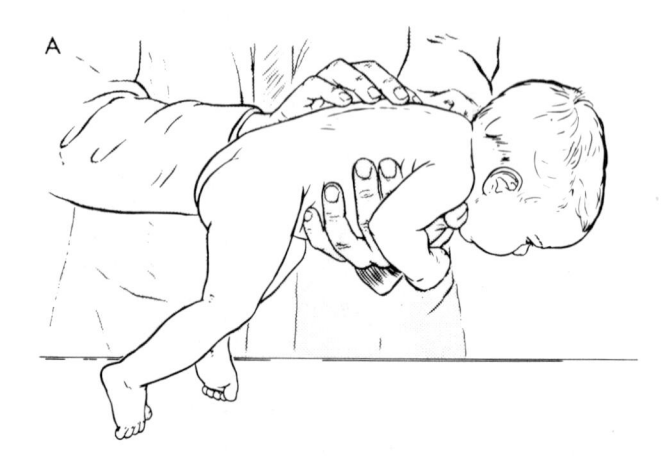

Fig 102

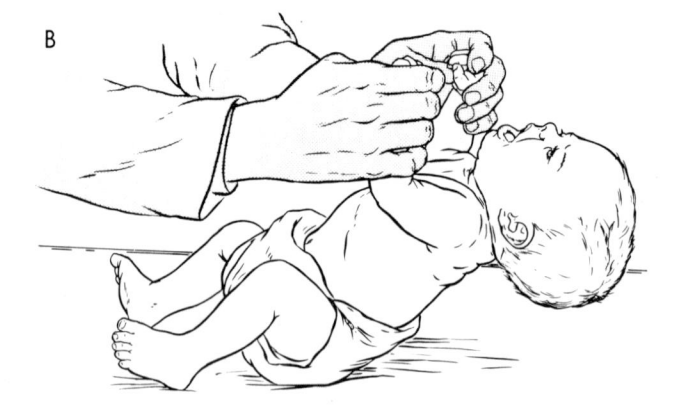

B

166 / *Infant at Six Weeks*

By the age of 6 weeks the healthy infant spends considerably more time awake. He will smile and often will follow his mother attentively with his eyes. The hands are held open more than before, and control of the head is better developed. While lying prone, the baby is able to elevate his head, keeping his chin off the table momentarily. When held up in the prone position, the child supports his head in the same plane as his trunk with his arms partly flexed at the elbows and legs partially extended as shown in Figure 102,A. Elevation from a supine position (Fig 102,B) demonstrates some ability to support the head though development is far from complete. When the infant is placed in the sitting position and supported as shown in Figure 103, his back is rounded and his head is only temporarily maintained in an upright position.

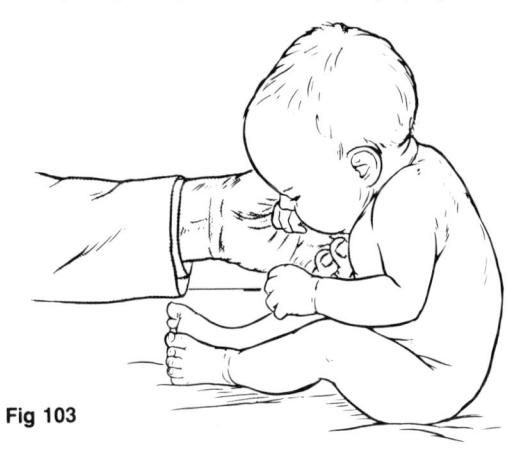

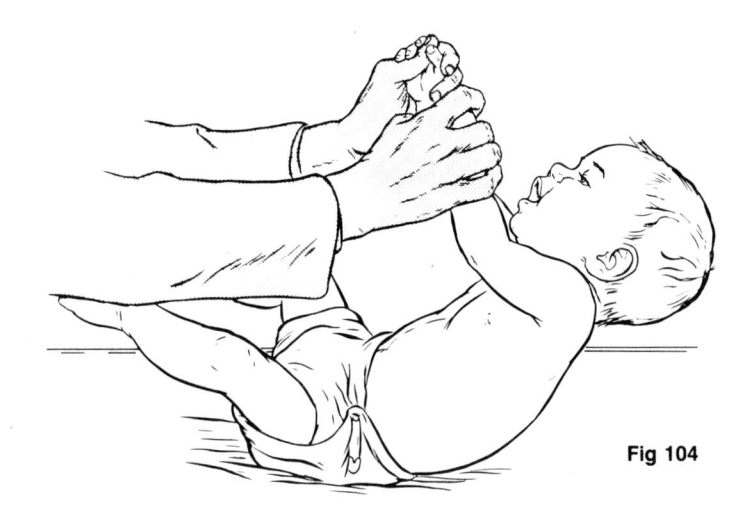

Fig 103

Fig 104

By 6 months of age the normal infant no longer shows the neonatal reflexes just described. His developmental progress is such that he supports the head well when he is pulled into a sitting position, as shown in Figure 104, and is able to roll over, to sit unsupported, and to support his weight on his feet if he is held upright. Hand and foot regard are often evidenced at this age by the child intently watching his hand or foot when it is extended over his face in the supine position. The eyes can follow a slowly moving object when tested as illustrated in Figure 105. Lying prone, he is able to elevate his chest and upper abdomen off the bed. He may hold his bottle, grasp his feet, and grasp a small cube in palmar fashion. An infant this age may imitate sounds and may exhibit displeasure at the removal of a toy from his environment. Other likes and dislikes may also be expressed.

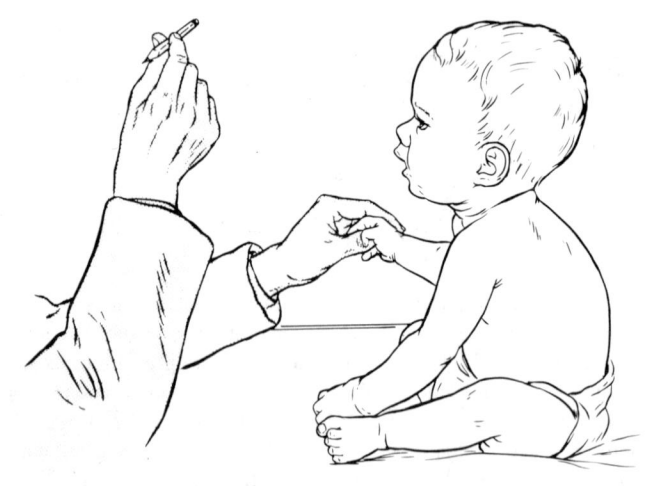

Fig 105

At 9 months of age the infant not only sits alone well but can pivot the trunk so as to reach an object partially behind him. He can reach with either hand and is able to grasp small objects by opposing the thumb to the index finger (Figure 106, A). Once grasped, objects can be transferred from hand to hand. He may now pull up from a sitting to a standing position and maintain this position by holding on with the hands (Fig 106,B). The child of 9 months is playful; he may pat an image of himself in a mirror. Soon he will wave "bye-bye" and respond appropriately to several words.

Fig 106

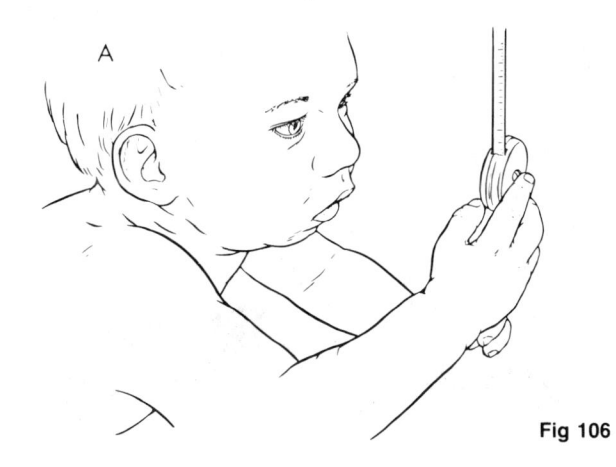

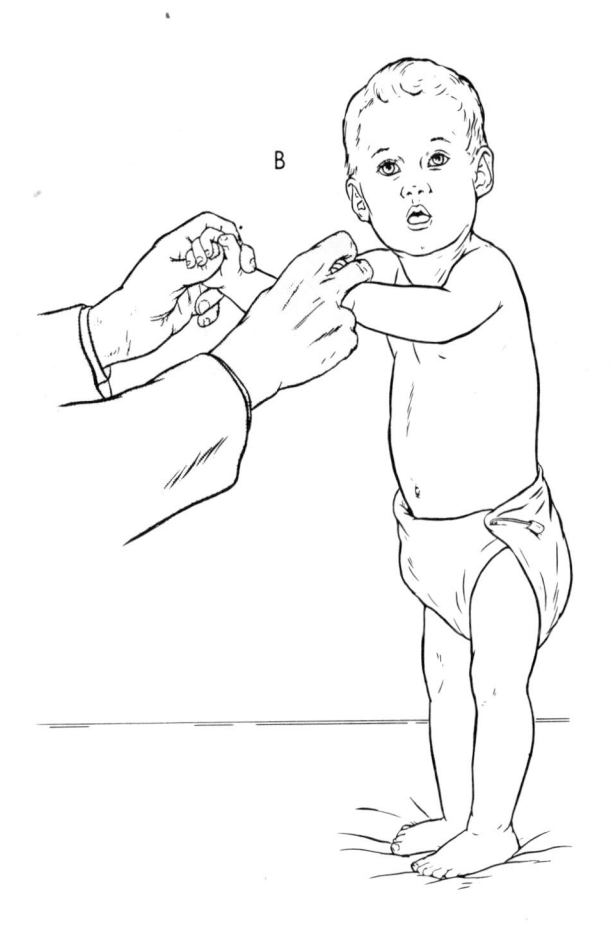

Infant Examination at Nine Months / 169

At 1 year, the normal child will often take steps alone if one hand is held (Fig 107). Independent walking usually develops between 12 and 15 months of age but may occur earlier. The year-old child will hand objects to the examiner, pick up a series of objects, and drop them in a container. He may show interest in pictures and will play games, such as pulling a blanket over his head. A word or two may be spoken at 12 months, several words at 15 months. By 1 year of age most children will assist in dressing themselves by holding out an arm for the coat sleeve or elevating a foot for the shoe. They do not yet have bladder control, nor are many able to manage a spoon effectively enough to feed themselves.

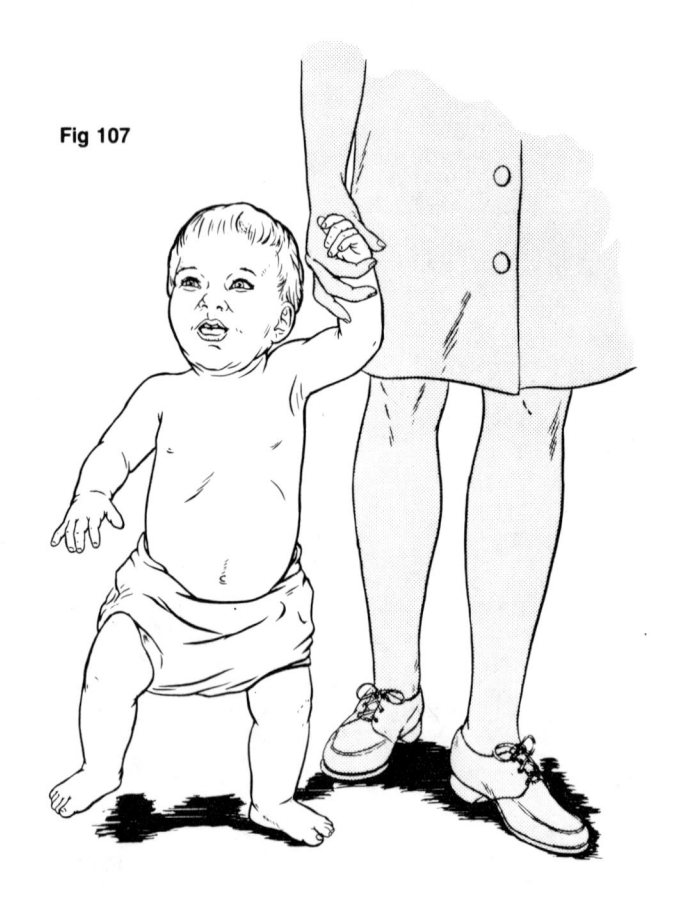

Fig 107

Examination and Measurement of the Head

Physical examinations of infants should always include measurement of head circumference. Measure from a point just above the supraorbital ridges to the farthest point in the occipital region (Fig 108). The largest circumference that can be obtained, using a centimeter tape, is recorded.

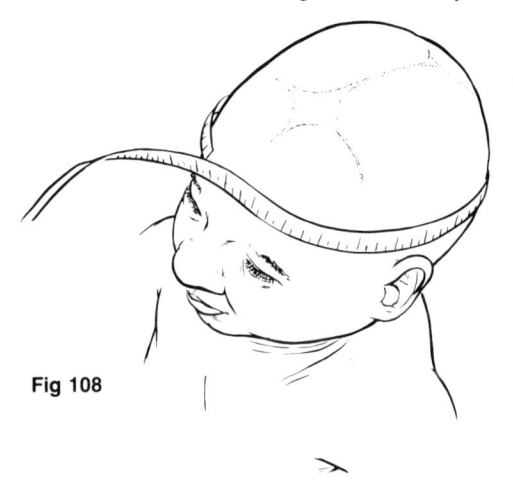

Fig 108

Fig 109

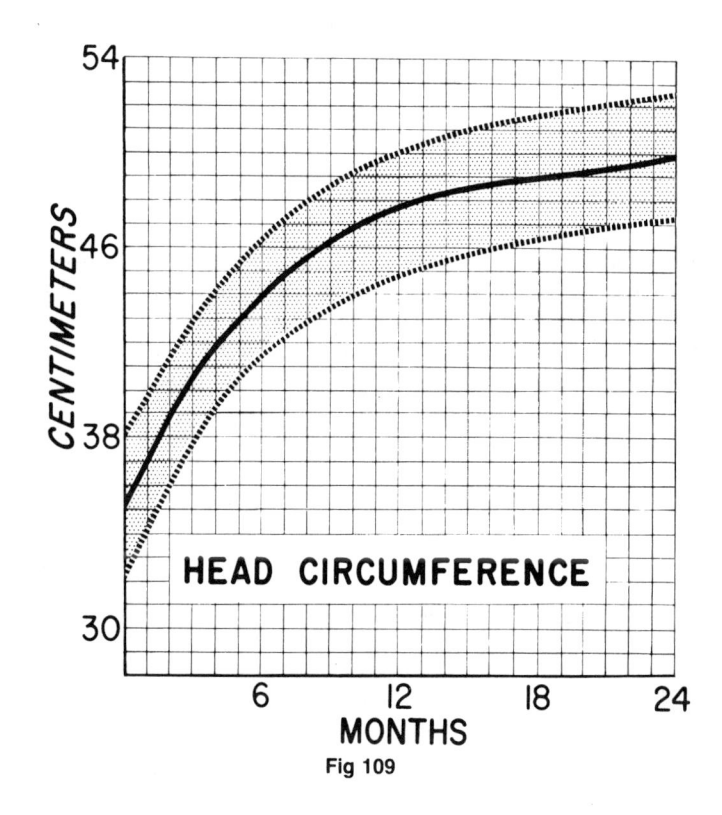

The circumference of the head should be greater than that of the chest for the first 6 months, but thereafter the chest circumference is the larger of the two. Plot the measurement on a chart as illustrated in Figure 109. This chart shows the normal range of circumference for a given age as well as the normal range of rate of growth. Serial measurements at different ages are more meaningful than a single determination. The rate of head growth is a reflection of growth or enlargement of the intracranial contents. An abnormally rapid rate of enlargement may occur with subdural hematoma or effusion, infantile hydrocephalus, or intracranial tumor. Abnormal delay in head growth signifies retarded growth of the brain. Universal premature closure of cranial sutures also may result in an abnormally small head.

Observation and palpation of the infant's head may yield additional information. Parietal cephalohematomas may distort the shape of the head. Premature suture synostosis usually results in characteristic deformities in the head shape, depending on the sutures involved. A palpable bony ridge may be felt in the region of the fused suture. Premature infants usually have a rather long and narrow head that appears disproportionately large for the rest of the body.

The anterior fontanelle should be palpated with the infant relaxed and placed in the sitting or upright position. The anterior fontanelle is palpably open until 15 to 18 months of age and serves as an index of intracranial pressure. A depressed or sunken fontanelle occurs with dehydration. A bulging or tense fontanelle indicates increased intracranial pressure. The anterior fontanelle fails to close when it should in conditions associated with increased pressure and in certain skeletal disorders, such as cleidocranial dysostosis, hypothyroidism, and hypophosphatasia.

Transillumination of the skull with a bright light is another technique that should be part of the physical examination of infants. Abnormal translucence will be found locally or generally wherever the cerebral mantle is severely thinned or absent or wherever there is a collection of fluid of a density that allows transmission of light—as in cases of advanced hydrocephalus, hydranencephaly, and subdural effusions. Such translucence is not found in acute subdural hematomas.

Laboratory Neurodiagnostic Aids

Electrophysiologic testing and neuroimaging procedures are important means of supplementing the clinical and anatomic formulation derived from a careful neurologic examination of the patient. In many instances, the clinical examination will have already established the anatomic location of a suspected lesion or the precise nature of the physiologic dysfunction resulting in the patient's symptoms. In these instances, neurodiagnostic procedures merely serve to confirm what the astute clinician already knows. In addition to this function, these tests can add an element of quantification to the clinician's findings. This can be extremely valuable in gauging improvement or decline in the patient's future course. For example, a neuroradiologic procedure can establish the actual size of a lesion for future comparison, or a neurophysiologic procedure such as nerve conduction velocity testing can establish the degree of conduction slowing to be used as a baseline for future comparison. Of equal importance is the fact that modern neurodiagnostic tests are often so sensitive that they reveal abnormalities of the nervous system that have not yet produced clinically apparent signs or symptoms. Clearly, neurodiagnostic tests can be a valuable *adjunct*, but it must be remembered that their interpretation is difficult in the absence of reliable data generated from a careful neurologic history and examination.

Electrophysiologic Tests

EEG.—Although classically used as a means of evaluating seizure disorders, the EEG has many other uses. It is used to aid the diagnosis and management of metabolic encephalopathy, mass lesions of the brain, and certain acute or chronic viral infections of the brain. It is also used to assess brain function during cerebrovascular surgery, to diagnose sleep disorders such as narcolepsy, and to help confirm brain death. The procedure carries virtually no serious risk. Typically, 20 electrodes are placed on the scalp covering both the right and left frontal, parietal, temporal, and occipital regions. After appropriate amplification and filtering, electrical activity originating in the cerebral cortex can be accurately recorded. This activity can be characterized according to its frequency (typically 8 to 13 cps and rhythmic in the awake patient in the occipital region, and slightly faster anteriorly), its amplitude (about 40 to 60 μV), and the morphology of the individual brain waves. Also, asymmetry in the activity recorded from the two hemispheres can be noted, as can any paroxysmal discharges that stand out against the ongoing background activity. A normal EEG is shown in Figure 110. Typical 10-cps posterior rhythm is seen on the first line and faster anterior activity on the fifth line.

The EEG is a critical part of the evaluation of seizures. It must be stressed, however, that seizures should be diagnosed on clinical grounds and not solely on the basis of an abnormal EEG, since approximately 10% of normal individuals have an EEG abnormality. Furthermore, patients with nonepileptic conditions such as migraine may also have abnormal EEGs. When there is clinical suspicion of seizures, the EEG can help confirm the diagnosis, identify the type of seizure, and determine the anatomic region in which seizure discharges are originating. In using the EEG for this purpose, it is important to remember that in patients with seizures the EEG may not be persistently abnormal in between seizures. Thus, a normal interictal EEG does not rule out a seizure disorder.

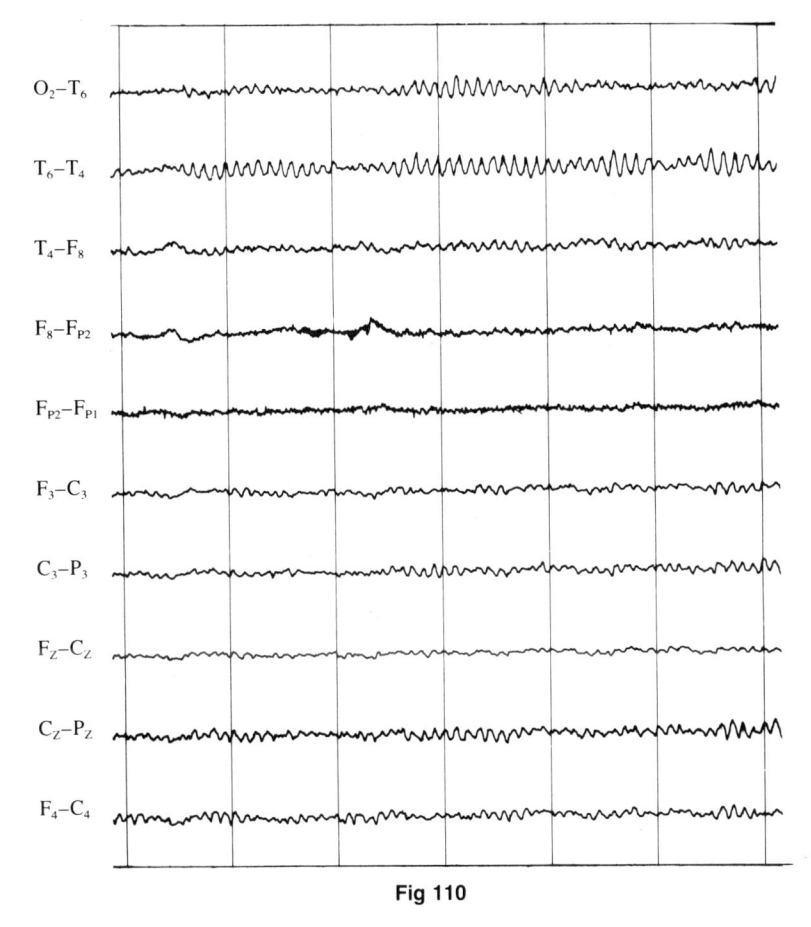

Several variations of the standard EEG technique are available to increase the likelihood of detecting an EEG abnormality. *Activation* techniques such as sleep, hyperventilation, or photic stimulation are often used. Also, specialized electrode placement can be employed. To enhance the detection of abnormalities arising from the medial surface of the temporal lobes, a common focus of abnormality in partial complex (psychomotor) epilepsy, electrodes are placed in the nasopharynx. Here, they are much closer to the involved portions of the temporal-lobe cortex than scalp electrodes and much more likely to detect abnormal discharges.

The 3-Hz spike-and-wave EEG abnormality typical of absence (petit mal) epilepsy is shown in Figure 111. In this case, the discharge contains waves that are slow and broad as well as those with a sharper configuration (spikes). This form of epilepsy is assumed to originate in deep midline structures of the brain, and the discharge is then projected to both hemispheres simultaneously. In focal epilepsy, abnormal discharges originate from a discrete area of the cerebral cortex and can be recorded best by

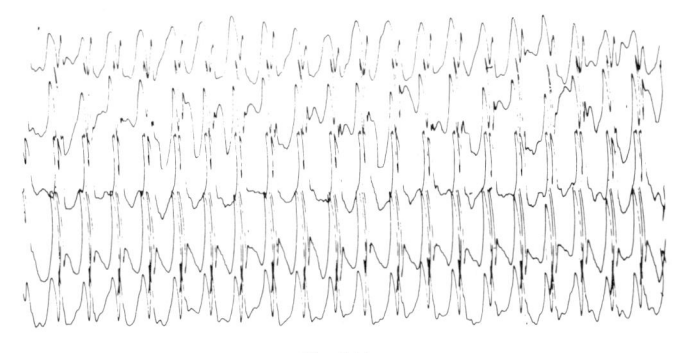

Fig 110

Fig 111

The EEG / 177

electrodes overlying that region. Sharp discharges arising in the *right temporal region* are shown in Figure 112. *(arrows)*. Such discharges can spread to involve adjacent regions of the brain and ultimately both hemispheres, resulting in a generalized seizure (p. 156).

The EEG is an imperfect guide to success in the treatment of epilepsy. The number and severity of clinical seizures is the most meaningful indication of the efficacy of treatment. However, in the treated patient, the presence of persistent epileptiform EEG activity, even in the absence of clinical seizures, is a valid reason to be very cautious about discontinuing or tapering antiepileptic drugs. Thus, an EEG is always performed before making this clinical decision.

The EEG is a critical component in the determination of cerebral death. A careful clinical evaluation of the patient and the circumstances, both medical and legal, surrounding the illness in question are essential to the intelligent interpretation and use of EEG data in this circumstance. In addition to the clinical demonstration of the absence of brain function, the legal definition of brain death in many jurisdictions requires the demonstration of cessation of critical physiologic activity such as cerebral blood flow or electrocerebral activity. The EEG determination of electrocerebral silence requires careful technique and expert interpretation. Considerations such as interelectrode distance, amplification of the EEG, and freedom from artifact are extremely important. In addition, before making an EEG diagnosis of brain death, the electroencephalographer must be certain that conditions capable of severely suppressing EEG activity, such as sedative intoxication or hypothermia, are not factors.

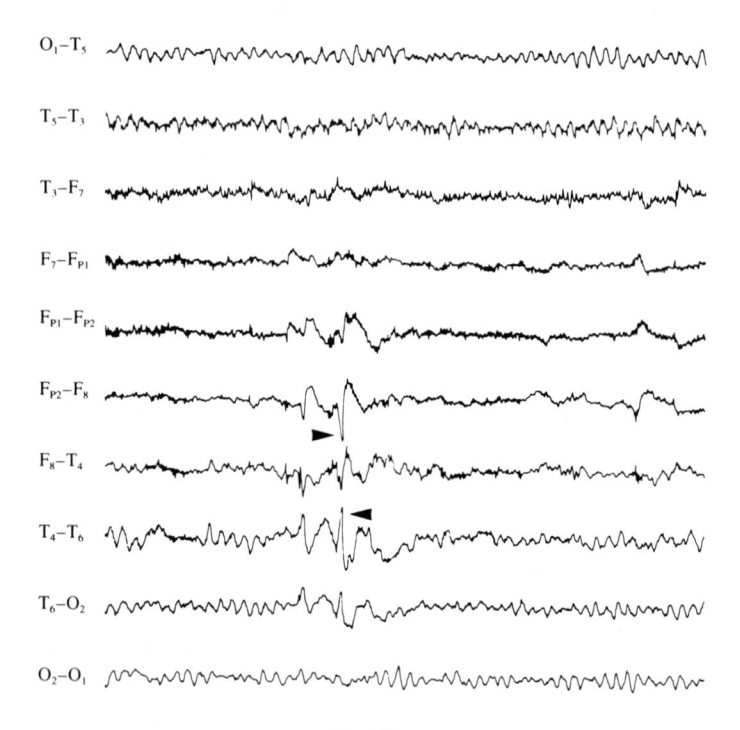

Fig 112

Intracerebral mass lesions such as tumor or abscess typically produce focal EEG abnormalities. Most often, a space-occupying lesion results in focal high-voltage waves that are much slower in frequency than the normal activity emanating from adjacent regions. Focal, slow EEG activity due to a brain tumor is illustrated in Figure 113 *(arrows)*. In truth, the EEG is seldom used to localize intrinsic mass lesions because modern noninvasive neuroimaging procedures can accomplish this so accurately. Yet, in some very early or slowly progressive neoplasms, focal EEG slowing, especially in the temporal region, may be present before imaging procedures become clearly abnormal. Lesions overlying the brain surface, such as subdural hematoma, not only cause focal slowing of EEG activity on the involved side but also suppression of the amplitude.

In toxic or metabolic encephalopathy, the EEG usually shows diffuse slowing, the severity of which parallels the clinical course. In this case, the EEG is a useful adjunct in objectifying clinical improvement or deterioration. The use of EEG in the evaluation of sleep disorders is based on the fact that each of the stages of sleep is characterized by a specific EEG pattern. The EEG can therefore be used to determine whether a patient is asleep at a given time and to plot the sequential stages of sleep. Correlating these data with the patient's sleep symptoms allows accurate diagnosis of conditions such as sleep apnea or narcolepsy.

Evoked Potentials.—Evoked potentials are useful in documenting subtle physiologic dysfunction in the visual, somatosensory, or auditory systems. The basic principle of each is similar: a sensory stimulus is delivered repetitively and the electrical activity it evokes in the nervous system is recorded at specified points en route to the cerebral cortex. Because the evoked electric response to each stimulus is so small, com-

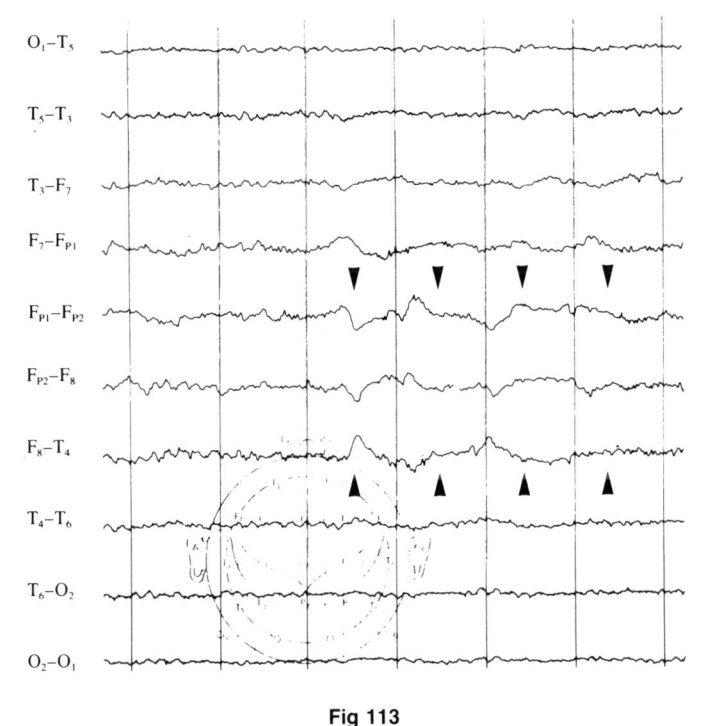

Fig 113

puterized averaging is employed to cancel out the random background EEG "noise" of the brain and summate the consistently occurring stimulus-related evoked potential. The final result is a series of upward and downward deflections called *waves* or *peaks*. Each wave or peak so recorded represents the electrical activity related to passage through or arrival at a specific anatomic way station as the evoked impulse travels to the cortex. By measuring the time required to arrive at each of these points and to travel between them, conduction through a sensory pathway can be assessed. One of the most important features of evoked potential testing is the ability to detect subtle abnormalities in the visual, auditory, or somatosensory systems *before* they produce clinical signs or symptoms, or *after* clinical signs or symptoms have improved and apparently disappeared.

Somatosensory evoked potentials (SEPs) are useful in identifying a lesion anywhere along the somatosensory pathway from the peripheral nerve to the cerebral cortex. An electric stimulus of the median or tibial nerve is typically used. Because a specific wave is produced as the proximally traveling evoked impulse traverses different anatomic points, SEPs can be useful in identifying peripheral nerve, plexus, spinal cord, brain-stem, and hemisphere lesions in the somatosensory pathway. In addition to helping localize lesions along the somatosensory pathway, SEPs can also be used in conditions such as multiple sclerosis to establish the extent of central nervous system involvement by demonstrating clinically silent lesions. The SEPs are sometimes used in evaluating suspected hysterical sensory loss or anesthesia, since some abnormality would be expected in the face of such symptoms. This is especially true if sensory loss involves vibration and joint position since the SEP largely reflects conduction in large fibers carrying these modalities. In Figure 114 the several waves found in a normal SEP recording are shown. The letters N and P refer to negative and positive polarity and the numbers to the latency of the wave in milliseconds.

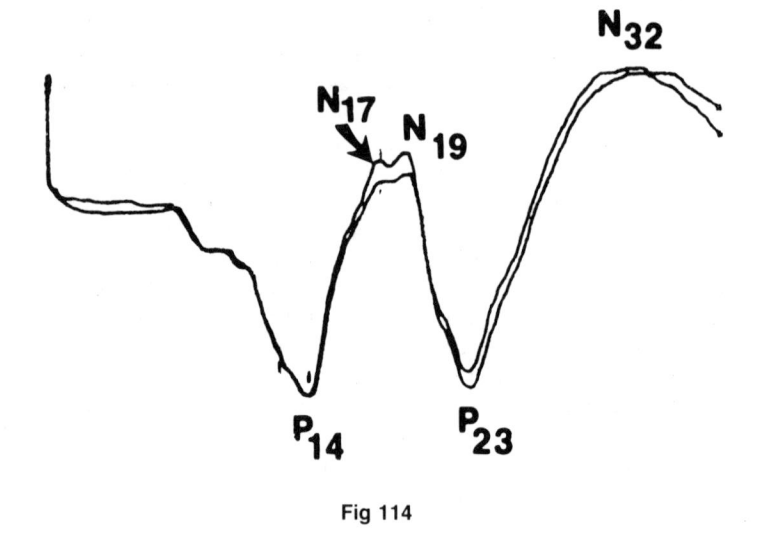

Fig 114

180 / *Somatosensory Evoked Potentials*

Brain-stem auditory evoked potentials (BAEPs) are used to assess conduction in the auditory nerve and its brain-stem connections. Using repetitive clicks as the stimulus, a series of 5 peaks can be recorded from scalp electrodes (Fig 115). These peaks are generated in the acoustic nerve and at several points in the brain-stem auditory pathways and then instantaneously conducted through the perfect electric conduction medium of the brain to recording electrodes on the scalp. Because the peaks

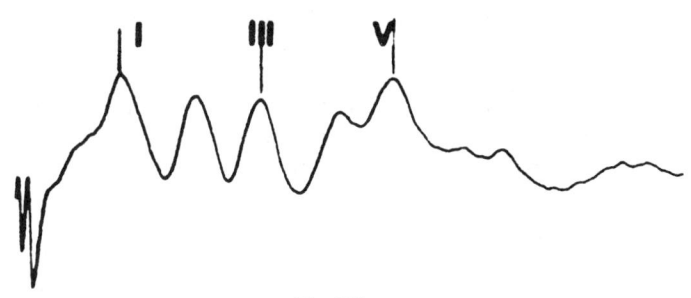

Fig 115

are recorded a great distance from their actual points of origin, they are referred to as *far field potentials*. The first peak is generated in the acoustic nerve, and its absence or delay is a good indication of dysfunction in this structure. The exact brain-stem structures responsible for generating each of the other four peaks are still not totally clear. Despite this limitation, the fact that the auditory pathways traverse a significant extent of the brain stem makes the BAEP a useful tool for identifying brain-stem damage or dysfunction in a general way, irrespective of whether auditory symptoms are present. In comatose patients or patients with severe closed-head trauma, for example, BAEP testing can help determine whether there is brain-stem involvement. In the presence of brain-stem pathology, one or more brain-stem-generated peaks are absent or there is a prolonged delay between peaks. Figure 116 shows an abnormal delay between the third and fifth peaks, indicating slowed conduction through the abnormal area. Like other types of evoked potential testing, BAEP can be used to identify subtle central nervous system involvement in suspected cases of multiple sclerosis.

Visual evoked potentials (VEPs) are used to test the visual pathways, particularly the optic nerves. Unlike some of the other forms of evoked potential testing, only a single wave is evaluated, the major positive wave occurring at approximately 100 msec after the stimulus (P_{100}). Both the amplitude and latency of this wave can be measured, a typical abnormality consisting of a delayed or absent response. Each eye is stimulated separately, and the latency and amplitude of the response on each side can be compared. An abnormality of the P_{100} wave is generally taken to

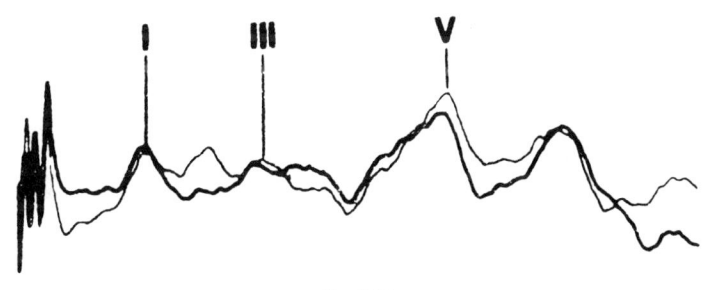

Fig 116

reflect a disturbance of function in the optic nerve on the side of stimulation. Figure 117 shows a normal VEP and a recording in optic neuritis. The P_{100} (*arrow*) on the right side (*OD*) is delayed compared with the left side (*OS*) suggesting right optic nerve dysfunction.

An important aspect of the VEP is its sensitivity to minimal pathology. This fact makes it extremely useful in looking for evidence of clinically inapparent demyelination of the optic nerve in multiple sclerosis. In optic neuritis, the VEP often remains abnormal even after clinical symptoms have resolved and vision has returned to normal.

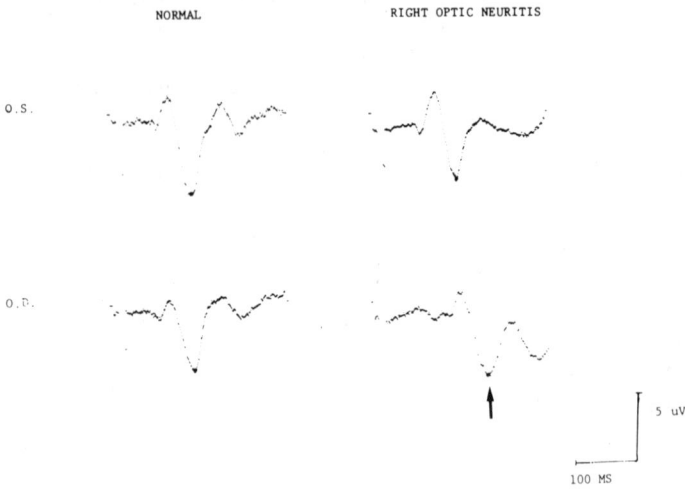

Fig 117

Nerve Conduction Studies.—Disorders of peripheral nerve are typically accompanied by clinical signs such as sensory loss, muscle weakness and atrophy, trophic skin and hair changes, and loss of stretch reflexes (p. 128). These signs result from nerve fibers having degenerated entirely and left their target organs (skin, muscle) denervated, or from abnormal conduction in diseased but anatomically intact nerve fibers. Nerve conduction studies provide a means of demonstrating conduction slowing or blockage. This helps establish which nerves are affected and identifies the point of involvement along the course of the involved nerves.

Nerve conduction velocity testing is based on the principle that an electric stimulus applied to a nerve through the skin initiates a self-propagating impulse that travels in both directions away from the point of stimulation. In a sensory nerve, the time of arrival of the impulse at a point distant from the stimulation site can be established by a pair of recording electrodes overlying the nerve at that point. When studying a motor nerve, electrodes are placed over a muscle it innervates, and the arrival of the nerve impulse is determined by the onset of muscle excitation. The time to muscle excitation from two different nerve stimulation points is determined, allowing calculation of the time required for the impulse to travel over the nerve between the two stimulation points. In both cases, the time required to travel a measured distance in a nerve is determined. The values determined in the way, i.e., conduction velocities, are compared with average values derived from a normal population. Nerve conduction velocity can only be determined in nerves that are accessible to stimulation through the skin. The nerves that are most commonly studied are the median, ulnar, and radial in the upper extremity and the peroneal, tibial, and sural in the lower extremity.

Nerve conduction velocity studies can help confirm the presence of peripheral nerve disease, provide some quantification of the severity of the disorder, determine whether the axon or the myelin sheath of the nerve are affected, and establish whether motor or sensory nerves or both are involved. Slowing of conduction velocity in either motor or sensory nerves is indicative of neuropathy. Because of the importance of the myelin sheath in rapid impulse conduction, demyelinating neuropathies (e.g., Guillain-Barré syndrome) result in very slow conduction velocity (less than 60% of the mean normal), whereas neuropathies that primarily effect the nerve axon (e.g., arsenic neuropathy) produce less prominent conduction slowing.

Nerve conduction studies are also useful in evaluating compressive or traumatic lesions of a single nerve. In this case, conduction velocities are found to be relatively normal proximal to the site of compression or trauma and either slowed across the point of involvement or totally blocked at that level. Common examples include the slowing of ulnar nerve conduction that occurs across the elbow in tardy ulnar palsy (see p. 132), and carpal tunnel syndrome with median nerve slowing across the wrist (p. 133).

Disorders affecting the most proximal segment of a peripheral nerve cannot be evaluated using standard nerve conduction techniques since recording and stimulating electrodes can only be placed on the extremities over a distal portion of the nerve. Two special techniques, the *F wave* and the *H-reflex*, allow the proximal segment of a nerve to be evaluated also. Both techniques depend on the fact that transcutaneous nerve stimulation initiates not only an impulse that travels distally in the extremity but also one that travels proximally to the spinal cord. In a motor nerve fiber this antidromic impulse arrives at the motor neuron cell body in the spinal cord and causes it to discharge, sending a recurrent impulse back toward the periphery and inducing a late muscle response called the F wave. The time required for the F wave to appear at recording electrodes in the originally stimulated extremity is therefore a reflection of the speed of conduction through the entire length of the nerve, including the most proximal portion, the spinal root. F-wave studies are sensitive to mild abnormalities of the peripheral nerve. The test is particularly useful in identifying abnormalities confined to the spinal roots, as may be the case in the early phases of Guillain-Barré syndrome.

The H-reflex is also elicited by stimulating the distal portion of a peripheral nerve. In this case, the sensory fibers of the stimulated nerve, specifically the group 1A fibers originating in stretch receptors of the muscle, carry the impulse back to the spinal cord, where, after a single synapse, motor neurons are excited, resulting in a peripherally directed impulse in the motor nerve. The time of arrival of this impulse in an extremity muscle is determined with a pair of surface electrodes on the muscle. The H-reflex is identical to the stretch reflex produced by tapping a tendon, except that the afferent impulse to the spinal cord is produced by an electric stimulation of the nerve rather than by a mechanical stimulation of stretch receptors. It is usually obtained by stimulating the tibial nerve and recording over the soleus muscle. In this circumstance, its absence or delay on one side suggests dysfunction of the first sacral spinal root. In a herniated disc involving this root, an abnormal H-reflex can be a sensitive and objective adjunct to the typical reflex, motor, and sensory findings.

The *blink reflex* is a means of assessing the facial and trigeminal nerves as well as their brain-stem connections. Electric stimulation of a branch of the trigeminal nerve near the eyebrow in the supraorbital notch initiates an impulse conducted centrally to the pons, where, after several synapses, there is a reflex response that travels through the facial nerve back to the orbicularis oculi muscle of the eyelid. The induced reflex contraction of the orbicularis muscle results in a visible blink. The actual time required for the impulse to travel to the pons and back to the eyelid is determined by a pair of electrodes on the eyelid that record the onset of the blink. An abnormality in either the trigeminal or facial nerve or their brain-stem connections can be detected by noting an absent or delayed blink reflex. Evaluation of disorders of these two cranial nerves is the most common use of the blink reflex. It is also useful in detecting brain-stem involvement in multiple sclerosis.

Electromyography.—Electromyography involves the recording of electric activity from muscle through a needle electrode placed directly through the skin. Most skeletal muscles can be easily reached using needle electrodes of varying lengths. The electric activity recorded is displayed on an oscilloscope screen, where it appears in characteristic wave-forms that are easily identified by an experienced electromyographer. The procedure is only slightly painful for those with an average pain threshold, but a small percentage of patients may have an aversion to needles. The purpose of electromyography is to detect evidence of dystrophic, metabolic, or inflammatory diseases of muscle, abnormalities of the muscle membrane, or evidence of muscle denervation. Electromyography therefore not only helps diagnose primary disorders of muscle but can also indirectly suggest abnormalities of the lower motor neuron.

Once the needle electrode is in place, recordings are made under three conditions: while the muscle is at rest, while it is being minimally contracted, and during strong contraction. In normal muscle, there is no activity at rest. In abnormal muscle, resting discharges may appear and usually take the form of fibrillations (Fig 118, *arrows*) or positive sharp

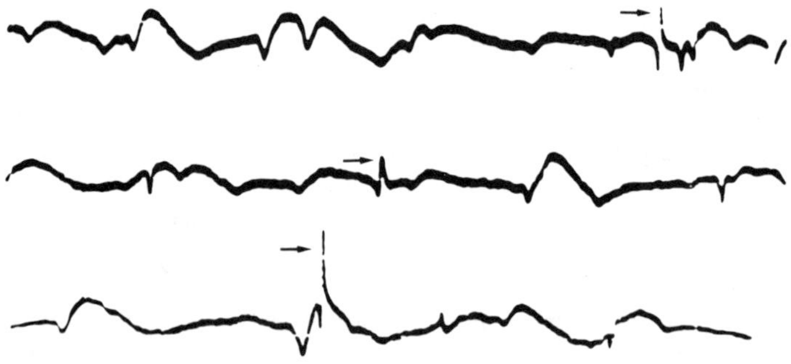

Fig 118

waves (Fig 119). Both are typically seen in muscle that has been denervated as a result of pathology of the lower motor neuron, such as motor neuron disease, axonal neuropathy, or traumatic nerve disruption. Occasionally, however, these spontaneous discharges can be seen in muscular dystrophy or myositis, presumably because involvement of the most distal portion of the nerve terminal within the diseased muscle effectively causes denervation.

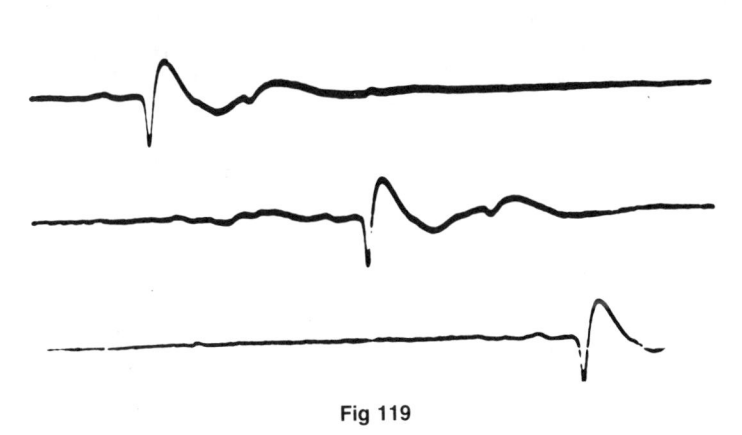

When a patient is asked to minimally contract the muscle being studied, a small number of motor neurons in the spinal cord discharge. All of the muscle fibers innervated by a single motor neuron discharge almost synchronously, and the sum of their electrical activity results in a typical triphasic wave, referred to as a motor unit action potential (Fig 120). The size and configuration of the motor unit potential provides a considerable amount of information about the muscle and its innervation. In

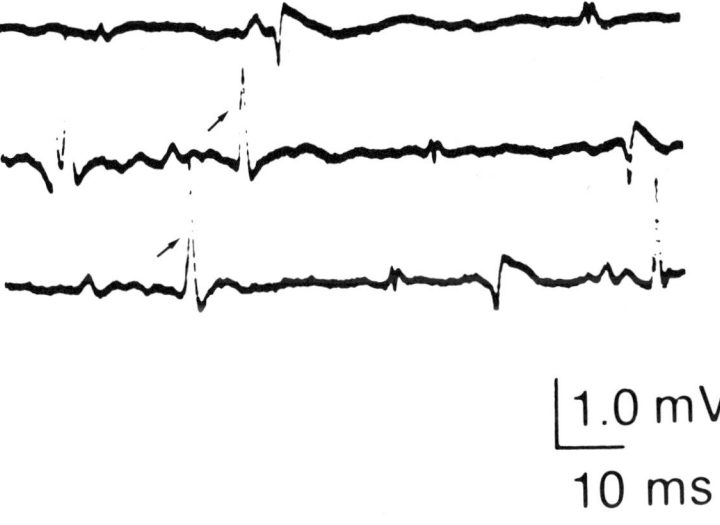

Fig 119

Fig 120

1.0 mV
10 ms

Electromyography / **185**

denervating disorders, surviving nerves sprout new branches to reinnervate once-denervated muscle fibers. This results in high-amplitude, long-duration motor unit potentials that are polyphasic rather than triphasic (Fig 121). On the other hand, in primary diseases of muscle such as muscular dystrophy, individual muscle fibers may degenerate, reducing the number of muscle fibers in each motor unit and producing a low-amplitude, short-duration motor unit potential with increased polyphasicity (Fig 122).

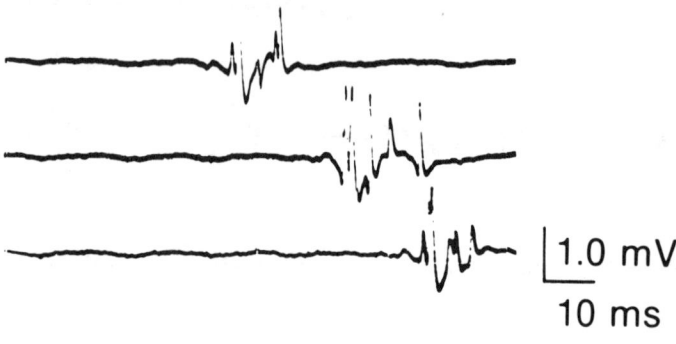

Fig 121

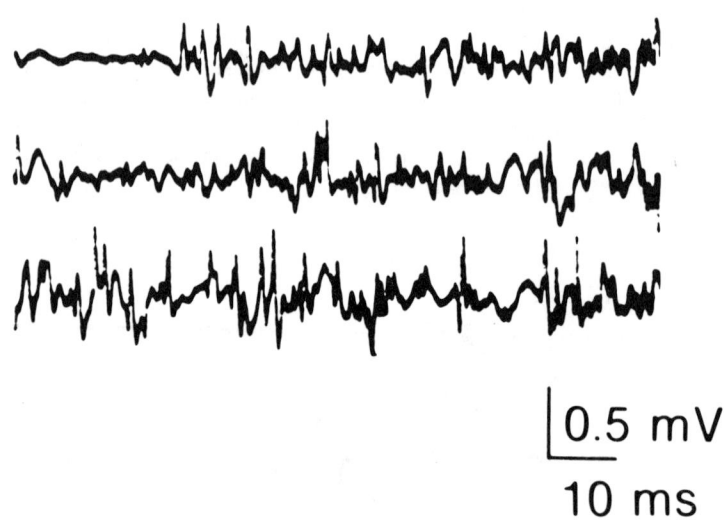

Fig 122

186 / *Electromyography*

When a muscle is contracted maximally, a large number of motor units are recruited for the effort, and the oscilloscope screen is filled with overlapping motor unit potentials (Fig 123) known as an interference pattern. In disorders of the lower motor neuron, fewer motor units remain and the interference pattern is sparse but of greater amplitude (Fig 124).

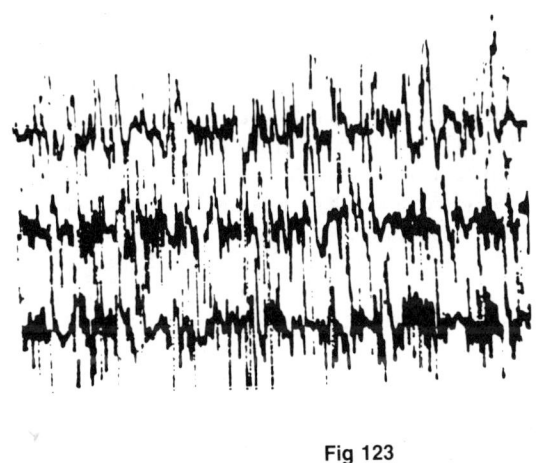

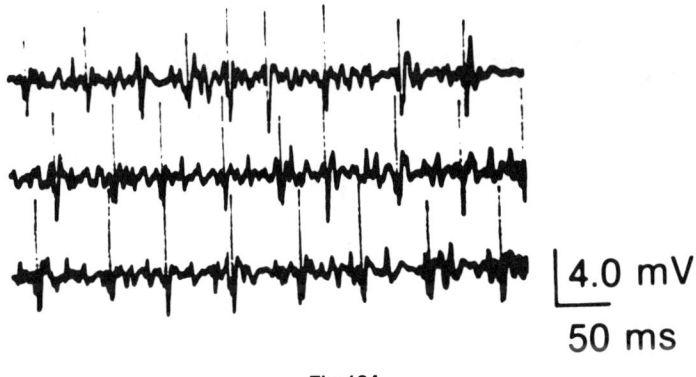

Fig 123

Fig 124

Fig 125

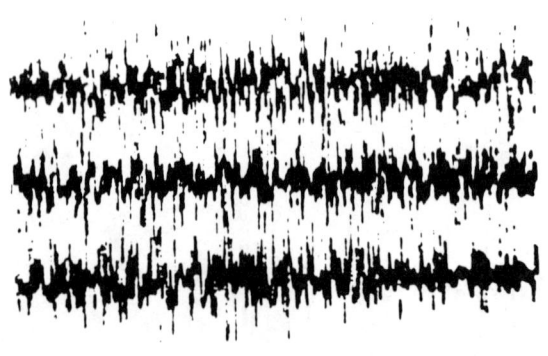

0.5 mV
50 ms

In primary muscle disorders, the interference pattern is smaller in amplitude (Fig 125) and produced much earlier in the course of a mild or moderate contraction. This later phenomenon is referred to as early recruitment.

Myotonic discharges are another abnormality that can be detected on electromyographic examination. True myotonic discharges are rapid, repetitive discharges seen in conditions characterized by clinical myotonia, such as myotonic dystrophy, myotonia congenita, and hyperkalemic periodic paralysis. When processed through a loudspeaker, the audio representation of myotonic discharges has a typical waxing and waning sound resembling that of a World War II dive-bomber or a modern motorcycle.

Fasciculations can also be detected by electromyography. Fasciculations are the spontaneous contraction of a group of muscle fibers innervated by a single motor nerve. They can be appreciated clinically as a brief muscle twitch under the skin, unlike fibrillations, an electromyographic finding (see above) that has no clinical correlate. Fasciculations are often, but not invariably, associated with denervating diseases, whereas fibrillations are always abnormal.

Repetitive Stimulation Studies.—Repetitive stimulation studies assess neuromuscular transmission. They are most commonly used in myasthenia gravis but are also helpful in the myasthenic syndrome (Lambert-Eaton syndrome) and in botulism. In this test, a nerve is stimulated repetitively at a specified frequency and the size of the evoked response in a muscle it innervates is recorded. In myasthenia gravis, it is important to choose a muscle that is clinically affected and easily studied. The median nerve and abductor pollicis brevis is a commonly used nerve-muscle combination for this purpose. If the hand muscles are clinically unaffected, however, the trapezius, deltoid, or facial muscles might be studied. In normal subjects, nerve stimulation at the rate of three per second produces an evoked muscle potential of consistent size (Fig 126). In myasthenia gravis, neuromuscular transmission gradually fails with repetitive stimulation at this rate, resulting in progressively smaller evoked potentials (Fig 127). A decrement of greater than 10% between the first and fifth evoked muscle responses suggests the diagnosis of myasthenia gravis. This electrophysiologic demonstration parallels the easy fatigability that myasthenic patients note with repetitive motor tasks (see p. 144). Cholinesterase inhibitors, such as pyridostigmine (Mestinon), may improve or totally reverse the electrophysiologic abnormalities of myasthenia gravis, so if at all possible, testing should not be carried out with the patient under anticholinesterase therapy.

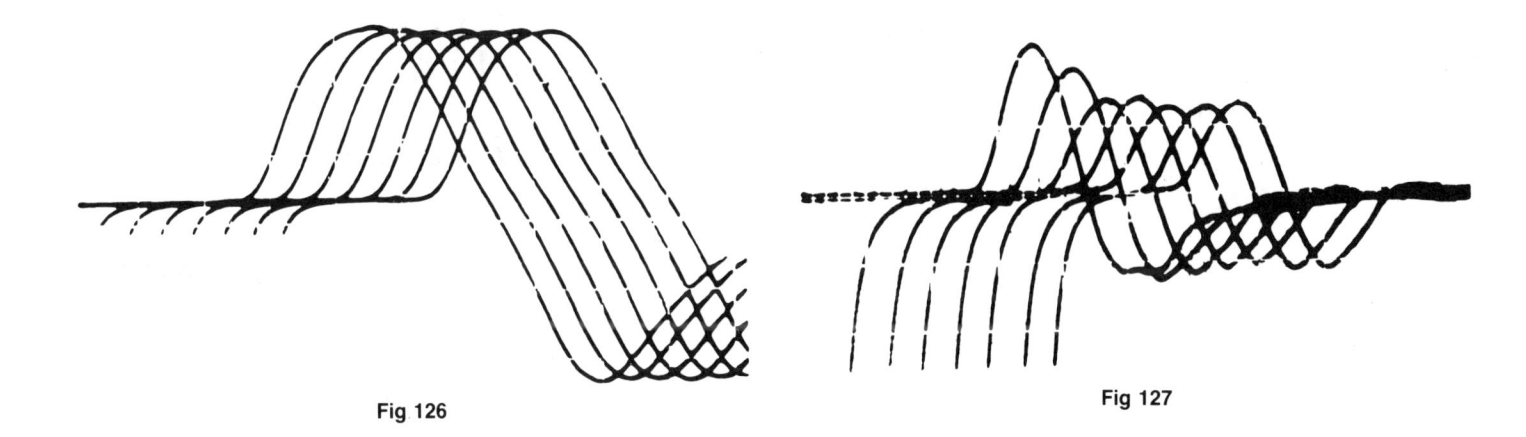

Fig 126

Fig 127

Repetitive Stimulation Studies / **189**

Single-fiber electromyography is another way of demonstrating abnormal neuromuscular transmission in myasthenia. It is a very sensitive and reliable test, but because of its technical complexity, it is not widely available.

In myasthenic (Lambert-Eaton) syndrome, repetitive stimulation studies reveal a very small first evoked muscle potential that *increases* in amplitude with repetitive stimulation at high rates (Fig 128). This is virtually the opposite of the decremental response seen in myasthenia and reflects the clinical observation that patients with this syndrome actually become stronger with repetitive efforts. In botulism, repetitive stimulation studies are similar to those in the myasthenic syndrome except that there is not quite as much facilitation with repetitive stimulation.

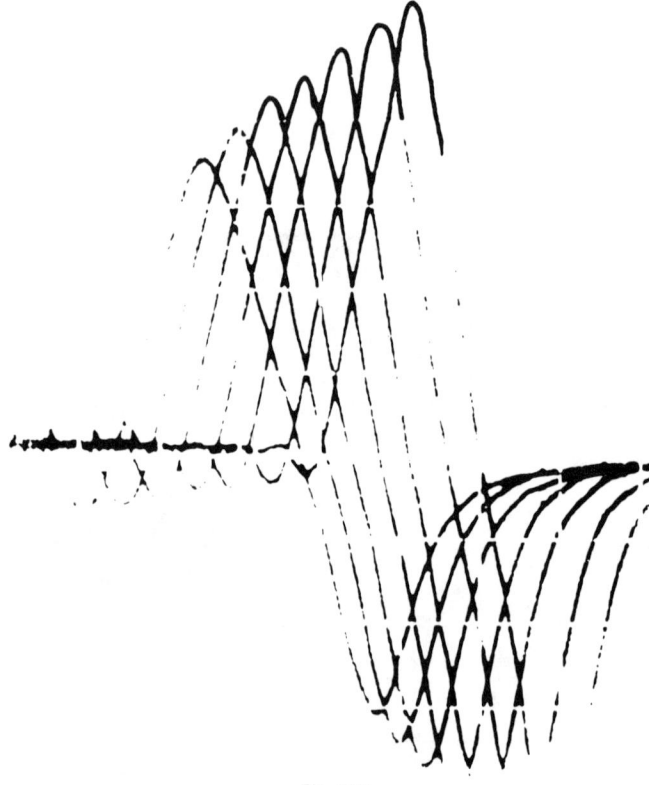

Fig 128

Neuroradiologic Tests of Skull and Brain

Skull Roentgenography.—Skull roentgenograms are used much less since the advent of more sophisticated neuroimaging techniques such as computed tomography (CT) or magnetic resonance imaging (MRI). Typically, routine skull roentgenograms consist of lateral, anteroposterior, posteroanterior, and basilar views. Depending on the area of specific interest, other specialized views are possible to show, in greater detail, the craniospinal junction, the foramen magnum, the optic foramina, the sella turcica, the orbits, or the internal auditory canals. Figure 129 is a normal lateral skull roentgenogram. Skull roentgenograms show only the bony cranium along with its foramina and fissures plus other densely calcified intracranial structures such as the normally calcified adult pineal gland. Pathologic structures, including some tumors, aneurysms, or vascular malformations, may become calcified and be seen as well. Skull roentgenograms are valuable in demonstrating conditions producing lytic or sclerotic changes in the skull, such as metastatic neoplasm or Paget's disease. Characteristic bony changes, particularly demineralization of the dorsum of the sella turcica, are seen in cases of chronically increased intracranial pressure. Local erosive or expansile bony changes are found

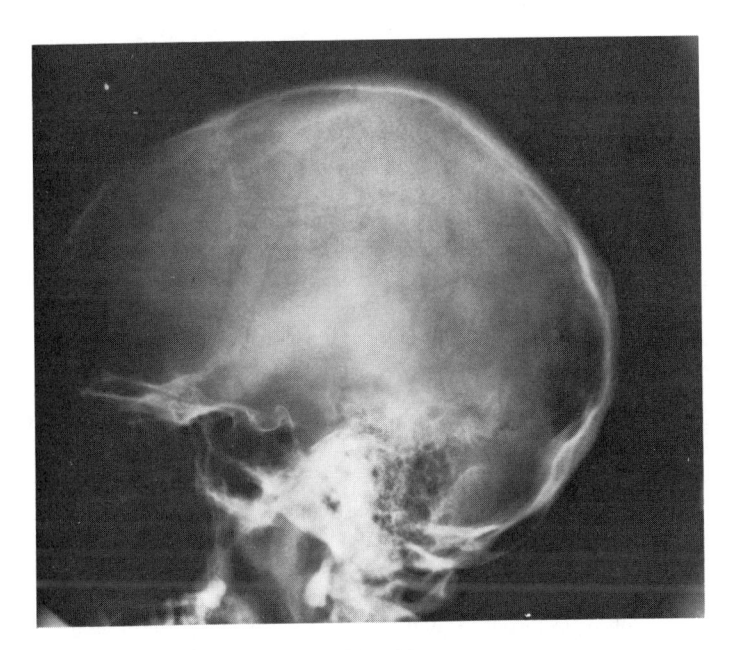

Fig 129

in the immediate vicinity of an expanding mass. For example, in Figure 130 the sella turcica has been enlarged by an expanding pituitary tumor (*arrows*). For uncalcified brain lesions not causing chronically increased intracranial pressure and not located in or adjacent to bone, the skull roentgenogram is usually not helpful. For identification of such lesions, CT, MRI, or cerebral angiography are usually required (see below).

In infancy and childhood some additional information can be gained from skull roentgenograms. Before suture closure, increased intracranial pressure can result in abnormal widening of the sutures. On the other hand, premature closure of the sutures can be detected by skull roentgenography (see p. 171), as can other developmental or congenital abnormalities of the cranial vault.

Skull roentgenograms are extremely important in the evaluation of cerebral trauma. They are particularly useful in identifying fractures of the skull.

Radionuclide Brain Scan.—The radionuclide (nuclear) brain scan, like the skull roentgenogram is used much less frequently than was the case before CT and MRI. By injecting a small amount of isotope (usually technetium 99) intravenously and then scanning the head to detect the passage of the isotope through the cerebral vasculature, several different types of clinical information can be obtained. The amount of isotope and its rate of passage in the right and left carotid arterial systems can be measured and compared. A delay in isotope arrival or decrease in total isotope passage on one side suggests the possibility of vascular stenosis or occulsion. Another situation in which a radionuclide cerebral blood flow study is used is in the determination of brain death. In this circum-

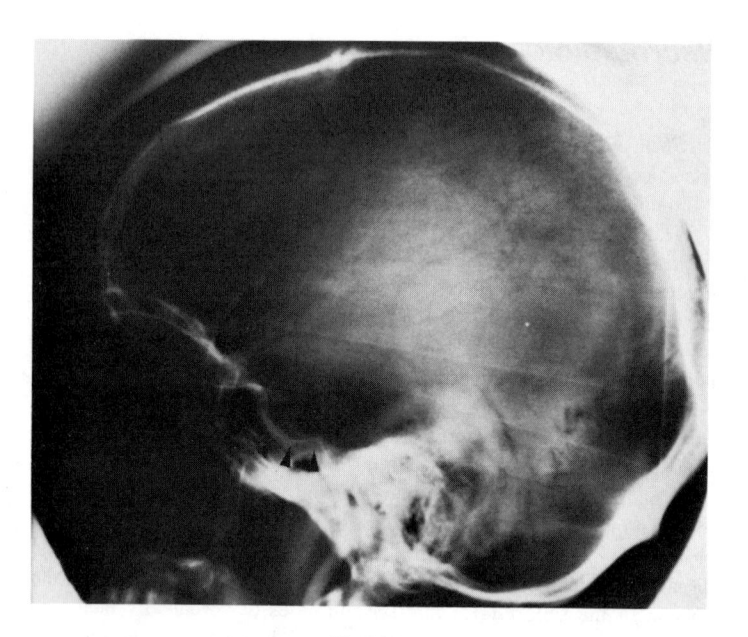

Fig 130

stance, a total absence of cerebral blood flow can be demonstrated.

The nuclear brain scan can also identify abnormalities of brain parenchyma in which there has been a breakdown of the blood-brain barrier. This includes abscess, tumor, focal encephalitis, or infarction. Here, the isotope concentrates in the abnormal area and is viewed as a "hot" spot on the scan. Again, CT or MRI are the preferred studies in such cases, but occasionally circumstances preclude the performance of either of these two imaging studies and the nuclear scan is used instead.

Typically, lateral, posteroanterior, and anteroposterior views are obtained. Figure 131 is a lateral brain scan depicting herpes simplex encephalitis of the temporal lobe.

Another procedure related to the brain scan is the isotope cisternogram. In this test, a small amount of isotope is injected into the lumbar subarachnoid space through a lumbar puncture needle. After a delay of several hours, the head is scanned to determine the distribution of the isotope in the cerebrospinal fluid circulating through the cerebral ventricles, basilar cisterns, and subarachnoid space overlying the surface of the brain. In normal-pressure hydrocephalus, a condition caused by obstruction of the cerebrospinal fluid absorptive pathways over the convexity of the brain, isotope-containing fluid can be visualized only within the ventricles and basilar cisterns.

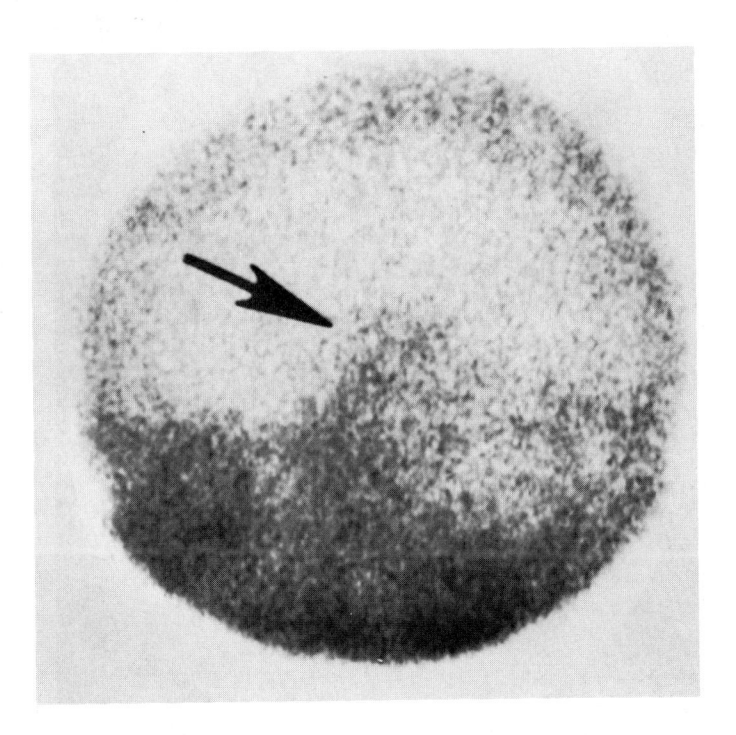

Radionuclide Brain Scan / 193

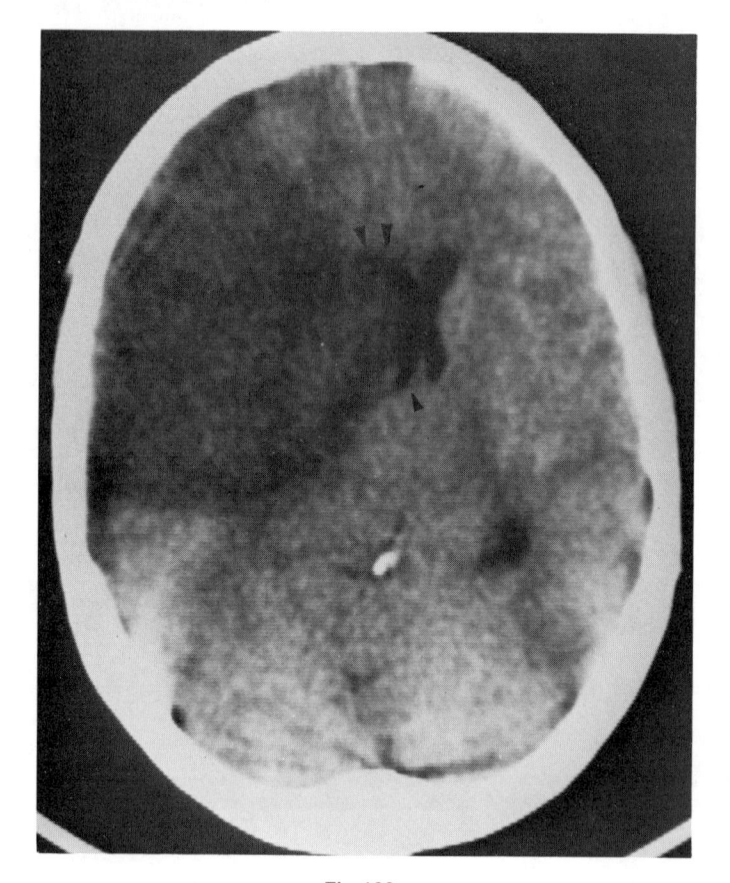

Fig 132

Fig 133

194 / *Computed Tomography of the Head*

CT of the Head.—Computed tomography of the head is capable of providing an image of the bones of the skull, the cerebral blood vessels, the cerebrospinal fluid-containing spaces, and the brain parenchyma. The images show the head in axial sections from the base of the skull to the vertex (see Fig 138). Abnormalities of the brain parenchyma often appear as an area of higher or lower density than the surrounding normal tissue. The CT scan allows a precise determination of the location and extent of intracranial pathology. In Figure 132 the low-density area corresponds to a recent cerebral infarction involving the perfusion territory of the middle cerebral artery. The ventricles (*arrows*) are compressed and displaced. In Figure 133 a glioblastoma is illustrated. Both can be compared with a normal CT scan (Fig 134).

Some forms of brain pathology, e.g., an infarction within a few hours of occurrence, may be *isodense* with surrounding brain and not be detectable. In such circumstances, *displacement* or *compression* of normal structures may be the only CT abnormality and help establish the diagnosis.

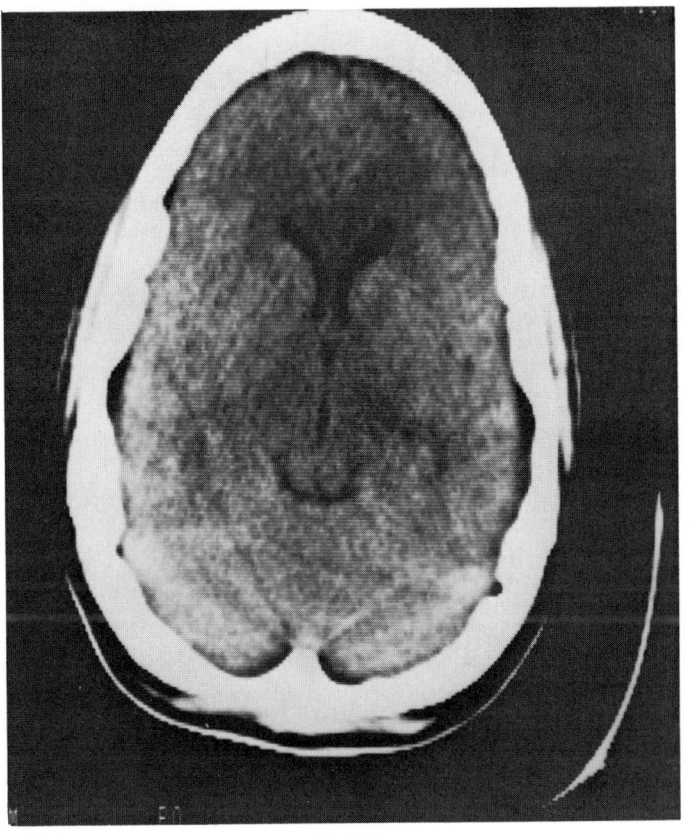

Fig 134

The intravenous injection of iodine-based contrast material often allows still more information to be obtained from a CT scan. The contrast concentrates in vascular structures, either normal or abnormal, and in areas where the blood-brain barrier has broken down. Figure 135 is a normal contrast-enhanced CT scan that illustrates the opacification of the blood vessels of the circle of Willis at the base of the brain. The basilar (*small arrow*), right and left middle cerebral (*triple arrows*), and posterior cerebral (*double arrows*), and the adjacent anterior cerebral anteries (*large arrow*) are shown. In Figure 136 an arteriovenous malformation has been opacified by intravenous contrast administration.

Fig 135

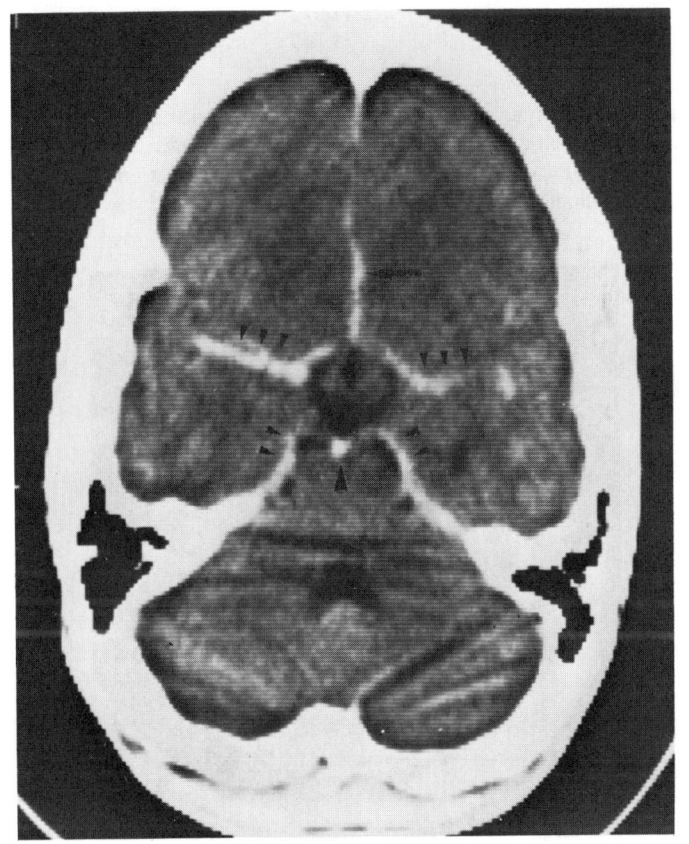

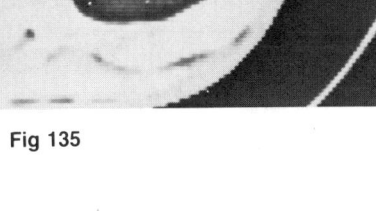

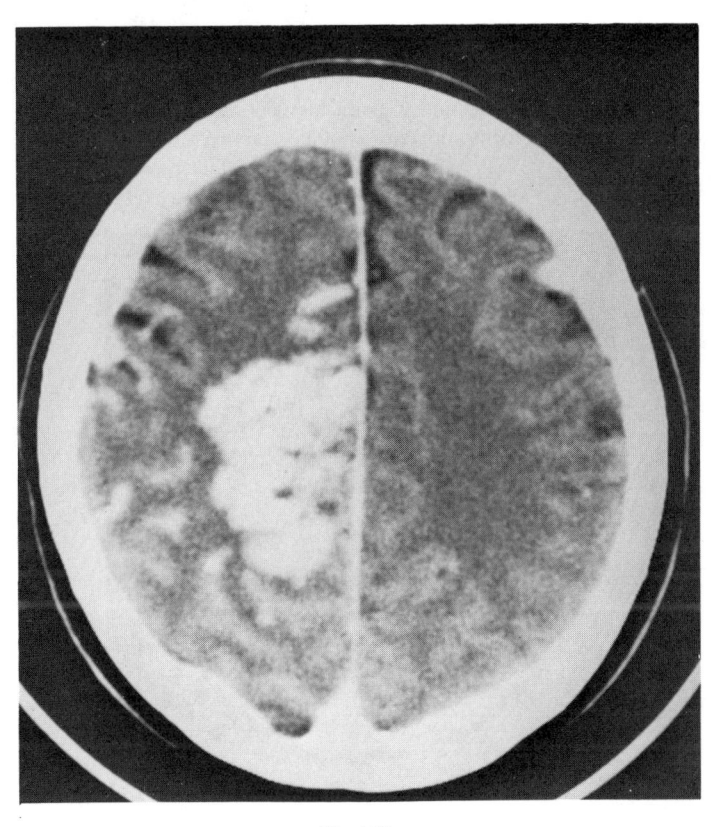

Fig 136

Computed Tomography of the Head / 197

Computed tomographic scanning is an effective means of detecting calcified intracranial structures. Calcification not sufficiently dense to be seen on plain skull roentgenograms is often seen easily on the CT scan. Normal structures, such as the pineal gland, the falx cerebri, and the chorid plexus, are often calcified and show up brilliantly on the unenhanced CT scan as a high (white) signal. Pathologic calcification, such as in the calcified meningioma shown in Figure 137,A, stands out as well. Because of the tumor's abnormal vascularity, it enhances after contrast administration (Fig 137,B).

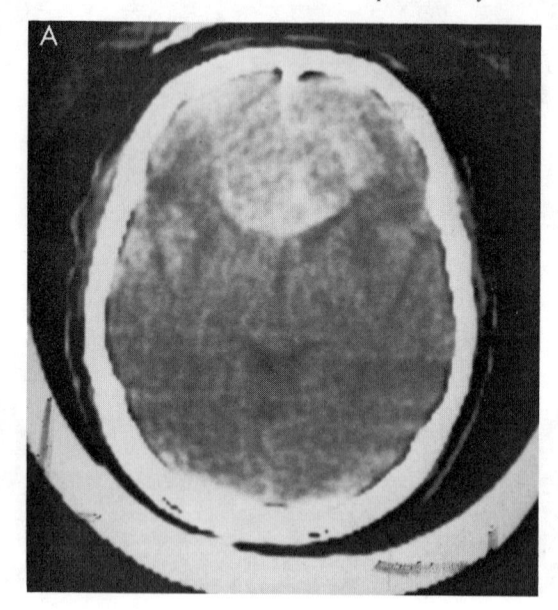

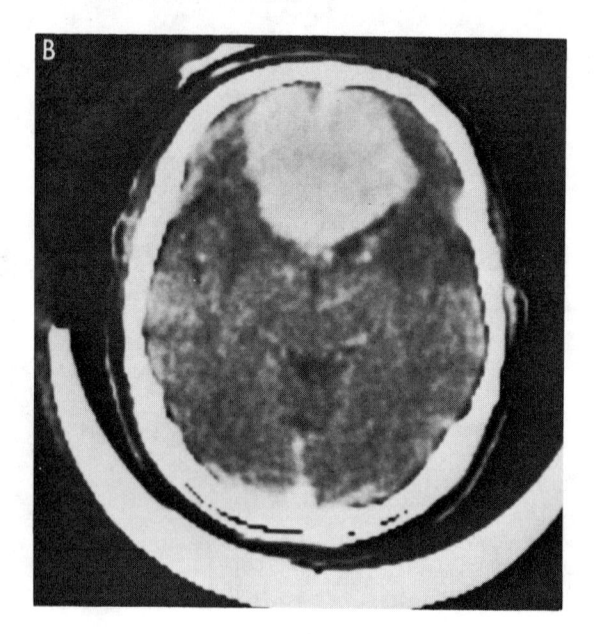

Fig 137

198 / Computed Tomography of the Head

Because CT demonstrates both the ventricles and the cortical sulci of the brain so well, it is an ideal way to detect hydrocephalus (Fig 138) or cortical atrophy (Fig 139).

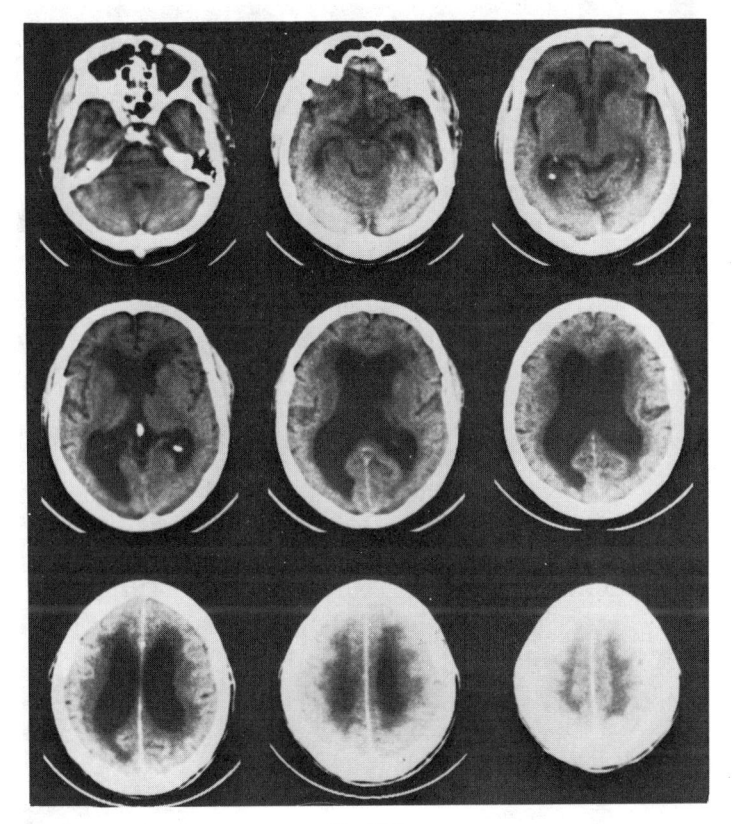

Fig 138

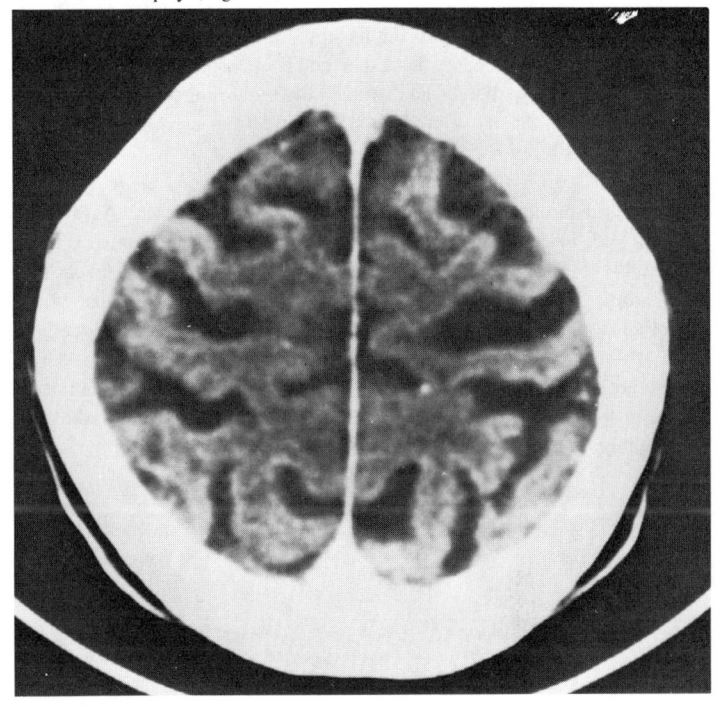

Fig 139

Computed Tomography of the Head / 199

The appearance of hemorrhage on a CT scan deserves special mention. Intraparenchymal or intraventricular blood takes on a high-density appearance. A hemorrhage into the basal ganglia is shown in Figure 140. When intracranial bleeding is suspected, it is customary to perform an *unenhanced* scan so there is no difficulty distinguishing the spontaneously appearing high-density abnormality of blood from a contrast-enhanced area of blood-brain barrier breakdown.

The CT scan is a discriminating, widely available procedure, but there are several circumstances in which it may be unreliable. As already mentioned, in cerebral infarction there may not be a detectable CT abnormality within the first 24 to 48 hours, sometimes longer. A subdural hematoma, in its subacute stage, may be isodense with normal brain, another potential pitfall of CT scanning. Because there is considerable CT artifact in areas of the brain adjacent to bone, scans of the posterior fossa are often seriously hampered by artifact resulting from the adjacent base of the skull. In each of these circumstances, other neuroradiologic procedures, such as angiography or MRI, may be more informative.

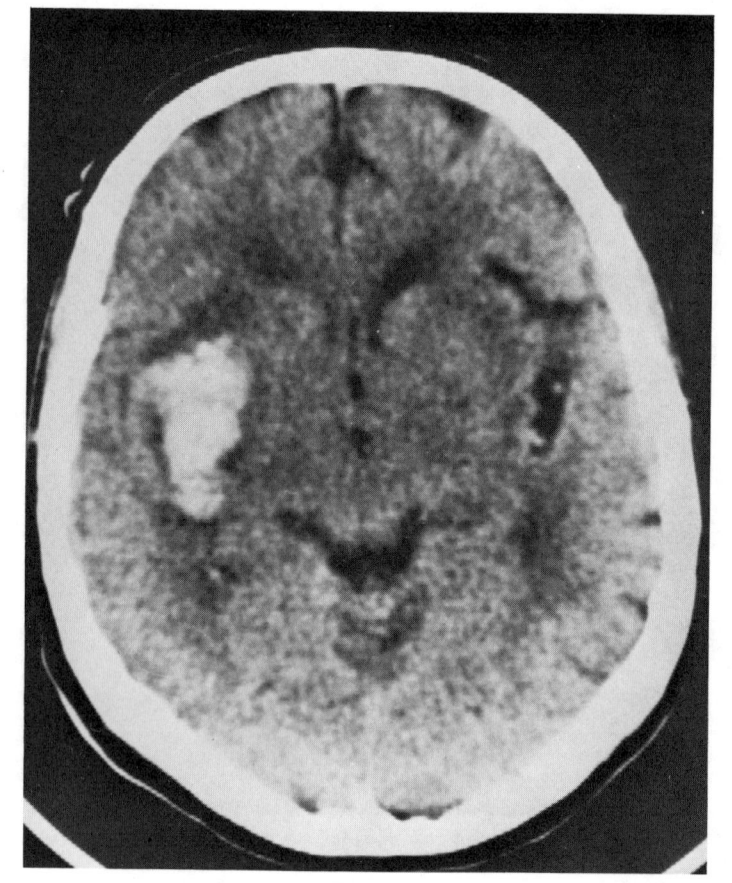

Fig 140

MRI of the Brain.—Magnetic resonance imaging is less widely available than CT. For imaging the brain, its advantages include the ability to show greater anatomic detail, better discrimination between white and gray matter, relative freedom from bone artifact, high sensitivity to cerebral edema, and the avoidance of intravenous iodinated contrast materials. In deciding whether to order an MRI, it is important to keep in mind that the patient must be able to tolerate being placed in a very confining space, which engenders claustrophobia in some individuals. Also, patients with cardiac pacemakers or implanted or attached ferromagnetic objects usually cannot be safely studied by this technique, since it employs a very strong magnetic field.

Keeping in mind the advantages listed above, there are several clinical circumstances for which MRI is a particularly useful diagnostic aid. Magnetic resonance imaging is the best means of imaging the brain stem and cerebellum because of freedom from the bone artifact that is so common in CT scans of this region. Because MRI scans are easily done in sagittal section, midline abnormalities in the corpus callosum, the suprasellar region, or the cerebellar vermis are particularly well demonstrated. Figure 141 shows a pituitary tumor (*arrow*). The sagittal MRI scan also nicely demonstrates the anatomic relationships at the cervical-cranial junction, allowing more precise diagnosis of conditions such as Arnold-Chiari malformation. In cerebral infarction, MRI complements

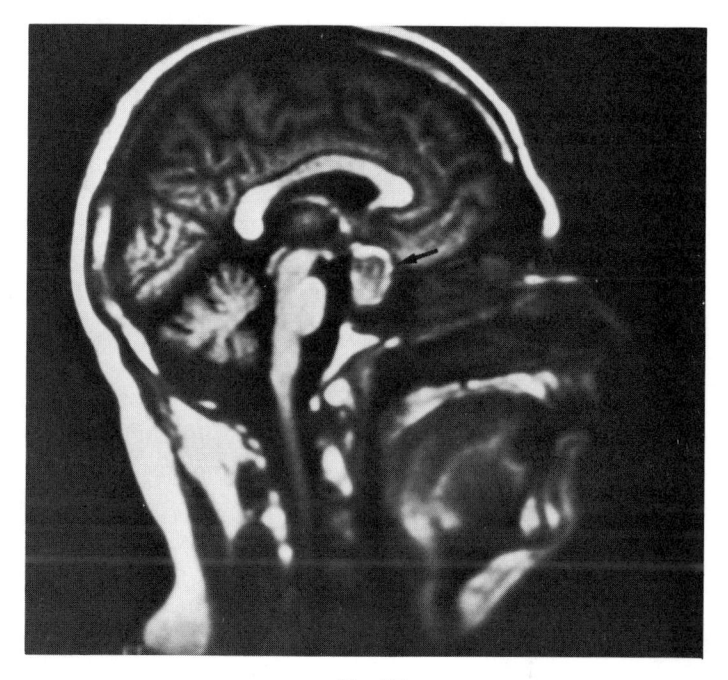

Fig 141

CT scanning because it shows small lacunar infarctions quite well and may demonstrate larger strokes during the very early phases when CT is still normal. Magnetic resonance imaging has proved to be especially valuable in multiple sclerosis (Fig 142), often showing multiple areas of demyelination, including those that are clinically asymptomatic.

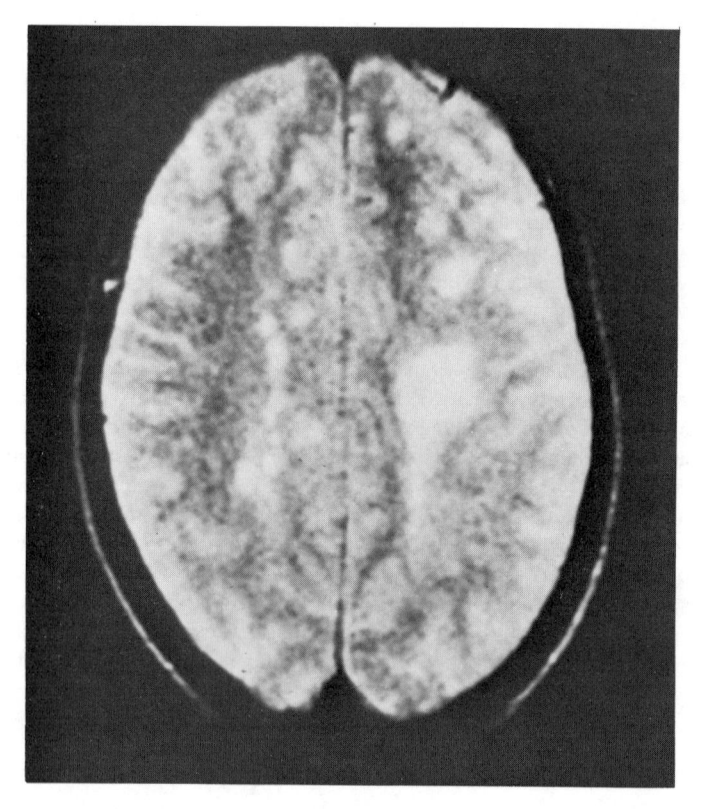

Fig 142

Cerebral Angiography.—Cerebral angiography carries a greater risk of morbidity or mortality than any of the procedures discussed above. Although this risk is still small, a decision to obtain this test should not be made without first carefully considering whether the same information can be gotten by less invasive means. The greatest utility of cerebral angiography is in evaluating primary disorders of the carotid and vertebral basilar arterial systems. These disorders include vascular occlusion or stenosis, inflammatory or infectious vasculitis, vascular malformations, and aneurysms. It is important to remember that the major cerebral veins and venous sinuses are also visualized, and their disorders can also be investigated by this technique.

Typically, the procedure is performed by injecting iodinated contrast material via a central arterial catheter that has been threaded into the aortic arch or the lumen of a carotid or vertebral artery. The origin and extracranial course of the carotid and vertebral arteries can be visualized to determine their patency. By following the course of the contrast material through the intracranial vessels, several other types of information can be gained. The presence of an intracerebral mass can be confirmed by demonstrating displacement of cerebral vessels or abnormal vasculature within the mass itself. In most cases, a mass such as a brain tumor or an abscess can be detected by CT or MRI scanning, making angiography unnecessary except in those instances where the precise blood supply of the mass must be known.

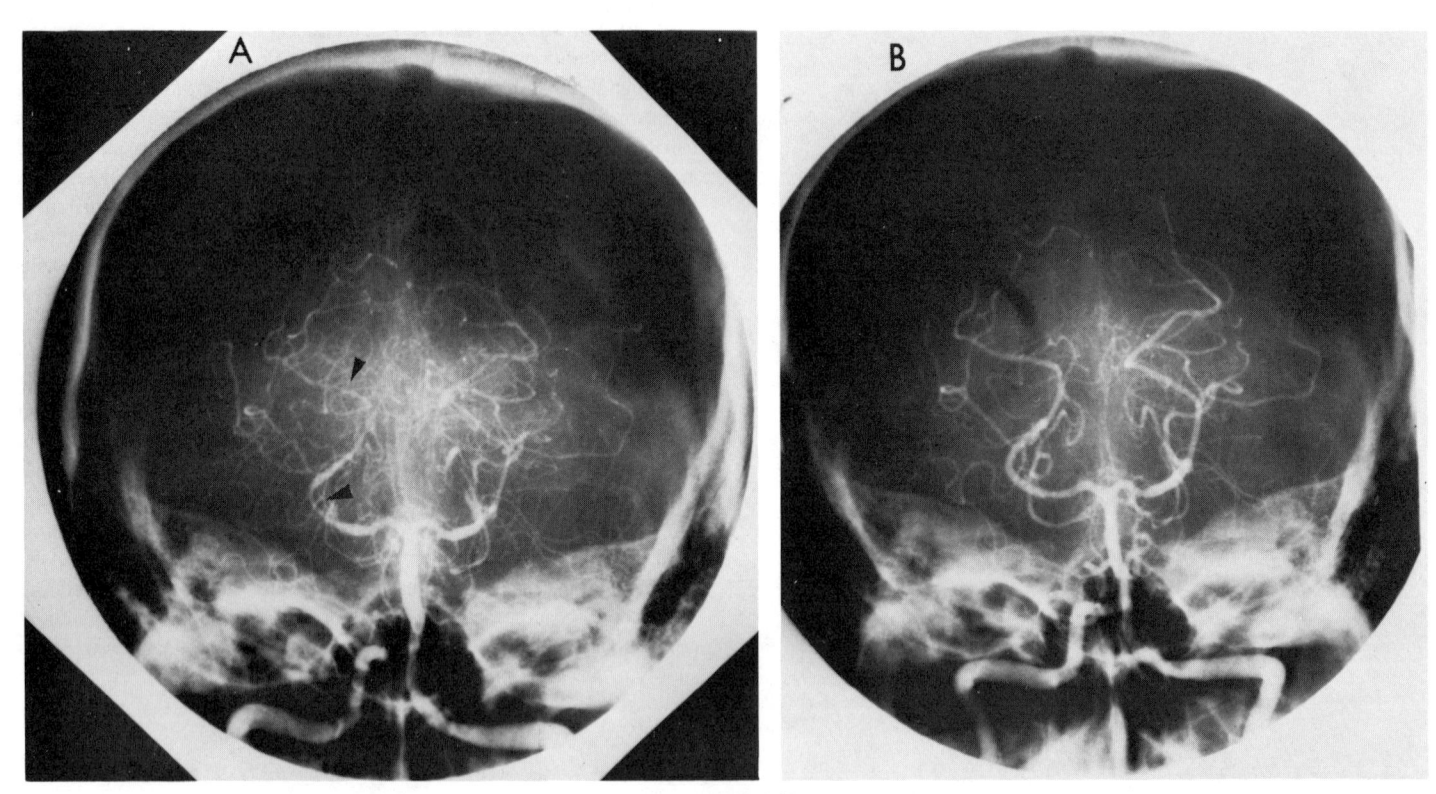

Fig 143

204 / *Cerebral Angiography*

Figure 143,A shows the typical beaded appearance and segmental narrowing of vessels in cerebral arteritis (*arrows*), compared with the more normal appearance after treatment in Figure 143,B. Figure 144 shows a large aneurysm arising from the middle cerebral artery. Modern scanning techniques have not yet surpassed angiography in demonstrating primary forms of vascular pathology such as these.

In another form of arteriography, the digital subtraction angiogram (DSA), images are reconstructed with computer assistance after either intravenous or intra-arterial contrast injection. In some situations, a DSA can be substituted for a standard arteriogram, especially for viewing the extracranial arterial vessels and the intracranial venous system. Advancing technology will likely enhance and broaden the use of DSA in the future.

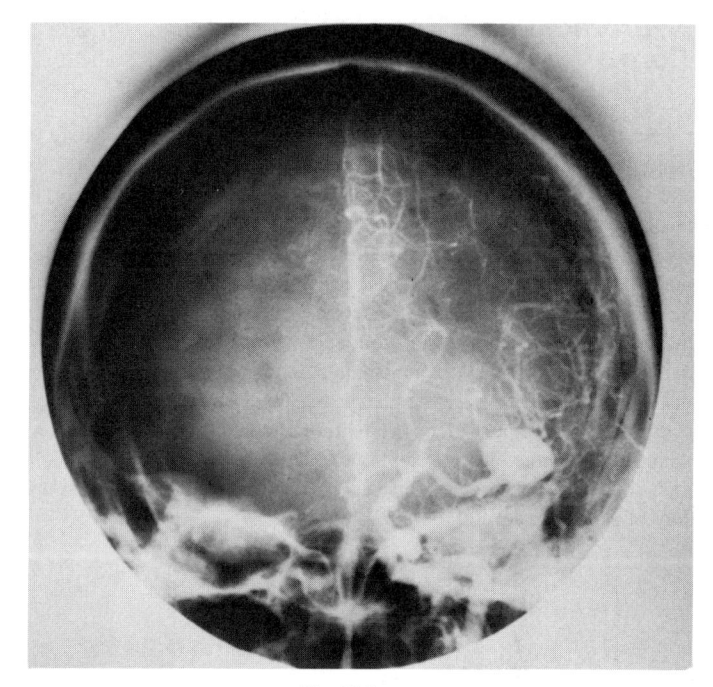

Fig 144

Neuroradiologic Tests of Spine and Spinal Cord

Spine Roentgenograms.—Spine roentgenograms show only the ossified elements of the spine, not the normal, noncalcified intervertebral disks or ligaments. These roentgenograms allow visualization of the anatomic relationships of spinal elements. Therefore, scoliosis, kyphosis, spondylolisthesis, fracture-dislocations, and vertebral fusion or nonsegmentation are usually clearly seen. Degenerative disk disease can often be inferred by a narrowed intervertebral disk space (Fig 145, *arrows*) or the presence of osteophytes. Although the spinal nerves cannot be visualized, an oblique view of the spine demonstrates the neural foramina through which they pass as they exit the spinal canal. Lytic or sclerotic neoplastic involvement of the vertebral column can often be seen on a plain spine roentgenogram, and though there are more sensitive tests for this, such as the isotope bone scan, it is a useful and relatively simple way of screening several vertebral levels.

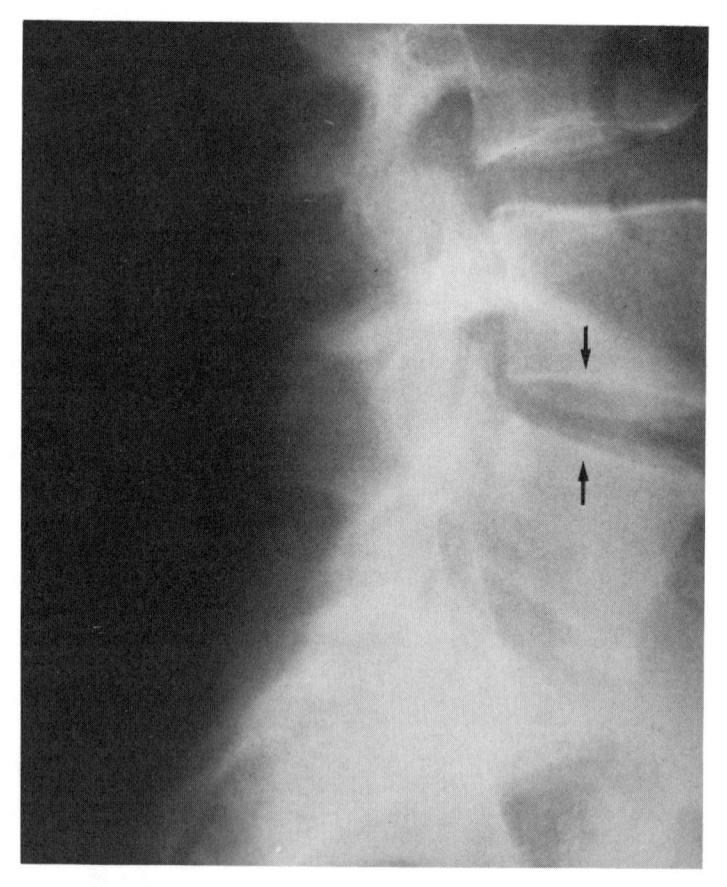

Fig 145

Myelography.—Myelography is performed by injecting a contrast agent into the lumbar or cervical subarachnoid space, the later via a cisternal puncture. The contrast agent fills the spinal nerve root sleeves and shows the spinal cord in relief within the spinal canal. Compressive lesions of the spinal root, such as a disk protrusion, prevent the normal filling of the nerve root sleeve by contrast (Fig 146; *arrow*). Compressive lesions of the spinal cord, such as tumors or centrally herniated intervertebral disks, result in an indentation of the column of contrast, or if very severe, a total block so that no contrast can pass beyond the point

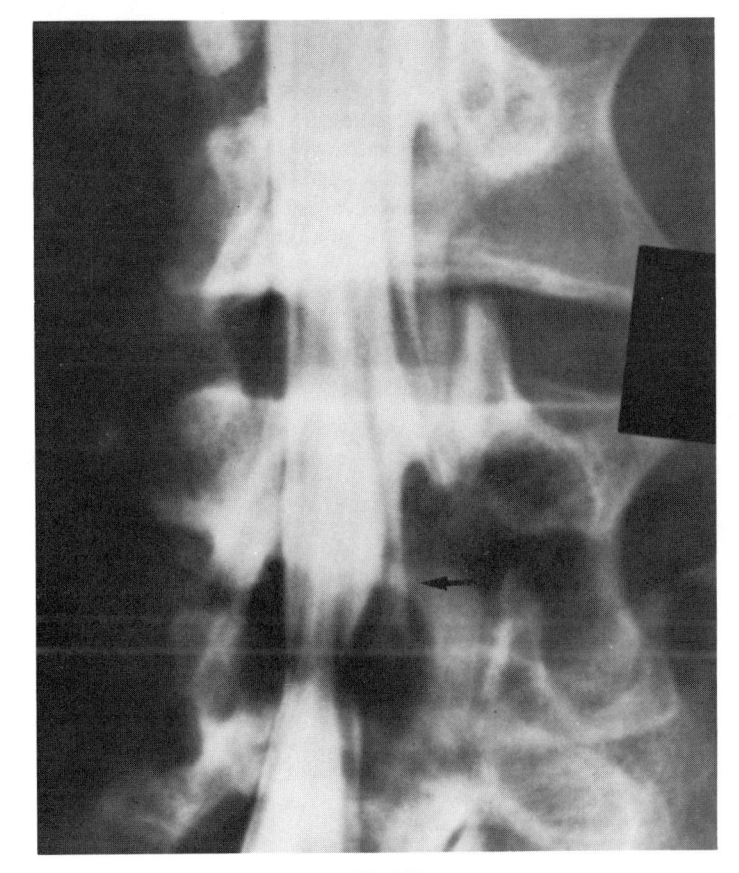

Fig 146

of involvement. In Figure 147 a metastatic tumor has resulted in the typical picture of an extradural spinal mass. A complete spinal block produced by an intradural spinal mass is shown in Figure 148. If a spinal block is demonstrated after a lumbar injection of contrast, additional contrast is often instilled above through a cervical injection to outline the cephalad extent of the block.

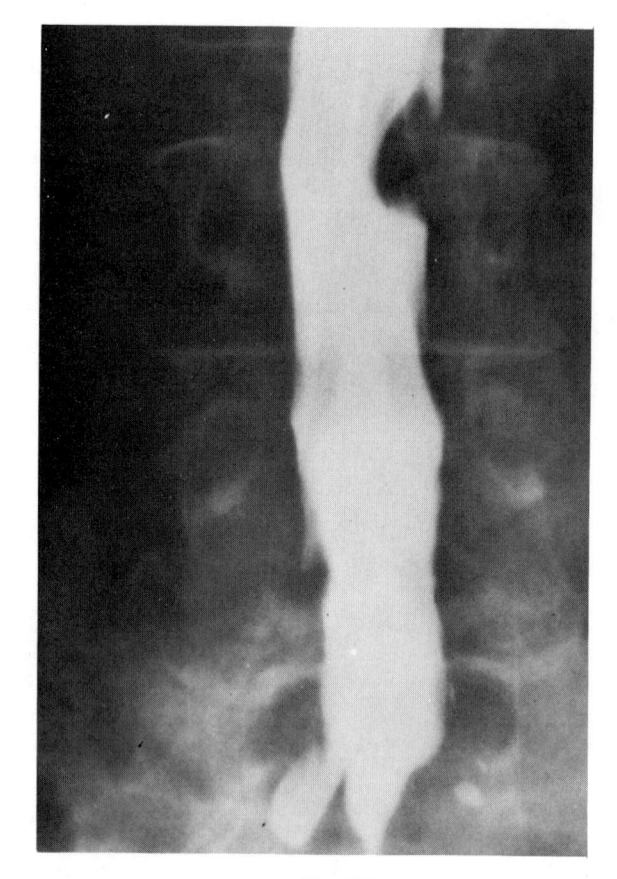

Fig 147

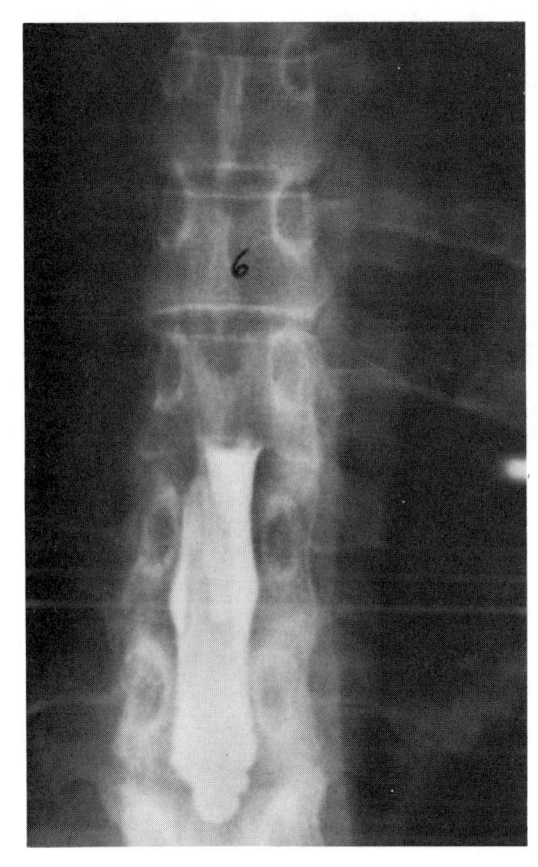

Fig 148

CT Scan of the Spine.—Computed tomography of the spine demonstrates the osseous vertebral structures as well as the intervertebral disks, spinal cord, nerve roots, ligaments, and epidural fat. Unlike in myelography, the spinal canal and its content are shown in axial sections. This makes CT an ideal way of viewing the shape and dimensions of the spinal canal and the anatomic relationships between the intervertebral disk, spinal roots, and spinal cord. One of the most common uses of spinal CT is in the diagnosis of disc disease. Disc protrusions can often be seen on CT, but often confirmatory myelography is done before considering surgical therapy. Often, CT and myelography are combined since the water-soluble contrast material used for myelography remains in the cerebrospinal fluid for up to 48 hours before being absorbed. The postmyelogram CT scan of the spine (Fig 149) then shows the herniated disc material (*single arrow*) in relief outlined by the vivid white, contrast-containing cerebrospinal fluid (*double arrows*). Another use of postcontrast CT scanning is in the diagnosis of syringomyelia. Because contrast material in the spinal fluid accumulates in a syrinx, a CT scan is often performed several hours after the completion of a myelogram when this condition is suspected.

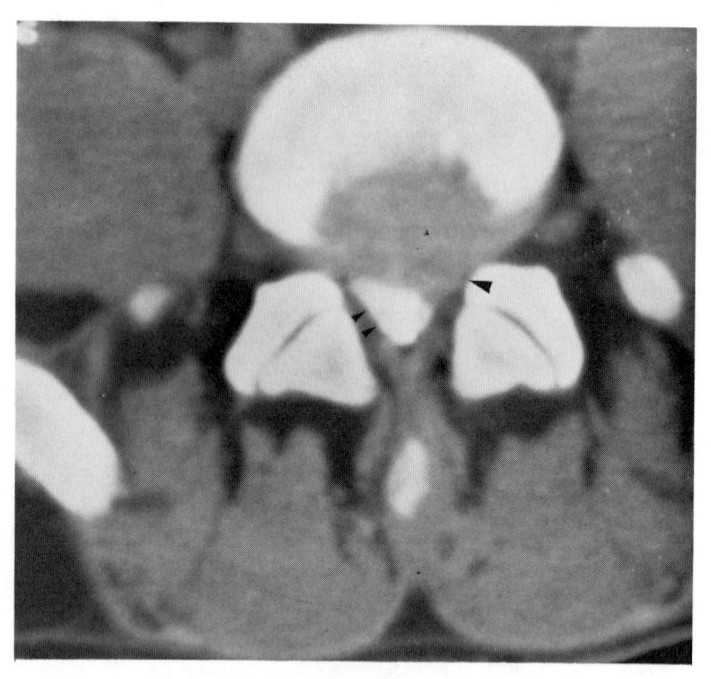

Fig 149

MRI of the Spinal Cord.—Magnetic resonance imaging of the spinal cord can be used to generate a sagittal or axial image. Herniated disks, primary or metastatic spinal-cord neoplasms, and syringomyelia can be demonstrated using this technique. Its role in diagnosing these conditions is still evolving, but with advances in technology it will become increasingly more important as a primary means of diagnosing spinal pathology. It has proved to be particularly useful in diagnosing syringomyelia (Fig 150, sagittal view) and, where available, should be considered the diagnostic procedure of choice for that condition. Also it is a very effective means of demonstrating cervical-cranial abnormalities, such as Arnold-Chiari malformation or neoplasms at the level of the foramen magnum.

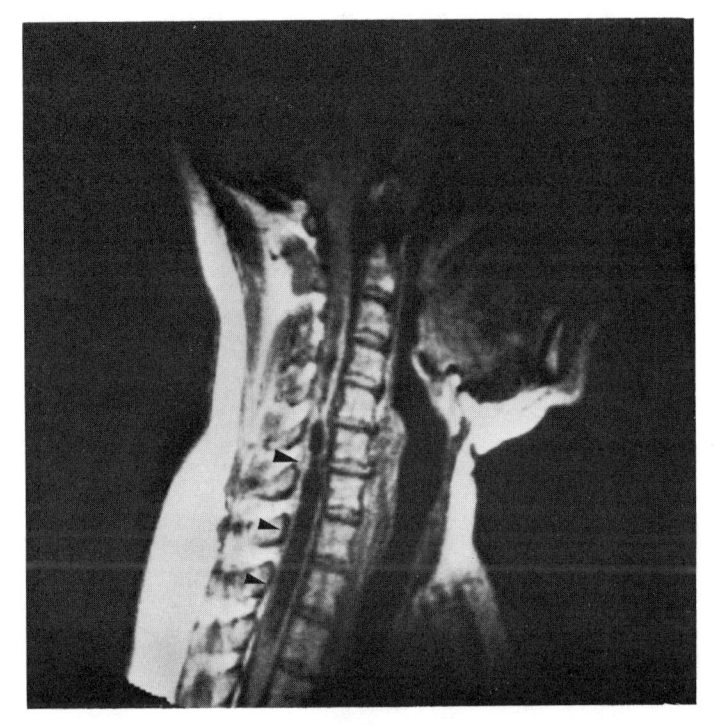

Fig 150

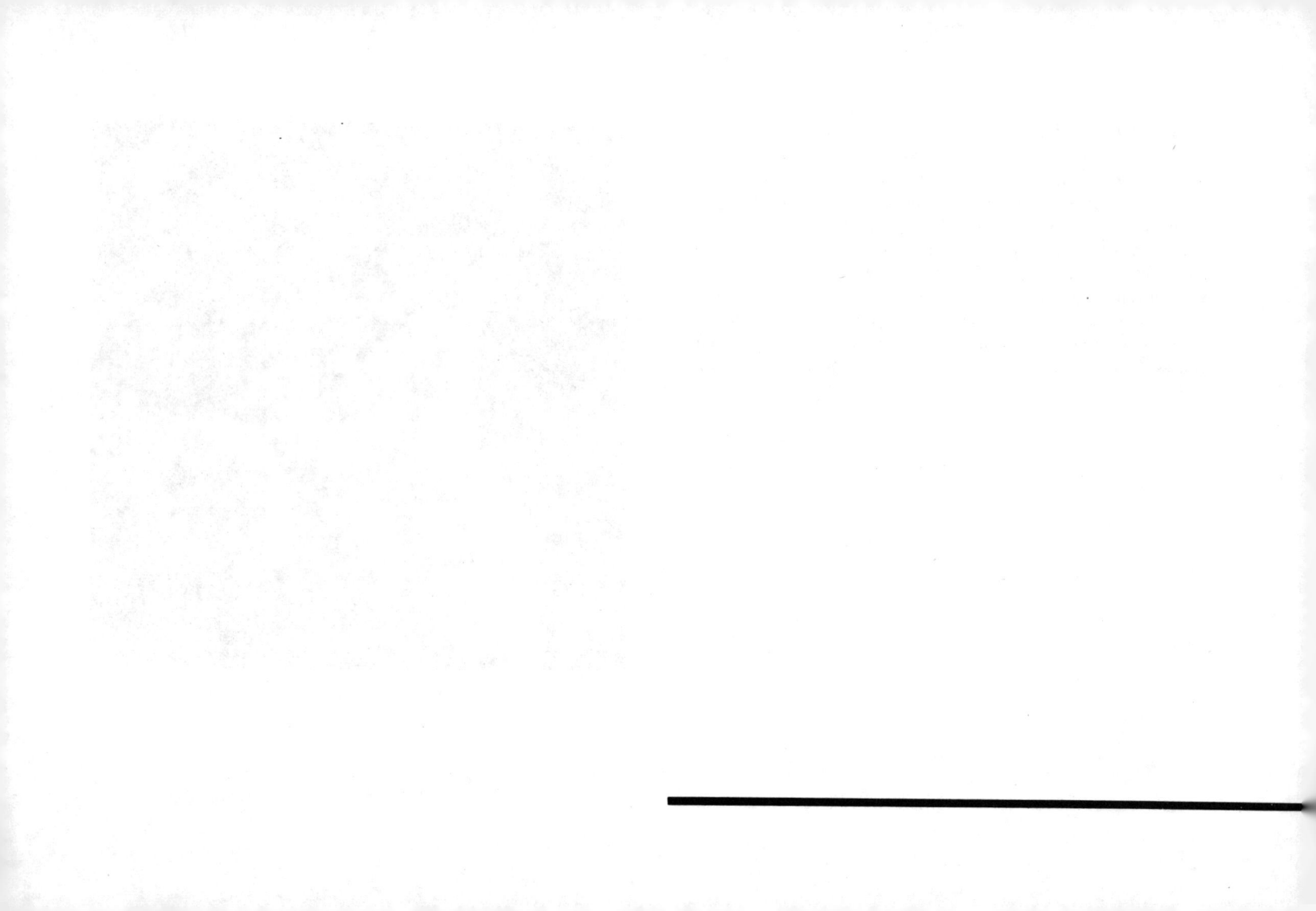

Supplemental Diagnostic Procedures

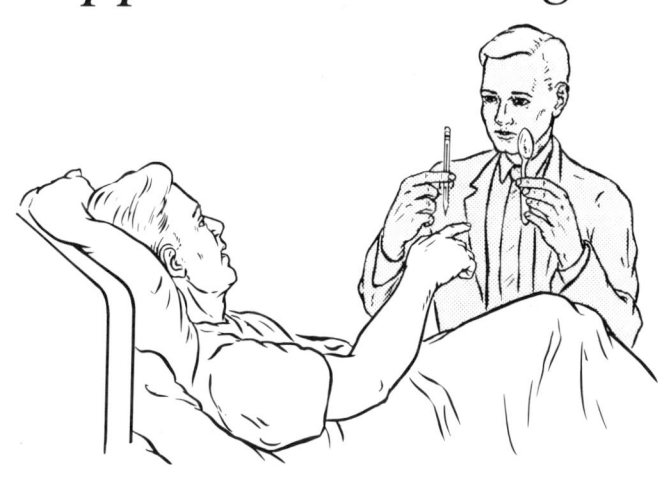

Brief Tests of Mental Status

Questions and conversation during the neurologic examination usually yield a valid impression of a patient's intellectual competence. His demeanor, his memory and orientation—as disclosed by his answers during the taking of the history—his understanding of questions and quickness in responding to them, and the language he uses all provide valuable indications of his mental status (see p. 2). The evidence is usually clearcut: either the patient shows he is alert and fully capable intellectually, or intellectual defects are so obvious that an "organic mental syndrome" is indisputable. Sometimes, however, an equivocal picture emerges wherein the patient shows indications of possible defect in one area or another (e.g., memory, retardation in response) without gross malfunctioning. To decide whether such a person is suffering from intellectual impairment as a result of cerebral disease may require objective tests of mental abilities to supplement the impressionistic findings of the clinical examination. A description of some brief and easily administered tests follows.

Memory is often the function that most readily betrays the existence of organic brain dysfunction. It is a process that consists of several components, the most important being registration, storage, and retrieval. Disturbance of one or a combination of these components gives rise to various types of memory deficit. Clinically, memory can be divided into three general types: immediate, recent, and remote, each of which can be tested separately.

Immediate memory is tested clinically by asking for recall after a very short time, generally several seconds to 2 minutes. Registration, the first step in the memory process, is essential for immediate recall, but the patient also must be able to concentrate sufficiently on the test material for registration to occur. Accordingly, attention is always tested as a prelude to the evaluation of immediate memory. In the digit span test, used to evaluate attention, the patient is instructed to repeat a series of numbers in exactly the same order as he hears them. The examiner recites numbers at the rate of one per second, being careful to avoid accentuation or grouping of numbers, either of which will simplify the task and invalidate the results. Beginning with the first four-digit series in the following list, the examiner continues testing until the patient fails two series in succession.

"Attention": Repetition of Digits

4-6-9-2	2-9-6-4-8-3
3-8-5-1	3-5-1-7-4-6
5-3-8-1-7	7-3-8-4-6-9-2
2-9-4-7-5	8-2-9-6-4-7-1

Interpretation of performance.—A patient less than 55 years old and of average intelligence should be able to repeat seven digits, and those in the 55 to 70 age range should be able to repeat six digits. If the patient is of dull-average intelligence, these criteria are reduced by one digit. Some notion of the difficulty of this test can be gained from developmental norms that indicate that repetition of seven digits is a 14-year-old performance, six digits a 10-year-old performance, five digits a 7-year-old performance, and four digits a 4-year-old performance. Performance below the specified level usually indicates a disturbance in "attention," i.e., an inability to screen out nonpertinent stimuli and to concentrate sufficiently on a series of presented events to be able to recall them in correct order. Such inattentiveness in the face of normal alertness is most commonly seen in acute confusional states caused by diffuse cerebral dysfunction such as toxic or metabolic encephalopathy, post-traumatic encephalopathy, or meningitis. Anxiety or depression also impair attention, and this possibility should be considered in interpreting defective performance. Since digit repetition also requires verbal processing, aphasic patients may be unable to perform this test.

Immediate memory is next evaluated by the digit reversal task. Tell the patient that you will say a series of numbers, but this time he is to repeat them backwards. Illustrate by saying that when you say "3-5" he is to say "5-3." Test understanding of instructions by giving another two-digit number. Give each series in the following list, beginning with the first three-digit series, until the patient fails two series in succession.

Immediate Memory: Reversal of Digits

4-1-9	3-1-8-5-9
8-2-5	5-9-2-7-4
9-2-6-4	3-8-1-4-2-7
2-7-3-5	6-2-5-7-3-1

Interpretation of performance.—A patient less than 55 years old and of average intelligence should be able to reverse five digits, and those older should be able to reverse four digits. If the patient is of dull-average intelligence, these criteria are reduced by one digit. Developmental norms indicate that reversal of five digits is a 12-year-old performance, four digits a 9-year-old performance, and three digits a 7-year-old performance. Reversal of digits is a more complicated process than simple repetition and implies the capacity for accurate short-term storage of a temporal sequence of impressions so that they can be manipulated. This storage is often accomplished by "visualization" of the digits, less often by "auditorization." The test provides a sensitive measure of cerebral dysfunction. As in repetition of digits, defective performance is more suggestive of either diffuse cerebral disease or left-hemisphere disease than of disease confined to the right hemisphere.

Recent memory involves the ability to recall information newly learned in the past minutes, hours, or as long as 1 or 2 days. The exact duration of recall that distinguishes recent memory from immediate recall and from remote recall is poorly defined, but the above definition is clinically useful. Intact recent memory implies not only normal registration but normal storage as well. Bilateral disease of limbic system structures such as the hippocampi, mamillary bodies, and dorsal median nucleus of the thalamus results in inability to store new information or retrieve that which was recently learned.

This function can be tested by asking the patient about events of the past day such as what was eaten at the most recent meal or how long he has been in the hospital or clinic. A relative or attendant may be required to verify the accuracy of the answer. An open-ended question such as "tell me about the recent headlines in the news" is often useful and has the advantage of requiring an answer that is easily confirmed by the examiner. New information provided by the examiner can also be used. Tell the patient you are going to name four objects such as a pencil, an orange, a book, and a shoe, then immediately ask him to repeat them, so that you can be certain they were properly understood and registered. Proceed with other portions of the neurologic or mental status examination so that constant rehearsal of the items is prevented. After five minutes have elapsed, ask the patient to recall the four objects.

Perhaps the simplest way to test recent memory is to assess temporal and geographic orientation since both depend on a continuous process of storing new information as the day progresses. It is important not to omit this portion of the examination out of fear of insulting the alert, glib, and seemingly oriented patient with such basic questions. In some conditions, such as transient global amnesia, short-term memory may be impaired out of proportion to other more readily apparent behavioral functions, and the deficit in this area may not be uncovered unless specifically sought. Orientation should be assessed by asking the following questions:

1. What is today's date? (Patient is required to give day, month, and year.)
2. What day of the week is it?
3. What time is it now? (Make sure the patient cannot look at a watch or clock.)
4. What is the name of this place? (Patient is required to name the hospital, clinic, or office he is in.)
5. What city are you in now?

Interpretation of performance.—A normal person is capable of recalling four objects after five minutes without difficulty. The patient who can recall only three may have impaired recent memory. Inability to recall more than two of four objects is clearly abnormal.

It is rare for normal people of average intelligence to miss the day of the month by more than 3 days, most make no error. An error of 4 to 5 days may reflect minor temporal disorientation, and an error of 6 or more days is indicative of severe disorientation. Any error regarding the year or the month is abnormal except when the answer reflects an error of less than 3 days, such as the end of a calendar month or year, e.g., December 1 instead of November 30. Disorientation for place or city suggests a severely impaired ability to learn and retain new information.

Remote memory involves retrieval of information that has been stored for a period of years. It is theorized that such storage occurs in the cerebral cortex, so cortical disease is possible if old memories cannot be summoned. This function may be tested by asking the patient about dates and other details of previous life events. The following questions are useful.

1. What is your birth date (day, month, and year)?
2. What is your wedding anniversary date?
3. In what year did you graduate from elementary school/high school/college?

Interpretation of performance.—Answers to questions pertaining to life events must be verified by a reliable source, usually a family member. Any error in this area suggests impairment of remote memory.

Higher Intellectual Function

The highest and most complex mental functions are those requiring arithmetic calculations, abstract thought, and synthesis of new ideas from previously learned information. These functions depend on the integrity of the cerebral cortex and consequently are impaired by cortical disease, particularly when diffuse. Disease confined to the dominant hemisphere may preferentially affect higher functions requiring verbal thought and reasoning, such as interpretation of proverbs or understanding of similarities. A decline in intellectual performance is often an early clue to the existence of brain dysfunction. It may be manifested by loss of ordinary social graces and judgment, inability to make change, or inability to appreciate the incongruity and absurdities of a humorous story. In testing a patient's intellectual functions at bedside, the examiner must be mindful of the patient's premorbid intellect, which can generally be estimated by his occupation and level of formal education. Poorly educated patients often have very little facility at abstract thought and calculation, whereas the highly educated individual should find such tasks easy. Specific testing for higher mental functions include (1) general information, (2) calculation, (3) proverb interpretation, (4) similarities, and (5) judgment.

Fund of information may be evaluated by questions pertaining to the patient's background and experience, his job, his place of residence, his interests. Examples of typical questions in these categories follow:

1. *Occupation*: A question asked of an automobile mechanic: What is the function of the carburetor?
2. *Place of residence*: A question asked of a resident of New York, City: What rivers border the island of Manhattan?
3. *Interests and hobbies*: A question asked of a sports enthusiast: What is the Heisman trophy?

Intrepretation of performance on background-related questions is sometimes difficult, but the examiner can usually gain an impression of the patient's level of information.

Arithmetic Calculation

Addition:	14 + 5	8 + 6	29 +13
Multiplication:	7 × 4	6 × 3	14 × 5
Subtraction:	19 − 7	17 − 8	43 −18
Division:	$3\sqrt{18}$	$4\sqrt{32}$	$12\sqrt{48}$

Administration of tests.—Present orally each of the problems in the list to the patient, noting errors or excessive slowness of response; questions may be repeated if the patient requests.

Interpretation of performance.—These 12 calculation problems constitute an easy test for normal people. Most patients of average intelligence perform perfectly. Patients with low-average intelligence may make one or two errors. Three or more errors represent defective calculation ability. If the failure occurs along with other evidence of mental impairment, it tends to confirm an impression of diffuse cerebral disease. Difficulty only in this area, however, without impairment of other intellectual functions, suggests a specific deficit (dyscalculia) and raises the possibility of disease of the posterior left hemisphere. Dyscalculia may occur independently of aphasia but is more often associated with a mild aphasic disorder.

Similarities.—The ability to perceive the similarities between different objects requires verbal reasoning and abstract thought. Give the patient each of the following pairs of words and ask him to describe how each pair is alike.

        pear—apple
        bicycle—automobile
        scarf—stocking
        table—chair

Interpretation.—These questions can be correctly answered on two levels. On the higher level the two objects are placed in the same class or category, e.g., *fruit* for pear and apple. A response at the lower level points out a common trait or function; e.g., both pear and apple are things to eat. Patients whose educational, occupational, and social background indicate at least average intelligence should provide answers at the higher level, whereas those with dull or low-average intelligence may give answers at the lower level. Failure to appreciate any similarity is indicative of impaired cognitive functioning.

Proverbs.—Ability to interpret proverbs requires understanding, social judgment, and preserved ability for abstract thought. Tell the patient that you are going to recite a saying that he may or may not have heard before. Ask him to explain the meaning of the saying in his own words. Patients often hesitate to interpret proverbs they have not heard previously but will proceed after a little encouragement. The following four proverbs are useful:

- People in glass houses should not throw stones.
- Don't cry over spilled milk.
- A bird in the hand is worth two in the bush.
- The tongue is the enemy of the throat.

Interpretation.—The retarded or demented patient will respond with a concrete interpretation such as "stones will break glass," whereas the patient of average intelligence is often, but not invariably, capable of an abstract interpretation. The patient must be of at least high-average intelligence, however, for a failing performance to signify disease.

Judgment.—Impaired judgment is often reflected in the daily activities of the demented patient. It can be formally tested by presenting the patient with hypothetical problem situations in which sound judgment is required to arrive at a satisfactory solution. The following two situations may be used for this purpose, presented in the form of a question.

1. What would you do if you found a sealed, addressed letter with an unused stamp on the ground?
2. What would you do if you smelled smoke while in a movie theatre?

Interpretation.—A response that reflects a lack of judgment in the first situation would be "I'd throw it away" or "I'd peel off the stamp," whereas normal judgment would suggest that the letter be dropped into the nearest mailbox.

The language function portion of the mental status examination focuses on the patient's expression and comprehension of both spoken and written language. It is meaningful not only because specific language deficits have distinct neuroanatomic correlates, but also because the functions tested here affect performance on other portions of the mental status examination, such as proverb interpretation and verbal memory.

As part of the evaluation of language functions, it is important to determine the patient's handedness and cerebral dominance. The left hemisphere is virtually always dominant for language in right-handed people and is dominant for about 60% of left-handed people. With more than 90% of the population right-handed, it follows that most cases of language dysfunction result from disorders of the left hemisphere. Be careful in determining handedness, though; many left-handed people are taught early in life to write with the right hand. Ask which hand is used for other skilled activities, such as throwing a ball, using a hammer, or cutting with scissors.

Listen to the patient's interaction with the examiner or family members, specifically for the rate, rhythm, intonation, quantity, and informational content of speech. Listen for word-finding pauses. Note any substitution of inappropriate words (paraphasia) or use of nonsensical words (neologisms). There are two forms of paraphasia. Verbal paraphasia is the substitution of an incorrect though closely related word, such as "hand" for "foot," whereas literal paraphasia is the substitution of an inappropriate sound within a word such as "foof" for "foot." A neologism is a well-articulated word, newly created by the patient and having no established meaning; e.g., "I drank a cup of *flen*."

Aphasic speech can be characterized as being fluent or nonfluent. Fluent aphasia is characterized by effortless, high-output speech with normal rhythm and intonation but with the inclusion of many meaningless phrases, paraphasias, and neologisms. When the neologistic and paraphasic content is extremely high, the speech is virtually incomprehensible and referred to as *jargon aphasia*. Fluent aphasia typically results from brain dysfunction posterior to the rolandic fissure. Wernicke's aphasia, resulting from a lesion in the posterior portion of the superior temporal gyrus, is an example of a fluent aphasia in which impaired verbal comprehension is also prominent.

Lesions anterior to the rolandic fissure are more likely to result in a nonfluent aphasia. Output is reduced and many connecting words eliminated, resulting in "telegraphic" speech. Articulation is abnormal, intonation may be disturbed, and words are uttered haltingly and with frustration. Despite these abnormalities, the speech content is meaningful and appropriate. Broca's aphasia, resulting from a lesion in the posterior inferior frontal lobe, is an example of a nonfluent aphasia. In this syndrome, verbal comprehension is usually only moderately impaired. In addition to Broca's and Wernicke's aphasia, several other aphasic syndromes have been described. Some are believed to be caused by lesions that produce disconnection between component segments of the speech area or between the speech area and the remainder of the brain. Though the details of these forms of aphasia are beyond the scope of this discussion, it is worthwhile to note that these aphasias possess distinctive features, especially pertaining to repetition, that set them apart from the more typical Broca or Wernicke type of aphasia.

Often, the evaluation of spontaneous speech alone will lead to correct identification and characterization of the expressive component of an aphasic syndrome. A more formal evaluation of speech is necessary to evaluate more subtle cases and is essential for adequate evaluation of comprehension.

The spoon-pencil test is a screening procedure used to probe for the presence of expressive and receptive aphasic disorders. It was originally designed for use with the bedridden patient but can be used whenever the question of aphasic deficit arises. The only materials required are a teaspoon and a full-length sharpened pencil with an eraser.

Administration of test.—*Expressive language* is tested first, using the following schedule of questions. First, show the patient the spoon, pointing to its various parts when appropriate. Ask the questions slowly, articulating clearly. The patient should be given plenty of time to give his verbal response. If the patient does not respond, repeat the question. Then show the patient the pencil and ask the questions listed in the schedule. Record the patient's response and note whether repetition of the question was required.

Schedule of Questions—Expressive Language

(Spoon)
1. What do you call this?
2. What color is the spoon?
3. What is the spoon made of?
4. What do you do with a spoon?
5. What do you call this part of the spoon? (handle)

(Pencil)
6. What do you call this?
7. What color is it?
8. What is the pencil made of?
9. What do you call this part of the pencil? (eraser)
10. What color is the eraser?
11. What is the eraser made of?
12. What do you call this part of the pencil? (point)
13. What color is the point of the pencil?
14. What do you do with a pencil?

Receptive language is tested by presenting both the spoon and the pencil as in Figure 151 and asking the following questions, which call for only a pointing response.

Schedule of Questions—Receptive Language

1. Show me (point to) the pencil.
2. Show me (point to) the spoon.
3. Which is yellow? (color of pencil)
4. Which is longer?
5. Which is harder?
6. Which do you eat with?
7. Which is made of wood?
8. Which do you write with?
9. Which has a handle?
10. Which is softer?
11. Which has an eraser on it?
12. Which is made of metal?
13. Which do you use in a dining room?
14. Which is shorter?
15. Which do you use in a schoolroom?
16. Which do you use with a notebook?
17. Which do you feed a small child with?
18. Which has a part that is made of rubber?

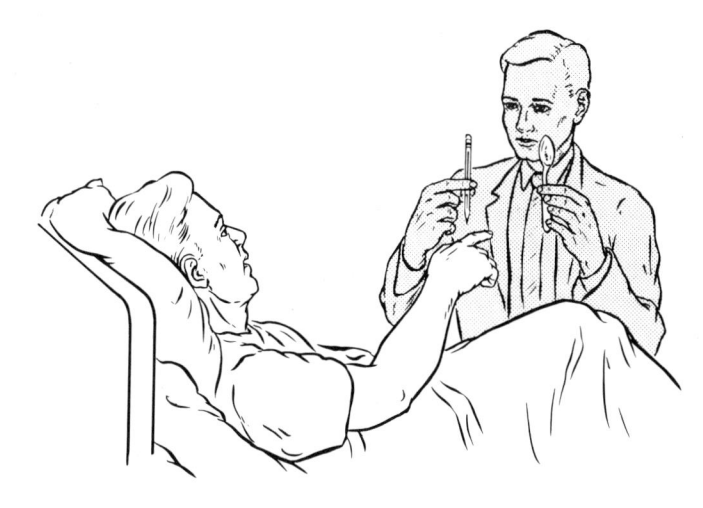

Fig 151

Examination for Aphasia—Spoon-Pencil Test / **221**

Interpretation of performance.—A nonaphasic, fluent person who is not mentally defective or mentally obtunded should perform perfectly on both the expressive and receptive aspects of the test. A patient with general mental impairment may make one or two errors because of a lack of attention, but three or four errors are strong evidence of a language deficit, and more than four errors indicate a severe deficit.

Performance on the expressive language test often reveals whether the impairment is of a nonfluent (Broca's) aphasia or a fluent type. Close to consistent failure, with difficulty in articulation, suggests a Broca type of aphasia (frontal-lobe damage), whereas a less consistent performance, with word-finding difficulties and paraphasic errors, is more likely due to Wernicke's aphasia (temporal-lobe damage). The levels of performance on the expressive and the receptive aspects of the test should be compared. If there is severe impairment in both areas, the patient has *global* aphasia. This is usually due to a large lesion, often an infarction, involving both the anterior and posterior speech areas. Severe expressive impairment with relatively mild receptive impairment indicates the classic motor (Broca's) aphasia. Severe expressive impairment with completely intact receptive capacity may indicate dysarthria rather than a true language disturbance in the sense of impairment of symbolic understanding and formulation. Defective reception with retained expressive capacity indicates a pure "word-deafness" with central involvement of the auditory system rather than a language disturbance in the strict sense just defined.

Patients with disturbances limited to reading or writing (alexia, agraphia) or higher-level language functions (agrammatism, impoverishment in spontaneous speech) perform on a perfect or near-perfect level on this test. Therefore, the procedure permits the inference of an aphasic disorder when performance is imperfect but does not exclude the possibility of a special or high-level language deficit when performance is perfect.

Though most aphasic syndromes are due to impairment of the cortical speech areas, it is important to remember that infarction or hemorrhage into subcortical structures, such as the caudate, putamen, or thalamus, can on occasion cause aphasia. Subcortical aphasia often has the additional feature of a soft voice with poor articulation and an abnormality in the rate of speech.

Writing.—Evaluation of the ability to write is important because all aphasic people have some degree of agraphia. Test spontaneous writing by asking the patient to write a short sentence describing the weather or the room he is in. Writing letters, words, or phrases to dictation should be tested in patients who are unable to perform the first task. Look for abnormalities such as spelling errors, grossly incorrect punctuation or capitalizations, and word substitutions. Rarely, with lesions in the dominant parietal lobe, agraphia appears in the absence of aphasia. The opposite situation, however—the absence of agraphia in the face of apparent aphasia—should raise the suspicion that the disorder of speech is not truly aphasic but is a dysarthric disorder.

Reading.—*Alexia* is impairment of reading ability due to a brain lesion. It is a common accompaniment of aphasia, particularly when verbal comprehension is abnormal. It may be present without significant aphasia when the causative lesion is confined to either the angular gyrus in the dominant hemisphere or to the visual cortex in the dominant hemisphere and adjacent splenium of the corpus callosum. In the former instance there is associated difficulty with writing, whereas a lesion in the latter region (which is almost always due to posterior cerebral artery thrombosis) results in the syndrome of alexia without agraphia.

Knowledge of the patient's educational background is essential for accurate evaluation of reading ability, lest an illiterate person be mistaken for an alexic one. The following test can be used to detect a severe abnormality of reading in patients with at least a fifth-grade education.

Administration of test.—Ask the patient to read each lowercase letter from the following aloud, noting the correctness of pronunciation of each. Next, ask the patient to read each word aloud.

```
        p   e   y   t   o   z   j
    somebody           daughter
    expression         background
    interested         situation
```

Interpretation of performance.—Inability to correctly identify and pronounce all of the lowercase letters is a performance below the third-grade level. Inability to correctly read all of the words in the list indicates a performance below the fifth-grade level. The greater the number of errors in either test, the more severely impaired is the patient's reading ability. For the patient with an expressive aphasia, one may need to resort to words that allow the patient to point to an object in the room corresponding to the word he just read. A poor performance under these circumstances should be interpreted cautiously.

Caloric Test for Vestibular Function

Function of the vestibular portion of the eight cranial nerve and its end organ can be tested by caloric stimulation of the semicircular canals. For most purposes, irrigation of the ear canals with icy water is adequate. The test is based on the fact that asymmetric stimulation of the vestibular end organs will produce tonic, conjugate, lateral deviation of the eyes. In the awake patient there is a rhythmic, correctional jerk of the eyes back toward the neutral position resulting in phasic nystagmus, whereas in the comatose patient this correctional phase is absent, leaving the eyes tonically deviated (p. 154). The test is principally used to discover whether the end organ and nerve are responsive to stimuli and whether the ves-

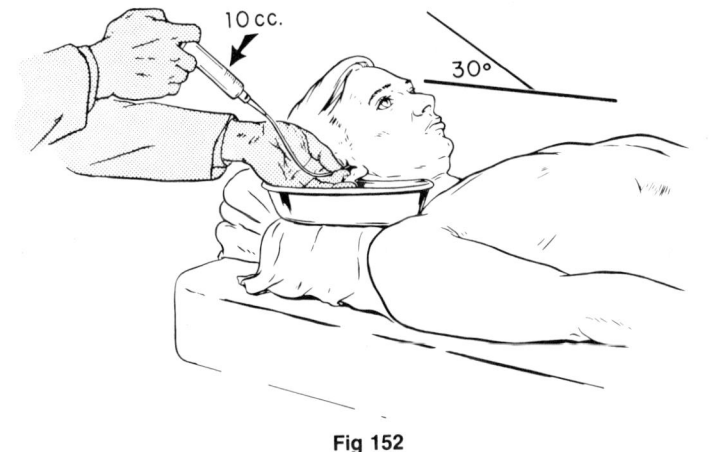

Fig 152

tibular nuclei maintain normal connections with the nuclei of the oculomotor nerves. Application of the test as shown in Figure 152 is particularly useful in the comatose patient because the conjugate eye movement that helps detect abnormalities of ocular movement and helps determine whether coma originates from a lesion of brain stem or cortex. It is also useful in determining whether spontaneous conjugate eye deviation in a comatose patient is secondary to involvement of the pontine gaze center or dysfunction above this level in the upper brain stem or frontal lobe, since in the former case the deviation cannot be overcome by caloric stimulation whereas in the latter it can.

First check the ear canals and inspect the eardrums. The canals should be patent and the eardrums must be intact. Position the patient as shown in Figure 152, with the head elevated 30 degrees so that the horizontal canal will be stimulated. Insert a soft plastic tube up to the eardrum (slightly painful) and withdraw it 1 to 2 mm. Then rather quickly (in 5 to 10 seconds) but gently inject 10 ml of icy water. This is mildly uncomfortable. The patient should not move his head and should gaze forward without fixing his eyes on anything. In the awake patient nystagmus will appear within 5 to 20 seconds. The fast component will be to the opposite side. In the stuporous or comatose patient the eyes will deviate to the side of stimulation. The other ear is stimulated after all symptoms have subsided.

Nystagmus is given directional designation on the basis of the fast component. The direction is reversed to the side of stimulation if warm water is used for stimulation. A useful mnemonic device is COWS: Cold Opposite, Warm Same. The nystagmus should be about the same on either side in duration and amplitude, and in symptoms of vertigo and nausea. Retest if no response is obtained. Persistent absence of response or greatly diminished response strongly indicates disease of the eight nerve, its end organ, or the central connections on that side. Asymmetric response of the eyes in relationship to each other, whether in the awake or comatose patient, suggests ocular-muscle paresis or a brain-stem lesion.

Lumbar Puncture

This procedure is simple in principle but often misapplied.

The term "lumbar puncture" means hollow-needle puncture of the meninges of the lumbar subarachnoid space. The puncture is done below the level of the end of the spinal cord (conus medullaris), i.e., below the L-2 vertebra in the adult and the L-4 vertebra in the infant.

Purpose

1. To determine the pressure of the cerebrospinal fluid as a reflection of intracranial pressure.
2. To determine the absolute amount and, when indicated, the electrophoretic pattern of protein in the fluid.
3. To determine the cellular content of the fluid.
4. To establish the presence of blood and to estimate the duration of its presence in the cerebrospinal fluid.
5. To determine the presence and nature of bacterial, spirochetal, viral, fungal, or rickettsial infection of the meninges by obtaining fluid for microscopic, serologic, and microbiologic examination.
6. To examine the fluid for malignant cells.

7. To introduce medications that do not cross the blood-brain barrier directly into the cerebrospinal fluid.
8. To introduce air or positive contrast materials for neuroradiologic procedures.

Contraindications

1. Elevated intracranial pressure, especially when a posterior fossa mass is suspected, contraindicates this procedure. The clinical assumption of elevated pressure is made when papilledema is present or when headache, vomiting, visual blurring ataxia, and lethargy, in any combination, are associated. Be especially circumspect when the patient is experiencing severe waves of headache with associated cardiovascular changes. In the more acute elevations, pulse rate may slow and blood pressure may climb. Sometimes, even though increased intracranial pressure is suspected, it is imperative to examine the cerebrospinal fluid to establish the presence of subarachnoid hemorrhage or meningitis. In such instances, unlike cases of intracranial hypertension caused by a focal mass lesion, lumbar puncture is much less likely to precipitate herniation, and the importance of the information gained greatly outweighs the risk. In the case of increased pressure due to intracerebral hematoma or abscess, lumbar puncture provides little information that cannot be obtained by other means (MRI or CT) and there is a risk of fatal herniation. If it is determined that a lumbar puncture is necessary in a patient with increased intracranial pressure, a small-gauge needle should be used (see p. xxx) so that the amount of spinal fluid escaping from the dural hole after the procedure is minimized. The concurrent use of anti-cerebral edema agents should also be considered.

2. Infection of the skin at the site of the puncture is uncommon. Such infection is, however, an absolute contraindication to a lumbar puncture since passage of the diagnostic needle through the infected area prior to its entry into the subarachnoid space carries a high risk of introducing infection into the central nervous system.

3. Anticoagulant administration or a pronounced bleeding tendency warrant concern, especially because of the possibility of initiating a spinal extradural or, occasionally, subdural hematoma. If a lumbar puncture must be performed in the face of severe thrombocytopenia, a platelet infusion should be given first. Special care must be taken to avoid unnecessary trauma by repeated attempts at passage of the needle. Accordingly, in such cases the task should be delegated to the most skilled or experience operator. Additionally, the use of a small (22-gauge) needle will help minimize trauma.

4. Emotional problems should occasionally stay one's hand when indications for the procedure are not compelling. The contentious, hostile, or passive-aggressive patient may complain greatly about symptoms that he attributes to the lumbar puncture; thus, it is wise to carefully assess the need for examining the fluid in such patients before proceeding.

5. When it is probable that myelography will be indicated, the lumbar puncture can often be delayed until this procedure is done to avoid duplication. Moreover, the low-pressure syndromes that frequently develop after lumbar puncture may result in technical failure of this radiologic procedure. However, lumbar puncture may be necessary to complete diagnostic studies before myelography is necessary. Then it should be delayed several days after the first lumbar puncture.

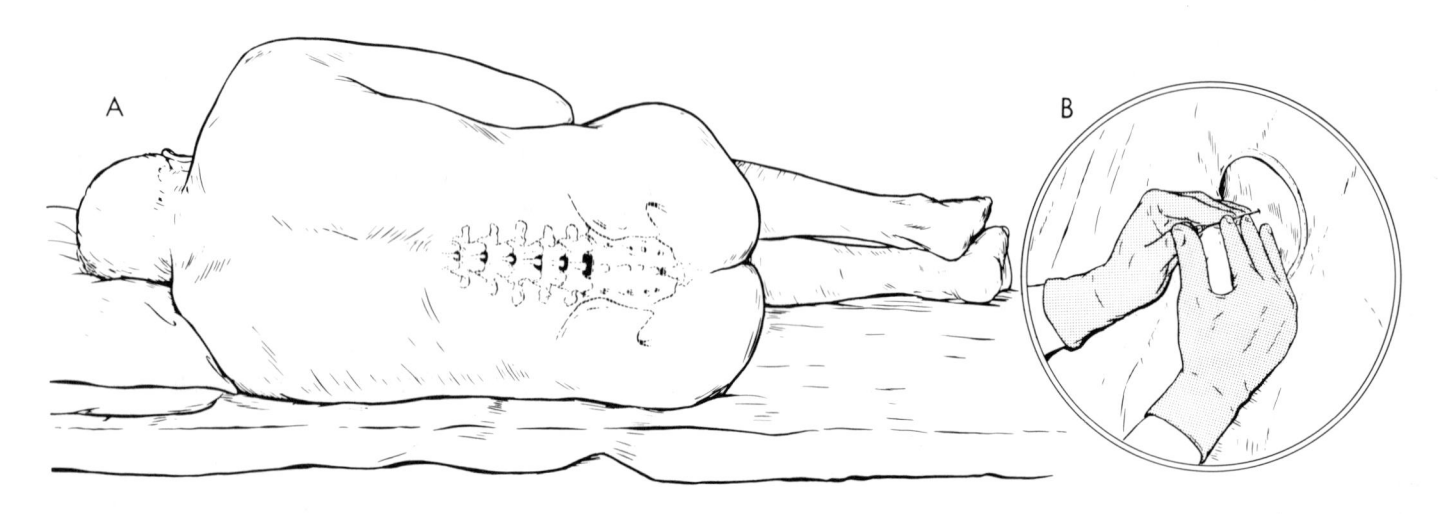

Fig 153

Essential is the proper positioning of the patient on a nonsagging surface—a firm mattress or a padded examining table. The proper flexed position, with the thighs well up on the abdomen and the neck moderately flexed, is shown in Figure 153,A. Find the lumbar spinous processes and then the process at the level of the iliac crest. This marks the L-4 vertebra. The puncture is done just above or below this process.

Be certain the area is clean to visual inspection; if not, scrub it with soap and water. Then prepared a radius of 8 to 10 inches with thimerosal (Merthiolate) or tincture of iodine. These solutions, unlike plain alcohol, stain the skin so that the extent of the area prepared will always be apparent to the operator. Drape sterile towels or a prepared sheet with an opening centered over the area. Have an assistant stand in front of the patient. Restraint should be avoided if possible. Then be seated behind the patient at a height such that his midback is at a natural working level for the hands. Use sterile gloves. Locate against the spinous processes and the interspinous space, then inject the skin over this area in a small wheal with 1% lidocaine solution. Use 1 to 2 ml and inject the projected needle tract for a distance of 2 cm.

226 / *Lumbar Puncture—Method and Interpretation*

Use a 20-gauge, sharp spinal puncture needle with stylet. If there is a possibility of significantly increased intracranial pressure, a smaller, 22-gauge needle should be used. Figure 153,B shows the proper position of the hands. Aim the needle in the midline—usually angulated cephalad 5 to 15 degrees—and advance slowly. If the needle meets bone, withdraw the tip to subcutaneous tissue and redirect. Be gentle and slow. Avoid flourishes and quick jabs. Reassure the patient as you proceed in a planned fashion to find the interspace, and avoid frantic, repetitive jabbings in the same area. As the needle goes deeper, withdraw the stylet every 2 to 3 mm of advancement to see if fluid flows. Usually, but not always, a "click" or "pop" will be felt when the needle pierces the dura. Advance the needle a few millimeters further and remove the stylet. Minor adjustments may be made to secure adequate flow, usually a rapid dripping. Lose as little fluid as possible before attaching a three-way stopcock and manometer. Even the most expert may fail at times, but this is usually because of spinal deformity, an uncooperative or disturbed patient, local intraspinal disease at the site of needle puncture, or low intraspinal pressure resulting from leakage after a preceding lumbar puncture.

More details of actual performance of the needle puncture are not efficiently given by essay. The student must learn from demonstrations and personal trials with expert advice. Study the lumbar spine on a skeleton, at surgery, and in the dissecting room if possible. Then study the lumbar meninges and the cauda equina lying in the dural sac. Once a reasonable understanding of anatomy is attained and the possible mechanical and hydraulic difficulties understood, the procedure may be

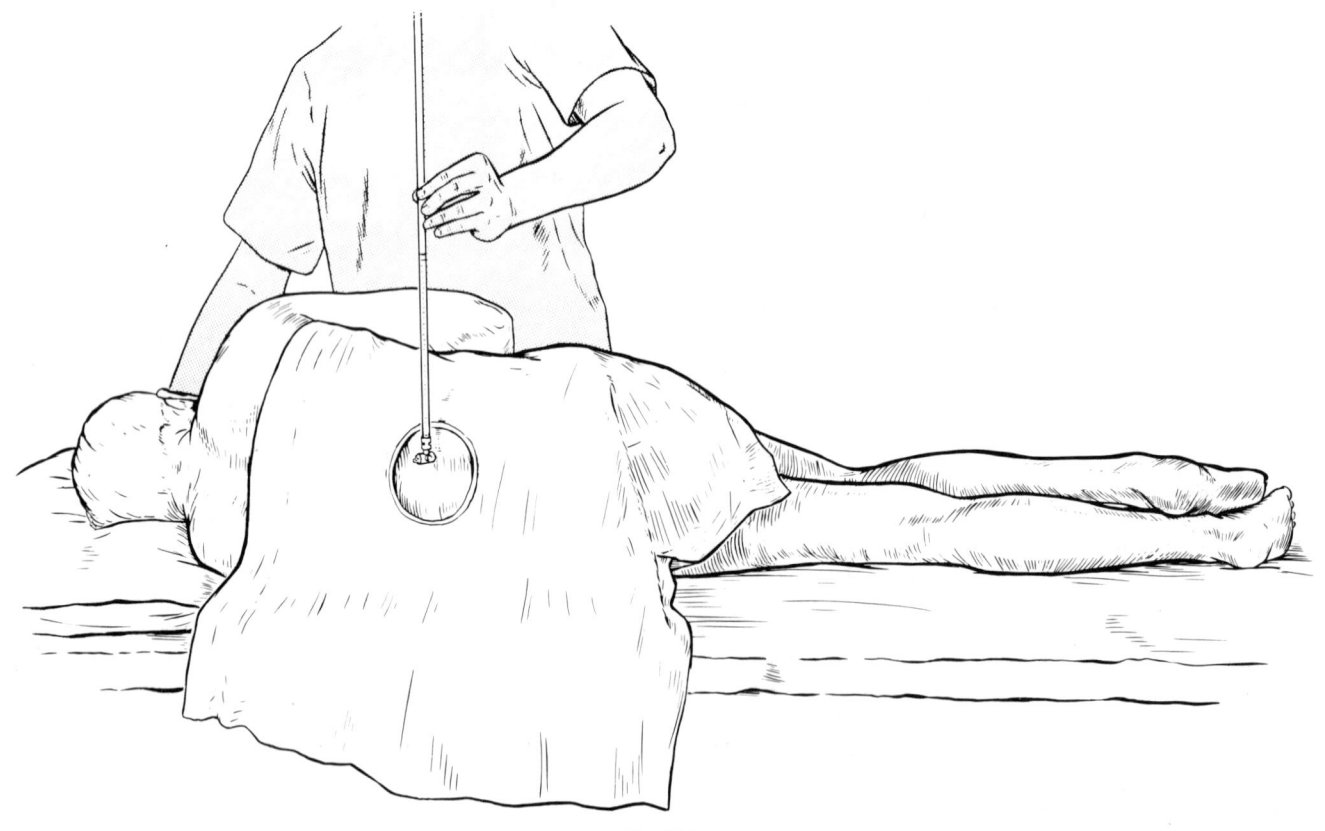

Fig 154

228 / *Lumbar Puncture—Method and Interpretation*

approached in an intelligent fashion and the mystery and cookbookery dispelled. Do this early in your career.

Once fluid drips from the needle, immediately attach the manometer. With the help of an assistant, have the patient extend the neck and rest the head on a pillow so that it does not deviate from the midplane of the body. Then have the patient, carefully avoiding movement of his back, extend his legs and assume as relaxed a posture as possible (Fig 154). Ask the patient to breathe quietly with mouth open and eyes closed. Do not ask the patient to breathe deeply, since hyperventilation is a potent means of lowering intracranial pressure and a falsely normal or low pressure reading may result. Be patient and watch the level of fluid in the manometer. Under these circumstances, the level of fluid in the normal subject will be less than 200 mm.

The level will fluctuate with each breath and slightly with each pulse. It is good to hold the butt of the needle firmly and tilt the manometer to one side, pivoting the stopcock in the needle. More fluid will flow into the manometer. When it is returned to a vertical position the fluid level should drop. If it does, be assured you are reading the maximum and proper pressure. Record the region of fluctuation of pressure, e.g., "130 to 145 mm," as the pressure reading.

If pressure is above 200 mm, wait; be certain the patient is relaxed and expelling his breath normally. When pressure is pathologically elevated, the range of fluctuation is often greater.

Collect the amount of fluid necessary for cell count, protein and glucose levels, serology, and any other tests indicated. If pressure is elevated, remove fluid for diagnostic studies slowly but do not compromise on the amount of fluid necessary to allow adequate microscopic, biochemical, cytologic, and bacteriologic analysis.

Send cerebrospinal fluid samples for cell count and for a serologic test for syphilis. Specimens should be sent to the laboratory for protein and glucose determinations. Fluid should be routinely sent for bacteriologic culture and sensitivity. If infection is suspected, or if cloudy cerebrospinal fluid is found, request Gram's stain, acid-fast stain, and, when appropriate, as in suspected cerebral abscess, special culture for anaerobic organism. Also, when clinically appropriate, tuberculosis and fungal cultures, India-ink preparation, and fungal antigen and antibody determinations should be requested. When multiple sclerosis is suspected, fluid should be sent for determination of immunoglobulin content and electrophoretic pattern. In cases of possible primary or metastatic neoplasm of the central nervous system, 5 to 10 ml of fluid should be sent to the cytopathology laboratory to determine if there are malignant cells.

When the studies are completed, withdraw the needle slowly. About 20% to 30% of patients will experience post-lumbar puncture headaches owing to internal seepage of cerebrospinal fluid around the needle hole in arachnoid and dura. This incidence can be reduced considerably by having the patient lay prone for 3 to 4 hours afterward. This position effects misalignment of the holes in the dura and arachnoid, thereby reducing leakage of cerebrospinal fluid. If a headache does occur, it can be relieved by the patient assuming the horizontal position. Treatment consists of keeping the patient flat in bed for a 24-hour interval, then allowing him to be up so long as he does not experience headache again. If he does, repeat this cycle until the headache is gone, if necessary for several days.

Blood in the cerebrospinal fluid is due either to trauma secondary to needle puncture or to spontaneous or traumatic bleeding within the cranial cavity or spinal canal. Trauma from needle puncture is usually due to the needle having been passed *through* the lumbar thecal sac into the rich plexus of veins in the ventral epidural space. It is imperative to determine whether blood in the fluid originated in this manner or represents spontaneous bleeding. One way to make this distinction is by drawing off equal amounts in three tubes and comparing the gross amount of blood in each. In a traumatic tap, there will be less blood in the third tube than in the first. If necessary, this can be quantified by determining the hematocrit of each tube. The most definitive and, unfortunately, most commonly omitted technique for identifying a traumatic tap is examination of the supernatant of a centrifuged specimen of spinal fluid. Hemoglobin, when admixed with cerebrospinal fluid, is converted to the pigments oxyhemoglobin and bilirubin, but only after at least 2 hours have elapsed for oxyhemoglobin and 10 hours for bilirubin. These pigments, when present, lend a distinct yellow or yellow-orange tint to the supernatant. The presence of such coloration, or *xanthochromia*, implies that blood found in the cerebrospinal fluid must have been present for at least 2 hours (and probably longer) and could not have resulted solely from the trauma induced by the spinal needle a few minutes before. If the amount of blood in the spinal fluid is minimal or if the supernatant is examined barely longer than 2 hours after bleeding, the intensity of staining of the supernatant may be barely perceptible. In order not to overlook such minimal xanthochromia, match the specimen against a comparable tube of plain tap water to see if, by comparison, a hint of pigment can be detected. Hold both tubes in bright light against a plain white background. Sensitivity can be increased further by "looking down the barrel" of both tubes, which, by providing a greater depth of fluid to look through, magnifies the difference between the colorless tap water and the xanthochromic fluid.

A yellowish cast to the fluid occasionally results from conditions other than bleeding. A protein content of greater than 150 mg/dl may produce mild xanthochromia due to the presence of albumin-bound bilirubin. Rarely, cerebrospinal fluid xanthochromia is found in patients with hyperbilirubinemia or meningeal melanoma.

The presence of blood in the cerebrospinal fluid must also be taken into account when interpreting the cell count and protein level. For every 700 red blood cells (RBCs) found per cubic millimeter of fluid, subtract 1 mg/dl of protein and 1 white blood cell (WBC) from the total amount found. Hence, a cerebrospinal fluid sample having 7,000 RBCs and 11 WBCs per cubic millimeter and 53 mg/dl protein can be corrected to one WBC per cubic millimeter and 43 mg/dl protein, both within normal limits (WBC count, 5/cu mm or fewer; protein level, 45 mg/dl or less).

BIBLIOGRAPHY

Adams RD, Victor M: *Principles of Neurology*, ed 3. New York, McGraw Hill Book Co, 1985.

Aminoff MJ: *Electrodiagnosis in Clinical Neurology*, ed 2. New York, Churchill Livingstone, 1986.

Asbury AK, McKhann GM, McDonald WI: *Diseases of the Nervous System*. Philadelphia, WB Saunders Co, 1986

Baker AB, Joynt RJ: *Clinical Neurology*. New York, Harper & Row, 1985.

Burde RM, Savino PJ, Trobe JD: *Clinical Decisions in Neuro-ophthalmology*. St Louis, CV Mosby Co, 1985.

Crosby EC, Humphrey T, Lauer EW: *Correlative Anatomy of the Nervous System*. New York, MacMillan Publishing Co, 1962.

Dawson DM, Hallett M, Millender LH: *Entrapment Neuropathies*. Boston, Little Brown & Co, 1983.

DeJong RN: *The Neurologic Examination*, ed 4. New York, Harper & Row, 1978.

Favill J: *Outline of the Spinal Nerves*. Springfield, Ill, Charles C Thomas, 1946.

Glaser JS: Neuro-ophthalmology. New York, Harper & Row, 1978.

Illingsworth RS: *The Development of the Young Child: Normal and Abnormal*, ed 8. New York, Churchill Livingstone, 1983.

Keegan JJ, Garrett FD: The segmental distribution of the cutaneous nerves in the limb of man. *Anat Rec* 1948; 102:409-437.

Kimura J: *Electrodiagnosis in Diseases of Nerve and Muscle: Principles and Practice*. Philadelphia, FA Davis, 1983.

Larsen HW: *Manual and Color Atlas of the Ocular Fundus*. Philadelphia, WB Saunders, 1969.

Medical Research Council: *Aids to the Investigation of Peripheral Nerve Injuries*, ed 4. London, Her Majesty's Stationary Office, 1982.

Plum F, Posner JB: *The Diagnosis of Stupor and Coma*, ed 3. Philadelphia, FA Davis Co, 1980.

Ramsey, RG: *Neuroradiology*. Philadelphia, WB Saunders, 1987.

Rowland, LP: *Merritt's Textbook of Neurology*, ed 7. Philadelphia, Lea & Febiger, 1984.

Sunderland S: *Nerves and Nerve Injuries*, ed 2. New York, Churchill Livingstone, Inc. 1979.

Index

A

Abdominal reflex, 56–57
Abducens nerve; see Sixth cranial nerve
Absence seizure, 156, 157
  electroencephalography and, 177
Achilles reflex, 52, 53, 126
Acoustic nerve tumor, 147
Action tremor, 112–113
Acuity, visual; see Visual acuity
Acute inflammatory polyradiculopathy, 120; see also Guillain-Barré syndrome
Adenoma sebacum, 146, 147
Agility of hand, 43
Agraphia, 222, 223
Akathisia, 114
Alexia, 222–223
Alternating motion rate, 42
  cellebellar signs and, 108
  hand and, 43
  hemiparesis and, 111
  legs and, 44
  tongue and, 104
Altitudinal hemianopsia, 82
Amnesia, transient global, 216
AMR; see Alternating motion rate
Amyotrophic lateral sclerosis, 13, 116
  pseudobulbar palsy and, 105

Anal wink, 149
Anesthesia, hysterical, 180
Aneurysm, 88
Angiography, 203–205
Angioma, spinal, 147
Angiomatosis, 147
Anisocoria, 18, 77
Ankle jerk reflex, 126
Anterior fontanelle, 152–153
Anticholinesterase agents, 145, 188–189
Anticoagulant, 225
Aphasia, 219
  global, 222
Apnea, sleep, 179
Argyll Robertson pupil, 77
Arithmetic calculation, 216, 217
ARM; see Alternating motion rate
Arm
  hemiparesis and, 108, 111
  peripheral nerve paralysis and, 130–133
  strength and function of, 36–39
Arnold-Chiari malformation, 211
Arteriovenous malformation, 196
Arteritis
  cerebral, 204, 205
  giant cell, 14
Artery
  carotid, 14, 203

  cerebral, 196
    arteritis and, 204, 205
  retinal, 80, 82
  vertebral, 203
Arthritis, cervical, 16
Artifact in computed tomography and, 201
Asterixis, 114
Asterognosis, 66
Ataxia, 10
Ataxic breathing, 153
Athetosis, 112
Atonic seizure, 157
Atrophy
  arm and, 40
  disuse, 12, 40
  facial, 141
  hypothenar eminence, 133
  leg, 135, 136
  optic, 25, 80
  peripheral nerve paralysis and, 128
  quadriceps and, 135
  root compression and, 121, 122
  sternocleidomastoid muscle and, 141
  tongue, 107
Atropine
  myasthenia gravis and, 145
  parasympathetic innervation and, 19

Audiometry, 31
Auditory nerve, 30–32
Aura, uncinate, 18, 157
Automatic reflex bladder, 148
Automatisms, 158
Autonomous bladder, 148
Axillary nerve paralysis, 130

B

Babinski sign, 50, 55
  hemiparesis and, 111
  hemiplegia and, 108
  seizure and, 157
  upper motor neuron paralysis and, 13
Balance, 108
Ballism, 112
Battle's sign, 14, 15
  coma and, 154
Becker variant of muscular dystrophy and, 138
Beevor's sign, 57
Bell's phenomenon, 100, 101, 102
Benedikt's syndrome, 89
Biceps, 124
Biceps stretch reflex, 50, 51
  musculocutaneous nerve paralysis and, 130
Bilirubin, 230
Biopsy, muscle, 138

Bitemporal hemianopsia, 83
Bladder, 148
Bleeding
  as contraindication to lumbar puncture, 225
  from ear, 14
Blepharospasm, 88
Blindness, monocular, 83
Blind spot, 82
Blink reflex, 183–184
Blood in cerebrospinal fluid, 224, 229–230
Bone tumor, 13
Botulism, 188, 190
Brachial neuritis, 129
Brachial plexus, 99
Bradykinesia, 113
  Parkinson's disease and, 114
Brain
  angiography of, 203–205
  herniation of, 88
  magnetic resonance imaging of, 201–202
  radiologic tests of, 191–205
  scanning of, 192–193
Brain death, 176
  electroencephalography and, 178
  radionuclide brain scan and, 192–193
Brain stem
  gaze paralysis and, 85–86
  pseudobulbar palsy and, 104
Brain-stem auditory evoked potentials, 181

Breathing, ataxic, 153
Brief tests of mental status, 214–223
Broca's aphasia, 219, 222
Brown-Séquard syndrome, 62
Brudzinski sign, 119
Bruit, 13, 15
  carotid, 17
  infant and, 14

C

Café au lait spots, 146, 147
Calcified intracranial structures, 147
Caloric test for vestibular function, 223–224
Carotid artery
  angiography and, 203
  occlusion of, 14
Carotid pulse, 17
Carpal tunnel syndrome, 133
Catatonic schizophrenia, 155
Causalgia, 136
Central nystagmus, 95
Cerebellar disorder
  coma and, 154
  extremity and, 36, 52
Cerebellar signs, 108
Cerebral arteries, 196
  arteritis in, 204, 205
Cerebral dominance, 219

Cerebrospinal fluid
　from ear, 14
　specimen of, 224, 229
Cerebrum
　angiography of, 203–205
　computed tomography scan and, 195
　death of, 178
　infarction of, 194, 195
　magnetic resonance imaging and, 201–202
　sensory examination and, 62
Cervical arthritis, 16
Cervical muscle, 14
Cervical root compression, 122–124
Cervical spine, 16
Chaddocks' sign, 56
Charcot-Marie-Tooth disease, 112
Chart
　head circumference, 171–172
　visual acuity, 20
Chest, 58
Cheyne-Stokes respiration, 153
Chiasm, optic, 82
Child, bruits in, 14; *see also* Infant
Cholinesterase inhibitors, 188–189
Chorea, 112
　Huntington's, 113
Circumduction, 7
　hemiplegia and, 109
Circumference, head, 171–172
Cisternogram, isotope, 193

Clonus, 54
Cogwheel ridigity, 16, 114
Coma, 152–155
　evoked potentials and, 181
　scalp lacerations and, 14
Complex partial seizure, 158
Compression
　carotid, 17
　root, 120–127, 207
　　cervical, 122–124
　　lumbar, 125–127
　sensory examination and, 59
Computed tomography
　of head, 194–200
　spine, 210
Concomitant strabismus, 22
Conduction, nerve
　hearing loss and, 31
　peripheral neuropathy and, 112
　studies of, 182–184
Congenital disease
　hemiparesis and, 147
　Horner's syndrome and, 99
　latent nystagmus and, 96
Consciousness, disturbances of, 152–158
Consensual light reaction, 18–19, 76
　swinging flashlight test and, 80
Contraction
　blepharospasm and, 88
　stretch and, 46

Contraindications to lumbar puncture, 225
Contusion, 14
Conus medullaris, 62, 72, 73
Convergence, 22, 23
Convergence-retraction nystagmus, 96
Coordination, 108
Cord
　spinal. *See* Spinal cord
　vocal, 32
Corneal stimulation, 26
Corticobulbar disease, 28
Corticospinal disease, 57
Cramp, writer's, 112
Cranial nerve, 76–107
　eighth, 30–32
　eleventh, 33, 106
　fifth, 26–28
　first, 17–18
　fourth, 91
　functions of, 17–34
　ninth, 32, 103
　second, 18–25; *see also* Second cranial nerve
　sixth, 92–93
　tenth, 105
　third, 89; *see also* Third cranial nerve
　twelfth, 34
Cranial suture, 172
　skull roentgenography of, 192
Craniotomy scar, 13

Cutaneous sensitivity, 59
Cystometry, 135–136

D

Dancing eyes, 96
Deadness of limb, 58
Deafness, 30–32
Death, brain
   electroencephalography and, 178
   radionuclide scan and, 192–193
Decerebrate posture, 152
Decorticate posture, 152
Déjà vu, 158
Deltoid
   paralysis of, 120
   strength and function of, 38, 39
Dermal sinus, 147
Dermatomyositis, 144
Dexterity, 43
Diabetes, 135
Diadochokinesia, 43; *see also* Alternating motion rate
Diaphragmatic paralysis, 128
Digital subtraction angiogram, 205
Digit span test, 214
Dilation, pupillary, 90, 91
Diplopia, 22
Disc, optic, 79
Disk, herniated
   computed tomography and, 210
   nerve conduction studies and, 183
   roentgenogram and, 206
   root compression syndrome and, 120, 121, 125
Disuse atrophy
   arm, 40
   quadriceps, 12
Dominance, cerebral, 219
Door-bell sign, 126
Dorsiflexion of wrist, 40, 41
Double simultaneous stimulation, 67
Downbeat jerk nystagmus, 96
Drainage from ear, 14
Drooping of eyelid; *see* Ptosis
Drug
   Horner's syndrome and, 98
   myasthenia gravis and, 145
   parasympathetic innervation and, 19
Duchenne's muscular dystrophy, 137, 138, 139
Dysarthria, 222
   tongue and, 104
Dysesthesia, 120
Dyskinesia, 36
Dyskinesis, 112–114
Dysmetria, 36
Dysphagia, 144
Dyssynergia, 36
Dystaxia, 9
Dystonia, 7, 112
Dystonic posture, 37
Dystonic toe, 56
Dystrophy
   eleventh cranial nerve and, 33, 107
   fascioscapulohumoral, 142
   loss of expression and, 26, 28
   muscular
      electromyography and, 138
      neck flexion and, 16, 17
   myotonic, 137
   ptosis and, 88

E

Ear, 30–32
   Battle's sign and, 154
   bleeding from, 14
   external, 28
   vestibular function and, 224
Ecchymosis, 154
Edrophonium chloride, 145
Eighth cranial nerve, 30–32
Elbow
   peripheral nerve paralysis and, 130
   strength and function of, 38
Electroencephalogram, 176–179
Electromyography, 184–188
   fibrillation and, 116–117
   muscular dystrophy and, 138

Electronystagmography, 31–32
Electrophysiologic tests, 176–190
    electroencephalogram, 176–179
    electromyography, 184–188
    evoked potentials, 179–180
    nerve conduction studies, 182–184
    repetitive stimulation studies, 188–190
Eleventh cranial nerve, 33, 106
Embolism, retinal artery, 80
Encephalopathy, metabolic, 176
    electroencephalography and, 179
Encephalotrigeminal angiomatosis, 147
Epilepsy; *see* Seizures
Essential tremor, 113
    Parkinson's disease and, 116
Evoked potentials, 179–182
Expression loss, 28, 115
External ear canal, 28
Extradural mass, 208
Extremity, strength of function of, 35–57
Eye, 17–25
    coma and, 152
    cranial nerves and, 76–97
    nystagmus and, 94–96
    vestibular function and, 223
Eyelid
    facial nerve and, 28, 29
    ptosis of; *see* Ptosis

F

Face
    atrophy of, 141
    muscular dystrophy and, 140, 141
    weakness of, 28
Facial-eye synkinesis, 102
Facial nerve, 28–29
    paresis and, 108, 110
        Horner's syndrome and, 98–99
Facioscapulohumeral dystrophy, 142
Familial tremor, 113
Far field potentials, 181
Fasciculation
    electromyography and, 188
    eleventh cranial nerve and, 107
    motor neuron lesion and, 116
    muscle and, 13
Femoral nerve, 134–135
Festination, 115
Fibrillation, 116–117
Fifth cranial nerve, 26–28
Fifth thoracic segment, 68
Finger
    agility, 43
    sensory examination and, 67
Finger drop, 131
Finger-to-nose test, 36–37
First cranial nerve, 17–18
Fixation nystagmus, 95–96
Flaccid extremities, 108
Flexion
    of knee, 44
    neck, 16, 17
        signs of meningitis and, 119
    of thigh, 44, 45
Floppy extremities, 108
Focal motor seizure, 157
Focal sensory seizure, 157–158
Fontanelle, anterior, 172
Foot, 64
Footdrop, 7, 12–13
    peroneal nerve paralysis and, 136
Forearm. *see also* Arm
    laceration of, 133
    peripheral nerve paralysis and, 131
Fourth cranial nerve, 91
Foville syndrome, 92
Fracture, neck, 16
Froment's test, 132–133
Frontalis, 28
Fund of information testing, 217
Funduscopic examination, 79
F wave reflex, 183

G

Gag reflex, 32, 104
Gait. *see also* Walking
    assessment of, 6–9
    hemiparesis and, 110
Gastrocnemius
    hopping and, 12

stretch reflex and, 52, 53
Gaze, 23, 85–86
  half, 87
  sixth cranial nerve and, 92–96
Giant cell arteritis, 14
Gilles de la Tourette's syndrome, 113
Girdle
  hip, 44, 45
  limb, dystrophy of, 142
Glaucoma, 80
Glioblastoma, 194, 195
Global amnesia, 216
Global aphasia, 222
Glossopharyngeal nerve, 103
Gower's sign, 138
Grand mal seizure, 156, 157
Graphesthesia, 66
Grasp reflex, 164
Grip, 40, 41
Guillain-Barré syndrome, 32
  nerve conduction studies and, 183
  paralysis and, 102
  peripheral neuropathy and, 120
  reflex and, 47

H

Half gaze, 87
Hamstring muscle, 44
Hand
  objects in, 66
  strength and function of, 40–43
  vibratory sense and, 64
Handedness, 219
Head
  infant, 171–172
  sympathetic nervous system, 97
Headache, 14
Head tilt, 22
Hearing, 30–32
Heel-to-knee test, 46
Heel-walking, 12
  lumbar root compression and, 126
Heliotrope rash, 144
Hematoma
  extracerebral, 88–89
  infant and, 172
  subdural; see Subdural hematoma
Hemianopsia, 82, 83
Hemiballism, 112
Hemiparesis, 108–112
  infant and, 163
  neurocutaneous syndrome and, 147
Hemiplegia, 108–112
Hemisensory stroke, 112
Hemispheric lesion, cerebellar, 108
Hemorrhage
  computed tomography and, 200
  corticobulbar pathway and, 104
  subarachnoid; see also Hematoma, subdural

Herniated disc
  computed tomgraphy and, 210
  nerve conduction studies and, 183
  roentgenogram of, 206
  root compression syndrome and, 120, 121, 125
Herniation, brain, 88
Herpes zoster, 68
Hip girdle, 44, 45
History, 1–2
Hoarseness, 32
  tenth cranial nerve and, 32
Hoffmann sign, 50, 51
Holmes-Adie syndrome, 77, 79
Homonymous defect, 24
Homonymous hemianopsia, 83, 84
Honeymoon palsy, 131
Hopping, 10
  gastrocnemius and, 12
  hemiparesis and, 110, 111
Horizontal gaze, 22
Horner's syndrome, 77, 99
H-reflex, 183
Humerus, 131
Hydrocephalus, 172
  computed tomography and, 199
  normal-pressure, 193
Hypalgesia, 58
Hyperkinesia, 113
Hypernephroma, 13, 15

Hyperreflexia, 108
Hypertension, 79
Hypothenar eminence
  atrophy of, 133
Hysteria
  dysmetria and, 37
  evoked potentials and, 180
  posture and, 7
  sensory examination and, 60
  swaying and, 8–9

I

Iliopsoas muscle, 44
Imaging. see also Radiological tests
  magnetic resonance, 201–202
  radionuclide, 192–193
Immediate memory, 214–215
Impingement, nerve root, 16
Infant, 162–172
  bruit and, 14
Infarction
  cerebral, 200
    computed tomography and, 194, 195
    magnetic resonance imaging and, 202
  corticobulbar pathway and, 104
Infection as contraindication to lumbar puncture, 225
Inflammation, spinal, 126
Inflammatory polyradiculopathy; see also Guillain-Barré syndrome

Infranuclear lesions, 99
Intention tremors, 43, 108
Intercerebral mass lesions, 179
Internal carotid artery, 14
Internuclear ophthalmoplegia, 86
Interossei, 133
Intervertebral disk. see Disk, intervertebral
Intracranial pressure, elevated
  as contraindication to lumbar puncture, 225
  skull roentgenography and, 192
Intracranial tumor, 172
Intradural mass, 208, 209
Ischemia of retinal artery, 82
Isotope cisternogram, 193

J

Jacksonian march, 157
Jamais vu, 158
Jargon aphasia, 219
Jaw jerk, 28, 104
Jendrassik's maneuver, 48, 49, 50
Jerk
  ankle, 126
  jaw, 104
  knee, 48, 49
Jerk nystagmus, 94
Judgment testing, 217, 218

K

Kernig sign, 119
Knee flexion, 44
Knee jerk, 48, 49
Knee-patting, 42

L

Laboratory diagnostic aids, 176–211
  electrophysiologic tests and, 176–190
  neuroradiologic tests
    of skull and brain, 191–205
    of spine and spinal cord, 206–211
Laceration
  forearm and wrist, 133
  scalp, 14
Lacunar stroke, 112
Lambert-Eaton syndrome, 188, 190
Lasègue's sign, 126
Lateral sclerosis, amyotrophic, 13, 116
  pseudobulbar palsy and, 105
Lead poisoning
  radial nerve palsy and, 131
Leg
  hemiparesis and, 111
  peripheral nerve paralysis and, 116–118, 135–136
  sensory examination and, 67

spastic, 7
Leprosy, 112
Lhermitte's sign, 16
Lid; *see* Eyelid
Light reflex, 76
   consensual, 18–19
   swinging flashlight test and, 80, 81
Limb girdle dystrophy, 142
Locked-in syndrome, 155
Lower motor neuron lesion, 12, 13
Lumbar puncture, 224–230
Lumbar root compression, 125–127
Lymphadenopathy, 17

M

Magnetic resonance imaging, 201–202
   spinal cord, 211
Masseter muscle, 26
Masseter-temporalis stretch reflex, 104
Mastication, 26–28
Mastoiditis, 28
Medial nerve, 40
   paralysis of, 133–134
Medulla, 62
Memory, 214–216
Meniere's disease, 31
Meningioma, 13, 198
   olfaction and, 18
Meningitis, 16

coma and, 154
olfaction and, 18
recurrent, 148
signs of, 118–119
Mental status, 2–3, 214–223
Meralgia paresthetica, 135
Metabolic encephalopathy, 176, 179
Metastatic carcinoma, 14
Midbrain displacement, 89
Middle ear, 30–32
Midline cerebellum, 108
Millard-Gubler syndrome, 92
Miosis, 19
Monocular blindness, 83
Mononeuritis, diabetic, 135
Mononeuritis multiplex, 119
Mononeuropathy, 119
Moro reflex, 163
Motor neuron lesion
   amyotrophic lateral sclerosis and, 116
   lower, 12, 13
   muscular dystrophy and, 16
   upper, 13
      alternating motion rate and, 42
      hand motion and, 43
Motor paralytic bladder, 148
Motor seizure, 157
Multiple myeloma, 13, 15
Multiple sclerosis
   abdominal reflex and, 57

antenuclear ophthalmoplegia and, 87
   evoked potentials and, 180, 182
   hopping and, 10
   Lhermitte's sign and, 16
   magnetic resonance imaging and, 202
   visual evoked potentials and, 182
Muscle
   atrophy of
      peripheral nerve paralysis and, 128
      root compression and, 122, 122–123
   cervical, 14
   disorders of, 137–143
   electromyography and, 184–188
   fasciculations of, 13
   serratus anterior, 129
   triceps, 130
   trigeminal nerve and, 26
   strength and function of, 35–57
Muscle contraction headache, 14
Muscle stretch receptor, 46
Muscular dystrophy; *see also* Dystrophy
   eleventh cranial nerve and, 107
   neck flexion and, 16, 17
Musculocutaneous nerve, 130
Myasthenia gravis, 144–145
   neck flexion and, 16, 17
   ptosis and, 88
   repetitive stimulation studies and, 188
Myasthenic syndrome, 188, 190

Myelography, 207–209
   as contraindication to lumbar puncture, 225
Myoclonus, 112
Myoedema, 143
Myopathy, 137–143
Myotonia, 141
Myotonic discharge, 188
Myotonic dystrophy, 137
   ptosis and, 88

N

Narcolepsy, 176
   electroencephalography and, 179
Nausea, 95
Near reflex, 18–19
Neck
   flexion of, 16, 17
   fracture of, 16
   innervation of, 68
   sensory examination of, 58
   signs of meningitis and, 119
   tonic reflex of, 164
Neologisms, 219
Neonatal Horner's syndrome and, 99
Neoplasm
   Horner's syndrome and, 99
   spinal, 126
      cord, 13

Neostigmine methylsulfate, 145
Nerve
   conduction of, 182–184
      peripheral neuropathy and, 112
   cranial; *see* Cranial nerves
   median, 40
   peripheral; *see* Peripheral nerves
   radial, 38
   sciatic, 44
   ulnar, 40
Nerve deafness, 31
Nerve root
   compression of; *see* Compression, root
   impingement of, 16
Neuralgia
   glossopharyngeal, 32
   trigeminal, 26
Neuritis
   brachial, 129
   optic, 79
      evoked potentials and, 182
Neurocutaneous syndromes, 146–148
Neurofibromatosis, 146, 147
Neuron, motor. *See* Motor neuron lesion
Neuropathy, peripheral
   reflex, 47
   stocking-glove pattern and, 60–62
   wrist and, 40
Neuroradiologic test; *see* Radiologic tests
Neurosyphilis, 77

Ninth cranial nerve, 32, 103
Nonfluent aphasia, 219
Normal-pressure hydrocephalus, 193
Nuchal rigidity
   coma and, 154
   meningitis and, 119
Nuclear brain scan, 192–193
Nuclear lesion, 92
Numbness, 58
Nystagmus, 22, 94
   vestibular function and, 200, 223, 224

O

Oblique muscle, 91
Occlusion
   carotid artery, 14, 17
   radionuclide brain scan and, 192
Oculocephalic reflex, 153
Oculocephalogyric reflex, 85–86
Oculomotor nerve; *see* Third cranial nerve
Oculovestibular reflex, 140
   coma and, 155
Olfaction, 17–18
   uncinate seizure and, 158
Ophthalmoplegia, 86
Ophthalmoscopy, 25
Oppenheim's sign, 56
Opsoclonus, 96
Optic atrophy, 25

Optic disc
  pallor of, 80
  swelling of, 79
Optic nerve, 18–25
  atrophy of, 80
  neuritis of, 79, 80
    evoked potentials and, 182
Optic radiation, 84
Optic tract lesion, 83
Optokinetic nystagmus, 95
Oscillatory movement, 94
Oscillopsia, 96
Otosclerosis, 28
Oxyhemoglobin, 230

P

Pain
  cervical spine and, 16
  loss of sensitivity to, 62
  root compression and, 120
  scalp and, 14
  sensation of, 63
  sensory examination and, 58–59
Pain-touch dissociation, 65
Palatal myoclonus, 105
Palate, 32, 105
Pallesthesia, 64
Pallor of optic disc, 80
Palsy
  Bell's, 100, 101
  gaze, 85–86
  honeymoon, 131
  pseudobulbar, 104
    amyotrophic lateral sclerosis and, 105
    eleventh cranial nerve and, 104
    loss of expression and, 28
  tardy ulnar, 133
Papilledema, 78, 79, 80
Paralysis
  Bell's, 100, 101
  bladder, 148
  corticobulbar pathway and, 104
  gaze, 85
  Guillain-Barré syndrome and, 102
  peripheral nerve, 128–136
  postictal, 157
  sixth cranial nerve and, 92, 93
  soft palate, 105
  superior oblique muscle, 91
  supranuclear, 99
  third-nerve, 77, 88
  tongue and, 107
  upper motor neuron, 13
  vocal cord, 105
Paraphasia, 219
Paraplegia, 117
Paresis
  facial, 108, 110
    Horner's syndrome and, 99
  radial nerve, 40
  sixth cranial nerve and, 92, 93
  third nerve, 87
  ulnar nerve, 40
Paresthesia, 58
  hand, 122
  peripheral neuropathy and, 120
  root compression and, 121
Paretic nystagmus, 94
Parietal-lobe disorder, 66–68
  optokinetic nystagmus and, 95
  visual field and, 84
Parinaud's syndrome, 85
Parkinson's disease, 7, 114–116
  cogwheel rigidity and, 16, 114
  definition of, 114
  extension of great toe and, 56
  hemiparesis and, 112
  knee-patting and, 42
  posture and, 7
Parosmia, 18
Partial seizure, 157
  electroencephalography and, 177
Patches, Shagreen, 146, 147
Patellar reflex, 52, 53
Pectoral muscle, 123
Pelvic examination, 148–149
Pendular nystagmus, 94, 95
Percussion, 128

Peripheral nerves
　lesions of, 59
　neuropathy of, 119–120
　　reflex and, 47
　　stocking glove-pattern and, 60–62
　　wrist and, 40
　　paralysis of, 128–136
Peroneal nerve. 136
Petit mal seizure, 156, 157
　electroencephalography and, 177
Phalen's sign, 134
Pharmacologic testing
　Horner's syndrome and, 98
　myasthenia gravis and, 145
Pharynx
　eleventh cranial nerve and, 107
　ninth cranial nerve and, 32
Phonation, 32
Phrenic nerve, 128
Physiologic blind spot, 82
Physiologic nystagmus, 94
Pill rolling tremor, 113
Pinhole test, 21
Pinprick test, 60, 62–63
Pituitary tumor, 192
　magnetic resonance imaging of, 201
Platysma, 28, 29
Poliomyelitis, 47
　motor neuron disease and, 116
Polymyositis, 144

Polyradiculopathy, acute inflammatory; see
　Guillain-Barré syndrome
Position; see also Posture
　for lumbar puncture, 226
　peripheral neuropathy and, 40
　sense of, 62, 65
Posterior column lesion, 9
Postictal paralysis, 157
Postmyelogram computed tomography scan
　of spine, 210
Posture, 8–10, 114; see also Position
　coma and, 152
　dystonic, 37, 112
　lumbar root compression and, 125
　Parkinson's disease and, 114
Premature closure of cranial sutures, 172
　skull roentgenography and, 192
Protrusion of tongue, 34
Proverbs test, 217, 218
Pseudobulbar palsy, 104
　amyotrophic lateral sclerosis and, 105
　eleventh cranial nerve and, 104
　loss of expression and, 28
Pseudohypertrophic dystrophy, 138
Pseudopapiledema, 79
Psychogenic unresponsiveness, 154–155
Psychomotor seizure, 158
　electroencephalography and, 177
Pterygoid muscle, 26
Ptosis

　common conditions with, 87–88
　myasthenia gravis and, 144, 145
　third cranial nerve and, 22
Puncture, lumbar, 224–230
Pupil
　coma and, 152
　light reflex and, 76
　signs of, 77
　swinging flashlight test and, 80
　third nerve palsy and, 90, 91

Q

Quadrantanopsia, 84
Quadriceps
　atrophy of, 135
　disuse atrophy and, 12
　stretch reflex and, 52

R

Radial nerve
　elbow and, 130
　paralysis and, 131–132
　triceps and, 38
Radiation, visual, 84
Radiologic tests
　of skull and brain, 191–205
　　cerebral angiography, 203–205
　　computed tomography of head, 194–200

magnetic resonance imaging of brain, 201–202
   radionuclide brain scan, 192–193
   skull roentgenography and, 191–192
  of spine and spinal cord, 206–211
Radionuclide brain scan, 192–193
Rash
  coma and, 154
  heliotrope, 144
Reading, 222
Recent memory, 214, 215–216
Recklinghausen's disease, 147
Rectal examination, 148–149
Red sensitivity, 24
Reflex
  abdominal, 56–57
  achilles, 52, 53
  ankle jerk, 126
  blink, 183–184
  to corneal stimulation, 26
  extremity and, 46–57
  F wave, 183
  gag, 32, 104
  H, 183
  infant and, 162–165
  light, 76
    swinging flashlight test and, 80, 81
  Moro, 163
  near, 18–19
  oculocephalic, 153

oculocephalogyric, 85–86
oculovestibular, 140
paraplegia and, 117
patellar, 52, 53
snout, 104
stretch
  biceps, 124
  masseter-temporalis, 104
  musculocutaneous nerve paralysis and, 130
  peripheral nerve disorder and, 120, 128
  root compression and, 121
superficial, 56
triceps, 50, 51
Reflex bladder, automatic, 148
Reflex stepping, 165
Refractive error, 21
Remote memory, 214, 216–217
Repetitive stimulation studies, 188–190
Resonance imaging, magnetic, of brain, 201–202
Respiration, coma and, 153
Respiratory nerve, 128
Rest tremor, 112–113
Retina
  abnormality of, 25
  hypertension and, 79
Retinal artery
  embolism of, 80
  occlusion of, 82

Retrobulbar neuritis, 80
Rigidity
  cogwheel, 16, 114
  decerebrate
    coma and, 152
  nuchal
    coma and, 154
    meningitis and, 119
Rinne test, 28
Roentgenography
  skull, 191–192
  spine, 206
Romberg test, 8, 9
Root, spinal
  compression of; *see* Compression, root
  distribution of, 68, 69
  nerve conduction studies and, 183
Rooting reflex, 164

S

Sacral root, 62, 72, 73
Sacral sparing, 117
Saddle-area sensory loss, 62
Saturday night palsy, 131
Scalp, 13–15
Scan
  magnetic resonance imaging, 201–202, 211
  radionuclide brain, 192–193

Scapular winging, 38
  eleventh cranial nerve and, 106
  muscular dystrophy and, 142
  peripheral nerve paralysis and, 129
Scar, head, 13, 14
Sciatic nerve, 44
  paralysis of, 136
Sclerosis
  amyotrophic lateral, 13, 116
    pseudobulbar palsy and, 105
  multiple; see Multiple sclerosis
  tuberous, 147
Scotoma, 82
Second cranial nerve, 18–25
  atrophy of, 80
  neuritis of, 79, 80, 182
See-saw nystagmus, 96
Seizures, 156–158
  electroencephalography and, 176
  uncinate, 18, 157
Semicircular canals, 223
Sensitivity to red, 24
Sensory examination, 58–73
  cervical root compression and, 122
Sensory paralytic bladder, 148
Sensory seizure, 157–158
SEPS; see Somatosensory evoked potentials
Serratus anterior muscle, 129
Serratus anticus, 38, 39
Seventh cranial nerve, 28–29

Shagreen patches, 146, 147
Shock, spinal, 117
Shoulder, 68
Sign
  Babinski; see Babinski sign
  Battles, 14, 15
    coma and, 154
  Beevor's, 57
  Brudzinski, 119
  cerebellar, 108
  door-bell, 126
  Gower's, 138
  Kernig, 119
  Lermitte's, 16
  of meningitis, 118, 119
  Phalen's, 134
  Trömner, 50, 51
Simultaneous stimulation, 24
  double, 67
Sinus, dermal, 147
Sixth cranial nerve, 92–93
Skin, 154
Skull
  radiologic tests of, 191–205
  transillumination of, 172
Sleep disorder, 176
  electroencephalography and, 179
Smell, 18
  uncinate seizure and, 157
Snout reflex, 104

Soft palate, 105
Soleus stretch reflex, 52, 53
Somatic sensory examination, 58–73
Somatosensory evoked potentials, 180–181
Sparing, sacral, 117
Spasm
  dystonic, 112
  hemiparesis and, 108, 109
    infant and, 164
  torticollis and, 112
Spastic leg, 7
Spastic paresis, 110, 111
Speech, 2–3
  aphasic, 219
  tongue and, 104
Spinal accessory nerve; see Eleventh cranial nerve
Spinal cord
  neoplasm and, 13
  radiologic tests of, 206–211
  sensory deficits and, 68
Spinal root
  compression of; see Compression, root
  conduction studies and, distribution of, 68
Spinal segment distribution, 68, 69
Spinal shock, 117
Spine
  angioma of, 147
  cervical, 16
  paraplegia and, 117

radiologic tests of, 206–211
Spondylosis, 122
Spoon-pencil test, 220
Spot
  blind, 82
  café au lait, 146, 147
Squat and rise, 11
Stenosis, vascular, 192
Sternocleidomastoid muscle
  atrophy of, 140, 141
  eleventh cranial nerve and, 33, 106–107
Sterognosis, 67
Stimulation
  corneal, 26
  repetitive, 188–190
  simultaneous, 24
    double, 67
Stocking-glove pattern, 60–62
  peripheral neuropathy and, 120
Strabismus, 22
Straight-leg raising, 126, 127
Strength
  extremity, 35–57
  hemiparesis and, 111
Stretch receptor, 46
Stretch reflex
  biceps, 50, 51
    root compression and, 124
  masseter-temporalis, 104
  musculocutaneous nerve paralysis and, 130

peripheral nerve paralysis and, 128
peripheral neuropathy and, 120
root compression and, 121
Striatal toe, 56
Stroke, 104
Sturge-Weber syndrome, 147
Subarachnoid space
  signs of meningitis and, 119
  sixth cranial nerve and, 92
Subcortical aphasia, 222
Subdural effusion, 172
Subdural hematoma
  computed tomography and, 200
  electroencephalography and, 179
  infant and, 172
  signs of meningitis and, 119
Sucking reflex, 164
Superficial reflex, 56
Superior oblique muscle, 91
Supranuclear disorder, 85
  Horner's syndrome and, 99
Suture, cranial, 172, 192
Swaying, 8–9
Sweating, loss of, 128
Swinging flashlight test, 80, 81
Sydenham's chorea, 113
Sympathetic nervous system, 97
Synkinesis, facial-eye, 102
Synostosis, premature suture, 172
Syphilis, 77

Syringomyelia, 210
  magnetic resonance imaging and, 211

T

Tabetic neurosyphilis, 77
Tandem walking, 9
Tap. *See* Lumbar puncture
Tardive dyskinesia, 114
Tardy ulnar palsy, 133
Taste, 103
  Horner's syndrome and, 99
  ninth cranial nerve and, 32
Temperature, 62, 63, 65
Temporal fields, 82, 83
Temporal lobe lesion
  vision and, 84
  seizure and, 158
Temporal muscle, 26
Tenderness of scalp, 14
Tendon
  Achilles, 126
  stretch and, 47
Tenth cranial nerve, 32, 105
Terminal tremor, 36
Thalamic disorder, 63
Thenar eminence, 141
Thigh flexion, 44, 45
Third cranial nerve, 89
  paralysis of, 77, 88

Third cranial nerve (cont.)
  paresis of, 87
Thrombocytopenia, 154
Thrombosis, retinal artery, 80
Thumb, 147
Thyroid, 17
Tibial nerve, 136
Tic, 113
Tilt, head, 22
Tinel's sign, 128
Tinnitus, 28
Toe, striatal, 56
Toe drop, 126
Tomography, computed
  of head, 192–200
  spine, 210
Tongue
  alternating movement rate and, 104
  glossopharyngeal nerve and, 103
  myotonia and, 140, 141
  ninth cranial nerve and, 32
  paralysis of, 107
  protrusion of, 34
Tonic neck reflex, 164
Tonoclonic seizure, 156, 157
Touch, 62, 65
Tourette's syndrome, 113
Transient global amnesia, 216
Transillumination of skull, 172
Trapezius muscle
  eleventh cranial nerve and, 33, 106
  headache and, 14
  muscular dystrophy and, 140, 141
  strength and function of, 38, 39
Trömner sign, 50, 51
Tremor, 37
  dyskinesia and, 112–113
  dystonic, 112
  intention, 43, 108
  Parkinson's disease and, 113, 116
Triceps muscle
  elbow and, 130
  root compression and, 123
  strength and function of, 38
Triceps reflex, 50, 51
Trigeminal nerve, 26–28
  blink reflex and, 183–184
Trochlear nerve, 91
Trunk, lower, 60, 61
Tuberous sclerosis, 147
Tumor
  bone, 13
  brain, 203
  eighth nerve, 31
  pituitary, 192
    magnetic resonance imaging of, 201
  spinal, myelography and, 207–208
Tuning fork test
  hearing and, 30–31
  vibratory testing and, 64

Twelfth cranial nerve, 34
Two-point discrimination, 67
Tympanum, 28

U

Ulnar nerve
  lesions of, 40
  paralysis and, 132–133
  paresis and, 40
Uncinate aura, 18, 157
Uninhibited bladder, 148
Unresponsiveness, psychogenic, 154–155
Upbeat jerk nystagmus, 96
Upper lid; *see* Eyelid
Upper motor neuron dysfunction
  hand motion and, 43
  slowed alternating motion rate and, 42
Urinary control, 148

V

Vagus nerve, 32, 105
Vascular stenosis, 192
VEPs; *see* Visual evoked potentials
Vermis, 108
Vertebra, 66, 68; *see also* Disk,
    intervertebral
Vertebral artery, 203
Vertical gaze, 22

Vertigo, 95
Vestibular nerve, 30
  caloric test and, 223–224
  nystagmus and, 95
Vibratory sense, 64
Vision
  acuity of, 19–21
  fixation nystagmus and, 95–96
  posture and, 8
  tandem walking and, 9
Visual evoked potentials, 181–182
Visual field, 82
  estimation of, 24
  papilledema and, 79
Visual radiation, 84
Vocal cord, 32

Voice fatigue, 145

W

Waddling gait, 7
Walking, 6–9
  heel, 12
    lumbar root compression and, 126
  hemiplegia and, 109–110
  peripheral nerve paralysis and, 136
Wallenberg's syndrome, 62
Weakness, 12, 13
  facial, 28
  loss of expression and, 28
  muscle, 35–57
Weber's syndrome, 83

Weber test, 30–31
Wernicke's aphasia, 219
Winging, scapular; *see* Scapular winging
Word-deafness, 222
Word-finding, 219
Wrist
  dorsiflexion of, 40
  laceration of, 133
Wristdrop, 131
Writer's cramp, 112
Writing, 222

X

Xanthochromia, 230